Dental Materials: Theory, Practice and Cases

Dental Materials: Theory, Practice and Cases

Editor: Gerard Keith

AMERICAN
MEDICAL PUBLISHERS
www.americanmedicalpublishers.com

AMERICAN
MEDICAL PUBLISHERS
www.americanmedicalpublishers.com

Cataloging-in-Publication Data

Dental materials : theory, practice and cases / edited by Gerard Keith.
p. cm.
Includes bibliographical references and index.
ISBN 978-1-63927-654-7
1. Dental materials. 2. Dental instruments and apparatus. 3. Dental technology.
4. Prosthodontics. I. Keith, Gerard.
RK652.5 .D46 2023
617.695--dc23

American Medical Publishers,
41 Flatbush Avenue,
1st Floor, New York,
NY 11217, USA

ISBN 978-1-63927-654-7 (Hardback)

Contents

Preface

Dental materials comprise natural tissues and biocompatible synthetic materials that are utilized for restoring damaged, decayed and fractured teeth. They can be categorized as preventive materials, auxiliary materials or restorative materials. The study of dental materials encompasses a wide variety of terms, properties, compositions and microstructures that are used to forecast or describe the functioning of restorative and preventive biomaterials. Natural tissues like bone, enamel, cementum and dentin, and biocompatible synthetic materials like composite structures, polymers, ceramics and metals are used in dental procedures. Furthermore, materials including ceramic, amalgam and resin can be used to create crowns, fillings and other tooth restorations. Each material is suitable for a variety of applications and circumstances, and has different advantages and disadvantages. Dental materials are utilized in a variety of treatments including the reconstruction of teeth, removal of plaque, aesthetic intervention, implants and the treatment of caries. This book is compiled in such a manner, that it will provide in-depth knowledge about dental materials. It will serve as a reference to a broad spectrum of readers.

This book is the end result of constructive efforts and intensive research done by experts in this field. The aim of this book is to enlighten the readers with recent information in this area of research. The information provided in this profound book would serve as a valuable reference to students and researchers in this field.

At the end, I would like to thank all the authors for devoting their precious time and providing their valuable contribution to this book. I would also like to express my gratitude to my fellow colleagues who encouraged me throughout the process.

Editor

1

Tooth-Colored CAD/CAM Materials for Application in 3-Unit Fixed Dental Prostheses in the Molar Area: An Illustrated Clinical Comparison

Angelika Rauch *, Sebastian Hahnel, Elena Günther, Wolfgang Bidmon and Oliver Schierz

Department of Prosthodontics and Materials Science, University of Leipzig, Liebigstr. 10, Haus 1, 04103 Leipzig, Germany; sebastian.hahnel@medizin.uni-leipzig.de (S.H.); elena.guenther@medizin.uni-leipzig.de (E.G.); wolfgang.bidmon@medizin.uni-leipzig.de (W.B.); oliver.schierz@medizin.uni-leipzig.de (O.S.)

* Correspondence: angelika.rauch@medizin.uni-leipzig.de

Abstract: The aim of this study was to compare the clinical properties of tooth-colored computer-aided design/computer-aided manufacturing (CAD/CAM) materials for the fabrication of a 3-unit fixed dental prostheses (FDPs) in the same clinical scenario. A 53-year-old female patient was supplied with a 3-unit FDP to replace a second premolar in the upper jaw. Restorations were fabricated from 3 mol%, 4 mol%, and 5 mol% yttrium oxide zirconia, zirconia with translucency gradient, indirect composite resin, polyetheretherketone (PEEK), and polyetherketoneketone (PEKK). Milling time, weight, and radiopacity were investigated. Esthetics were examined following the US Public Health Service criteria (USPHS). The milling time for zirconia was twice as high as for the indirect composite resin, PEEK, or PEKK. The latter materials had a weight of 2 g each, while zirconia restorations yielded 5 g. Zirconia presented intense radiopacity. PEEK and PEKK required veneering and an opaquer was applied to the PEKK framework. All FDPs showed acceptable esthetics. PEEK and PEKK restorations were featured by a grayish shimmering. A variety of CAD/CAM materials are available to fabricate 3-unit FDPs with esthetically acceptable results. In the esthetic zone, PEEK and PEKK require veneering and an opaquer might be applied. Milling time, weight, and radiopacity were relatively high for zirconia FDPs.

Keywords: clinical evaluation; dental prosthesis; fixed partial denture; monolithic zirconia; polymers

1. Introduction

The conventional wisdom in restorative dentistry is that the esthetic appearance of dental restorations has gained increasing importance in the last decades, which is why the application of tooth-colored materials is highly favored by both patients and dentists. Recent surveys revealed that dentists often recommend ceramics, especially lithium disilicate and zirconia, for anterior and posterior single crowns [1,2]. However, if it comes to multi-unit fixed dental prostheses (FDPs), the range of materials is limited, since most of the silica-based ceramics are not approved for the fabrication of multi-unit FDPs. Pressed zirconia-reinforced lithium silicate ceramics, and milled computer-aided designed/computer-aided manufactured (CAD/CAM) or pressed lithium disilicate ceramics are available for the fabrication of 3-unit FDPs, yet only up to the second premolar. In the molar area, none of the silica-based ceramics are recommended for the application in multi-unit FDPs. For these scenarios, ceramics with a polycrystalline structure are available, especially zirconia, which has been extensively used during the last years. The formulation of zirconia has been modified regarding its yttrium oxide dotation. Thus, different zirconia materials are available on the dental market and the amount of yttrium oxide relevantly influences the mechanical and optical properties [3]. While zirconia restorations with 3 mol% yttrium oxide (3 Y-TZP) present high flexural strengths, an endowment to 5 mol% yields lower values. The latter formulation is not recommended for the fabrication of FDPs with more than three units, but improved translucency may coincide with improved esthetics [4,5]. Indirect composite resins (CAD/CAM composite resins) are mostly recommended for partial restorations or single crowns. In comparison to ceramics, they are featured by high edge stability, lower brittleness, and a dentine-like elastic modulus [6]. Two composite resins (LuxaCam Composite, DMG, Hamburg, Germany; Trinia, SHOFU, Kyoto, Japan) are available for application in multi-unit FDPs [6]. In the recent years, polyetheretherketone (PEEK) and polyetherketoneketone (PEKK), which belong to the superordinate group of polyaryletherketone (PAEK), have been increasingly promoted for application in fixed prosthodontics. PAEK materials feature high biocompatibility and favorable mechanical properties. They are available in colors similar to that of teeth, e.g., dentine, whitish, universal, and in other colors such as grayish or pink [7–10].

Tooth-colored materials currently available on the market for the fabrication of 3-unit FPDs belong to different classes regarding their chemical structure and composition. It is therefore clear that their distinct properties may impact the individual esthetic appearance of the restoration. In addition, it has been highlighted that zirconia restorations may produce artifacts in X-ray examinations [11], which indicates that the radiopacity of the restorative material can be a relevant issue for later diagnostic procedures. In contrast, for resin-based composites, radiopacity has been described as a desirable property as it allows the differentiation of carious lesions below the crown margin or decalcified dentin from the restoration as well as the location of voids or other defects within the restoration [12].

The differences in chemical structure and composition of the materials available on the market account for differences in the individual material's density. With regard to this aspect, densities of 6 g/cm^3 have been reported for zirconia, while PAEK and composite resin materials feature far lower densities between 1.3 and 2.0 g/cm^3 [8,13,14]. From a clinical point of view, lower density of a restorative material results in less weight of the restoration, which might be favorable in patients requiring extensive restorations. Tooth-colored CAD/CAM materials are processed by using CAD software and can be milled with 4- or 5-axis CAM machines. The density of a CAD/CAM-processed restorative material could be a parameter that impacts milling efficiency, which suggests that denser restorative materials might require higher milling times.

Against this background, this clinical report illustrates the replacement of a second premolar by using a 3-unit fixed dental prosthesis fabricated from different restorative materials available on the market for this particular setting, comparing clinically relevant properties such as esthetics, radiopacity, and weight as well as parameters potentially relevant for the dental laboratory such as milling time. The working hypothesis was that there are no differences between the various materials and restorations regarding the properties investigated.

2. Materials and Methods

A 53-year-old healthy female patient introduced herself at the Department of Prosthodontics and Materials Science at Leipzig University (Leipzig, Germany). The second premolar in the left upper jaw was missing. The patient history revealed that she was supplied with a dental implant that had to be explanted a year before the appointment, due to an inflammation. Therefore, she was looking for an alternative to replace the missing premolar.

During clinical examination, healthy periodontal conditions were observed and a screening for temporomandibular disorders was negative. The patient denied being aware of bruxism, and during the clinical examination no signs of bruxism were identified. All teeth were naturally healthy or restored with sufficient restorations, except for a carious lesion in the left first molar of the upper jaw (Figure 1a,b).

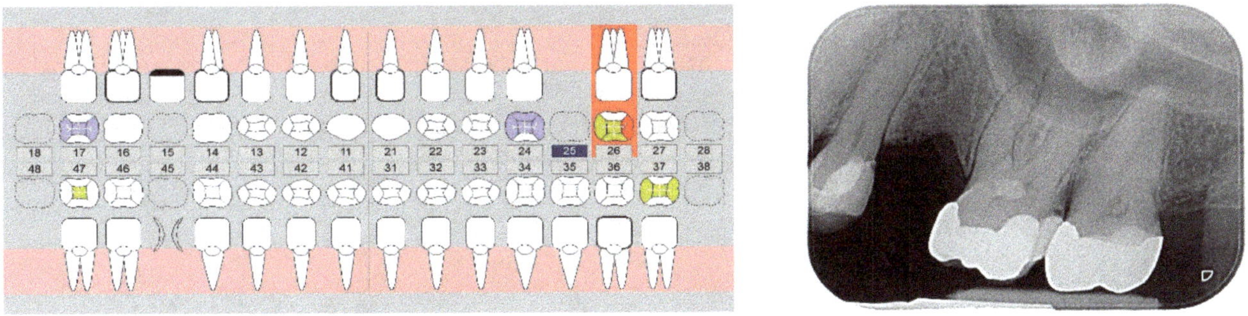

(a) (b)

Figure 1. Results of the (**a**) intraoral and (**b**) X-ray examination.

As the patient was not interested in any implant-supported restoration, the fabrication of a 3-unit FDP was proposed to replace the missing tooth. The patient agreed to the concept and gave her signed consent to be part of the clinical trial. For comparisons, 3 Y-TZP, 4 Y-TZP, and 5 Y-TZP supplied by the same manufacturer were chosen, and another zirconia with translucency gradient, one composite resin, one PEEK, and one PEKK material were selected (Table 1).

Table 1. Applied materials for the clinical report, product information according to instructions of manufacturers (Vita Zahnfabrik, Bad Säckingen, Germany; Ivoclar Vivadent, Schaan, Liechtenstein; DMG, Hamburg, Germany; Cendres Métaux, Biel, Switzerland) for posterior multi-unit fixed dental prostheses (FDPs).

Product Name, Company	VITA YZ HT White, Vita Zahnfabrik	VITA YZ ST Multicolor, Vita Zahnfabrik	VITA YZ XT Color, Vita Zahnfabrik	IPS e.max ZirCAD Prime, Ivoclar Vivadent	LuxaCam Composite, DMG	LuxaCam PEEK, DMG	Pekkton Ivory, Cendres Métaux
Material	3 Y-TZP	4 Y-TZP	5 Y-TZP	3 and 5 Y-TZP	indirect composite resin	polyether-ether-ketone (PEEK)	polyether-ketone-ketone (PEKK)
Available colors [a]	YZ HT White YZ HT Color (1M2, 2M2, 3M2, A1-A3)	YZ HT White YZ HT Color (A1-D4) YZ HT Multicolor (A1-D4)	YZ HT White YZ HT Color (A1-D4) YZ HT Multicolor (A1-D4)	BL1-BL4, A1-D4	Bleach 2, A1-A3, B1, C2, D2	universal	whitish
Minimum layer thickness–circular (mm)	0.5 (one pontic) 0.6 (two pontics)	0.6	1.0	1.0	0.6	0.6	0.6
Minimum layer thickness–occlusal (mm)	0.6 (one pontic) 0.7 (two pontics)	0.7 (one pontic) 0.8 (two pontics)	1.2	1.0	1.2	0.6	0.8
Minimum connector dimensions (mm^2)	9 (3-unit FDP) 12 (>one pontic)	12 (3-unit FDP) 15 (>one pontic)	12	9 (3-unit FDP) 12 (>4-unit FDP)	16	16	14
Others	maximum of two connected pontics	maximum of two connected pontics	only 3-unit FDP, no cantilever FDP	not with bruxism, maximum of two connected pontics	only 3-unit FDP	≤4-unit FDP	not with bruxism, only 3-unit FDPs, no cantilever FDPs

[a] please see latest product catalogue for available colors; yttria-stabilized tetragonal zirconia polycrystal ceramics (Y-TZP).

The abutment teeth were prepared according to preparation guidelines for ceramics (Figures 2a and 3a) and an impression was taken using the sandwich technique (Honigum heavy and light, DMG).

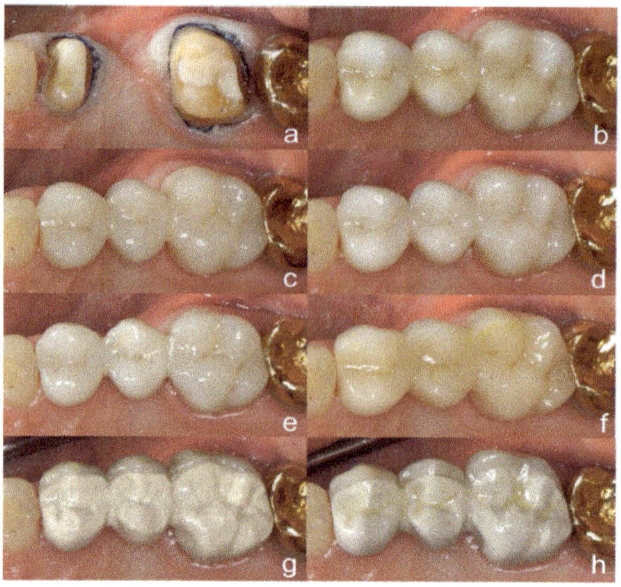

Figure 2. Design of the (**a**) abutment teeth and the 3-unit FDPs from an occlusal view; (**b**) 3 Y-TZP, (**c**) 4 Y-TZP, (**d**) 5 Y-TZP, (**e**) zirconia with transluency gradient, (**f**) indirect composite resin, (**g**) polyetheretherketone (PEEK), (**h**) polyetherketoneketone (PEKK).

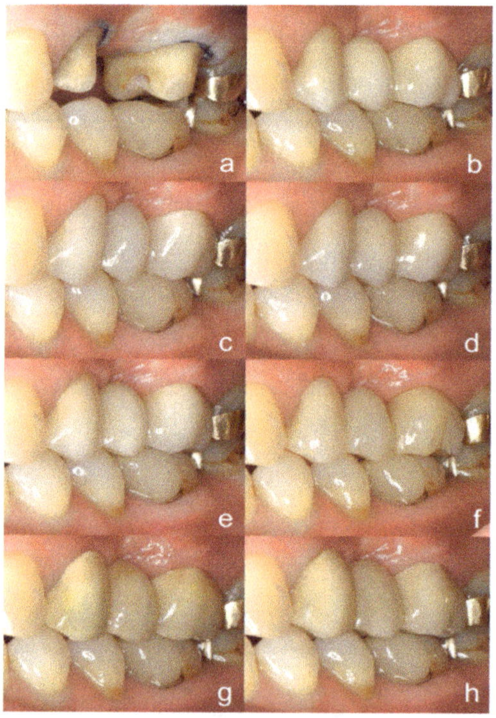

Figure 3. Design of the (**a**) abutment teeth and the 3-unit FDPs from a vestibular view; (**b**) 3 Y-TZP, (**c**) 4 Y-TZP, (**d**) 5 Y-TZP, (**e**) zirconia with transluency gradient, (**f**) indirect composite resin, (**g**) PEEK, (**h**) PEKK.

The tooth color was D3, which was determined by using the Vita classical shade guide (Vita Zahnfarbrik, Bad Säckingen, Germany). Working casts were prepared and digitalized with a laboratory scanner (inEos X5, Dentsply Sirona, Charlotte, NC, USA). Afterwards, the FDPs were designed (ceramill mind 2.4, Amann Girrbach, Pforzheim, Germany) in accordance with the manufacturer's instructions (Table 1) and milled (inLab MC X5, Dentsply Sirona). The approximated milling time issued by the CAM software (inLab CAM SW 20.0.1, Dentsply Sirona) for the individual restoration was recorded. The 3 Y-TZP zirconia material was only available as white material from the manufacturer and needed to be colored with coloring liquids (Figure 4).

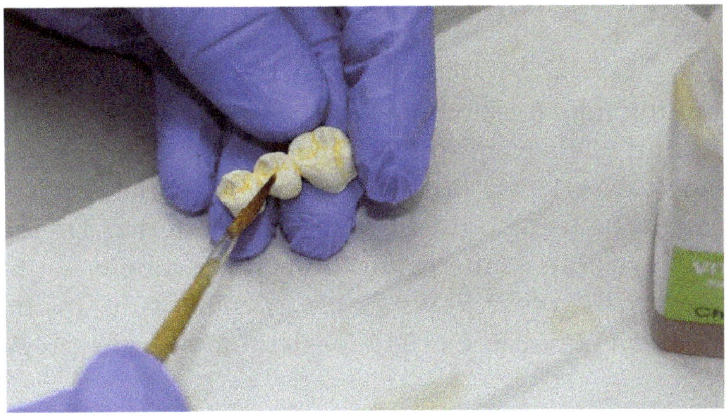

Figure 4. Manual coloring of the milled and white 3 Y-TZP restoration to achieve tooth color D3.

The FDPs fabricated from PEEK and PEKK materials were facially veneered with a composite resin using a conventional technique. For PEKK, an opaquer was priorly applied to mask the grayish framework.

To keep tooth hard tissue removal to the necessary minimum and to better compare the original colors, the occlusal and oral sides of all FDPs were fabricated in a monolithic approach. Only PEEK and PEKK restorations were facially veneered. All materials were characterized with stains to imitate the adjacent teeth (Table 2).

Table 2. Features of the fabricated 3-unit FDPs to replace the second premolar in the upper jaw.

Product Name, Company	VITA YZ HT^{White}, Vita Zahnfabrik	VITA YZ ST^{Multicolor}, Vita Zahnfabrik	VITA YZ XT^{Color}, Vita Zahnfabrik	IPS e.max ZirCAD Prime, Ivoclar Vivadent	LuxaCam Composite, DMG	LuxaCam PEEK, DMG	Pekkton Ivory, Cendres Métaux
Material	3 Y-TZP	4 Y-TZP	5 Y-TZP	3 and 5 Y-TZP	indirect composite resin	Polyether-ether-ketone (PEEK)	Polyether-ketone-ketone (PEKK)
Approximated milling time (min)	51	51	51	62	32	33	34
Weight (g)	5.3	5.0	5.2	5.2	1.9	1.5	1.6
Mean gray value in X-ray [a]							
Pontic area (orange)	255	255	255	255	255	99	67
Premolar margin (green)	255	255	255	255	174	48	62
Molar margin (pink)	255	255	255	255	199	95	47
Surface characterization	VITA akzent plus effect stains, VITA akzent plus glaze LT (both Vita Zahnfabrik)	VITA akzent plus effect stains, VITA akzent plus glaze LT (both Vita Zahnfabrik)	VITA akzent plus effect stains, VITA akzent plus glaze LT (both Vita Zahnfabrik)	VITA akzent plus effect stains, VITA akzent plus glaze LT (both Vita Zahnfabrik)	Signum Composite (Kulzer), Optiglaze Color (GC)	Signum Composite (Kulzer), Optiglaze Color (GC)	Signum Composite (Kulzer), Optiglaze Color (GC)
Others	-	-	-	-	D2 individualized with Optiglaze Color (GC) to better fit D3	-	opaquer needed to cover the framework before veneering

[a] please see Figure 5, measured reference mean gray value revealed 114 for dentine; yttria-stabilized tetragonal zirconia polycrystal ceramics (Y-TZP).

The weight of the FDPs was measured (PCB 1000-2, Kern & Sohn, Balingen-Frommern, Germany). An X-ray was made (7 mA, 70 kV, 40 ms; Heliodent Plus, Dentsply Sirona) to evaluate radiopacity with gray values (ImageJ 1.52p, National Institutes of Health, Bethesda, MD, USA) of the dentine of a reference abutment tooth as well as three distinct locations of the individual restorations (central in the pontic area, mesial at the premolar margin, and distal at the molar margin). An intraoral try-in of the FDPs was performed (Variolink Esthetic Try-In neutral, Ivoclar Vivadent, Schaan, Liechtenstein) and the patient was asked to choose her favorite FDP. Finally, all FDPs were evaluated for the parameters 'anatomic form', 'marginal adaption', and 'color match' according to USPHS guidelines [15] by an independent and trained examiner.

3. Results

The approximated milling time for zirconia with translucency gradient was highest, while half the time was estimated to mill FDPs from PEEK, PEKK, and the indirect composite resin (Table 2). The PEKK material that was labeled as whitish by its manufacturer appeared to be grayish and did not meet esthetic requirements by using only the veneering material. Therefore, it was covered with an opaquer beforehand. The weight of the restorations ranged between 5.0 and 5.3 g for zirconia and between 1.5 and 1.9 g for the other FDPs (Table 2). The X-ray examination of the reference abutment tooth revealed a mean gray value of 114 for dentine near the preparation margin (Figure 5, blue rectangle).

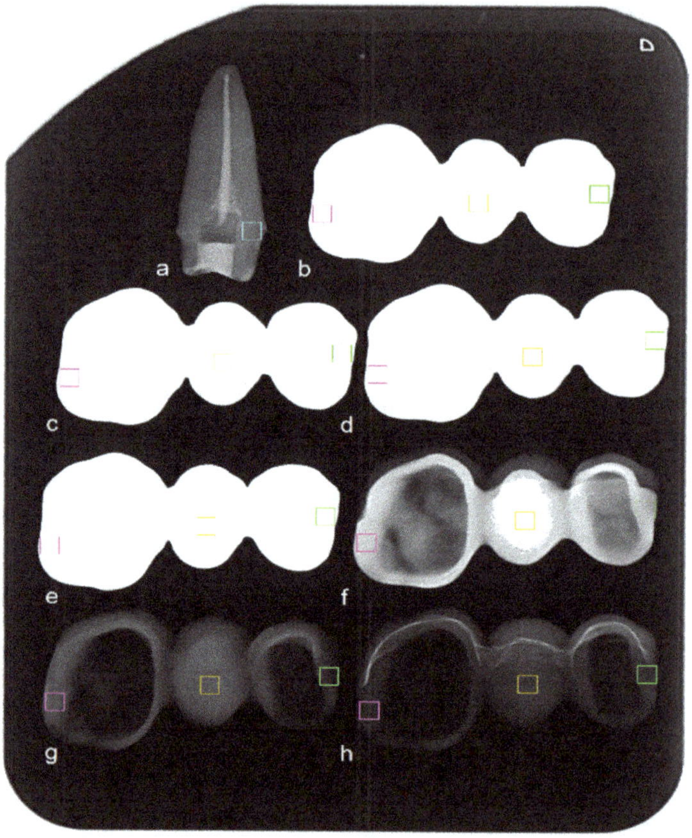

Figure 5. X-ray of (**a**) an extracted abutment tooth (reference) and the restorations (**b**) 3 Y-TZP, (**c**) 4 Y-TZP, (**d**) 5 Y-TZP, (**e**) zirconia with transluency gradient, (**f**) indirect composite resin, (**g**) PEEK, (**h**) PEKK with regions of interest (rectangles) for the measurements of gray values (Table 2).

Zirconia restorations presented intense radiographic opacity with highest gray values of 255 in all points of interest (Figure 5, Table 2).

According to US Public Health Service (USPHS) criteria, the clinical evaluation of all FDPs revealed rankings of Alpha for the categories 'anatomic form' and 'marginal adaption' (Figures 2 and 3). From the vestibular view, 'color match' of FDPs fabricated from PEEK and PEKK was rated as Bravo, since a relatively opaque and grayish shade was observed (Figure 3). The colors of restorations fabricated from zirconia and CAD/CAM composite resin were categorized as Alpha. The patient favored the zirconia FDP with translucency gradient, which was self-adhesively cemented (RelyX Unicem, 3M, St. Paul, MN, USA).

4. Discussion

Regarding the esthetic appearance of the 3-unit FDPs investigated in the current clinical report, the results suggest that a variety of CAD/CAM materials can be employed to supply patients with esthetically favorable 3-unit FDPs in the posterior area. However, PEEK and PEKK frameworks should be covered with an opaquer and require veneering with a composite resin or ceramic material to produce acceptable esthetic results. Moreover, the materials featured differences in their radiopacity, with the lowest radiopacity were identified for PAEK materials and highest radiopacity for zirconia. Regarding laboratory processing, approximated milling time was different between the various materials. Thus, the working hypothesis of this clinical report was rejected.

This clinical report illustrates that acceptable esthetical results in the posterior area can be achieved with various formulation of zirconia. Composite resins yielded similar favorable esthetic outcomes, ye for PAEK materials, veneering seems necessary in the esthetic zone. Even if PAEK materials are available in colors that are described as whitish or universal by the manufacturer, these are not similar to those of natural teeth. However, for the veneering of PEEK with CAD/CAM composite resins or ceramics, similar colorimetric properties might be achieved than for zirconia or metal frameworks [16]. Besides the CAD/CAM technique for veneering, PAEK materials can be veneered by using conventional techniques or with pre-fabricated composite resin veneers. Nonetheless, the veneering of PAEK materials is challenging. In vitro results revealed that conventionally fabricated or pre-fabricated composite resin veneers showed lower fracture loads than those milled with the CAD/CAM technique and adhesive failure was high for pre-fabricated veneers [17]. The technique of bonding composite resins to PAEK is controversially discussed. A systematic review concluded that restorations should be pretreated with mechanical and/or chemical methods, such as air abrasion or sulfuric acid etching. Finally, a bonding agent containing methyl methacrylate (MMA) or 10-methacryloyloxydecyl dihydrogen phosphate (MDP) should be applied [11].

Regarding cementation, it is possible that restorations fabricated from zirconia ceramics, PEEK, and PEKK are conventionally cemented. This might be beneficial in comparison to restorations fabricated from CAD/CAM composite resins that need to be adhesively cemented. Nonetheless, debonding of composite resins is still a frequently described complication; thus, the adhesive cementation technique should be processed with caution [6].

The mechanical properties of CAD/CAM composite resins, PEEK, and PEKK are featured by a relatively low elastic modulus of 3 to 5 GPa. This value is close to that of dentine (15 GPa), which might yield a cushioning effect on tooth-supported restorations and might also be interesting in implant dentistry. Stress transferred to the abutment tooth or abutment/implant might be reduced in comparison to restorations fabricated from other materials such as zirconia with 200 GPa [8,18]. Due to the low density of applied composite resins and PAEKs in the present clinical report, these restorations yielded lighter weight than restorations fabricated from zirconia, since volumes of the FDPs were similar. A decreased weight of restorations might be beneficial for patient satisfaction in cases with extensive restorative reconstructions, for instance in full-arch restorations [19]. Moreover, the low density can be one parameter that has an impact on milling time in the CAM machines. In the present clinical report, the low density of resin composites and PAEK materials correlated with shorter approximated milling times, which might be an advantage for the chairside application of, e.g., CAD/CAM composite resins.

In X-ray examinations, margins of the FDPs fabricated from PAEK and composite resins were less radiopaque than dentine. Radiopacity of zirconia was most intense, which corroborates previous investigations [11]. Judging from these observations, the application of PAEK or composite resins might be favorable in a clinical setting, as radiographic artifacts produced by zirconia can be avoided and a differentiation of, e.g., a carious lesion from a PAEK restoration margin might be easier.

Regarding microbiological parameters, favorable results have been reported in previous investigations focusing on biofilm formation on any of the CAD/CAM materials investigated in this clinical report. For implant surfaces, zirconia showed a significant reduction in biofilm formation in comparison to titanium, while biofilm formation on PEEK was equal or lower than on zirconia or titanium [20,21]. Lower biofilm formation was identified for milled CAD/CAM composite resins in comparison to direct composite resins [22].

To date, clinical investigations focusing on tooth-colored CAD/CAM materials for multi-unit FDPs are sparse. Only short-term investigations for monolithic zirconia are available, which revealed a survival rate of 96.7% after three years [23]. The strength of this clinical report is the comparison of various contemporary CAD/CAM materials for the fabrication of 3-unit FDPs in the same prosthetic scenario. While this clinical report presented esthetical aspects as well as information on weight, radiopacity, and milling time, its results should be corroborated by clinical trials with a large number of patients using validated instruments for the patient's esthetical perception such as the Orofacial Esthetic Scale [24].

5. Conclusions

Zirconia, composite resins, PEEK, and PEKK were available to fabricate 3-unit FDPs that replace a second premolar. Milling time and weight of zirconia was twice as high as for the other investigated materials. Radiopacity of zirconia restorations was intense at restoration margins and the gray values reached 255. All fabricated restorations achieved acceptable esthetics; yet, PEEK and PEKK required veneering and an opaquer was additionally used to cover the PEKK framework. However, the observations should be supported by clinical trials that use validated instruments for the estimation of esthetical perception.

Author Contributions: Conceptualization and methodology, A.R., S.H. and O.S.; validation, E.G.; investigation, A.R., E.G. and W.B.; writing—original draft preparation, A.R.; writing—review and editing, S.H.; O.S. and E.G.; visualization, W.B. and A.R. All authors have read and agreed to the published version of the manuscript.

Acknowledgments: The authors acknowledge support from Leipzig University for Open Access Publishing.

References

1. Makhija, S.K.; Lawson, N.C.; Gilbert, G.H.; Litaker, M.S.; McClelland, J.A.; Louis, D.R.; Gordan, V.V.; Pihlstrom, D.J.; Meyerowitz, C.; Mungia, R.; et al. National Dental Practice-Based Research Network Collaborative Group, Dentist material selection for single-unit crowns: Findings from the National Dental Practice-Based Research Network. *J. Dent.* **2016**, *55*, 40–47. [CrossRef] [PubMed]
2. Rauch, A.; Schrock, A.; Schierz, O.; Hahnel, S. Material selection for tooth-supported single crowns-a survey among dentists in Germany. *Clin. Oral. Investig.* **2020**. [CrossRef] [PubMed]
3. Stawarczyk, B.; Keul, C.; Eichberger, M.; Figge, D.; Edelhoff, D.; Lümkemann, N. Three generations of zirconia: From veneered to monolithic. Part I. *Quintessence Int.* **2017**, *48*, 369–380. [PubMed]
4. Stawarczyk, B.; Keul, C.; Eichberger, M.; Figge, D.; Edelhoff, D.; Lümkemann, N. Three generations of zirconia: From veneered to monolithic. Part II. *Quintessence Int.* **2017**, *48*, 441–450. [PubMed]
5. Kontonasaki, E.; Rigos, A.E.; Ilia, C.; Istantsos, T. Monolithic Zirconia: An Update to Current Knowledge. Optical Properties, Wear, and Clinical Performance. *Dent. J.* **2019**, *7*, 90. [CrossRef]
6. Jovanovic, M.; Zivic, M.; Milosavljevic, M. A Potential Application of Materials Based on a Polymer and CAD/CAM Composite Resins in Prosthetic Dentistry. *J. Prosthodont. Res.* **2020**. [CrossRef]
7. Papathanasiou, I.; Kamposiora, P.; Papavasiliou, G.; Ferrari, M. The use of PEEK in digital prosthodontics: A narrative review. *BMC Oral Health* **2020**, *20*, 217. [CrossRef]
8. Alexakou, E.; Damanaki, M.; Zoidis, P.; Bakiri, E.; Mouzis, N.; Smidt, G.; Kourtis, S. PEEK High Performance Polymers: A Review of Properties and Clinical Applications in Prosthodontics and Restorative Dentistry. *Eur. J. Prosthodont. Restor. Dent.* **2019**, *27*, 113–121.
9. Amelya, A.; Kim, J.E.; Woo, C.W.; Otgonbold, J.; Lee, K.W. Load-Bearing Capacity of Posterior CAD/CAM Implant-Supported Fixed Partial Dentures Fabricated with Different Esthetic Materials. *Int. J. Prosthodont.* **2019**, *32*, 201–204. [CrossRef]

10. Najeeb, S.; Zafar, M.S.; Khurshid, Z.; Siddiqui, F. Applications of polyetheretherketone (PEEK) in oral implantology and prosthodontics. *J. Prosthodont. Res.* **2016**, *60*, 12–19. [CrossRef]
11. Gama, L.T.; Duque, T.M.; Özcan, M.; Philippi, A.G.; Mezzomo, L.A.M.; Gonçalves, T. Adhesion to high-performance polymers applied in dentistry: A systematic review. *Dent. Mater.* **2020**, *36*, e93–e108. [CrossRef] [PubMed]
12. Sur, J.; Endo, A.; Matsuda, Y.; Itoh, K.; Katoh, T.; Araki, K.; Okano, T. A measure for quantifying the radiopacity of restorative resins. *Oral Radiol.* **2011**, *27*, 22–27. [CrossRef]
13. Cokic, S.M.; Vleugels, J.; Van Meerbeek, B.; Camargo, B.; Willems, E.; Li, M.; Zhang, F. Mechanical properties, aging stability and translucency of speed-sintered zirconia for chairside restorations. *Dent. Mater.* **2020**, *36*, 959–972. [CrossRef] [PubMed]
14. DMG Safety Data Sheet LuxaCam Composite. Available online: https://uk.dmg-dental.com/fileadmin/user_upload/shared/MSDS/en/MSDS_CPF_LuxaCamComposite_6600_EN.pdf (accessed on 1 December 2020).
15. Cvar, J.F.; Ryge, G. Reprint of criteria for the clinical evaluation of dental restorative materials. 1971. *Clin. Oral Investig.* **2005**, *9*, 215–232. [PubMed]
16. Stawarczyk, B.; Schmid, P.; Roos, M.; Eichberger, M.; Schmidlin, P.R. Spectrophotometric Evaluation of Polyetheretherketone (PEEK) as a Core Material and a Comparison with Gold Standard Core Materials. *Materials* **2016**, *9*, 491. [CrossRef]
17. Taufall, S.; Eichberger, M.; Schmidlin, P.R.; Stawarczyk, B. Fracture load and failure types of different veneered polyetheretherketone fixed dental prostheses. *Clin. Oral Investig.* **2016**, *20*, 2493–2500. [CrossRef]
18. Zhang, Y.; Kelly, J.R. Dental Ceramics for Restoration and Metal Veneering. *Dent. Clin. N. Am.* **2017**, *61*, 797–819. [CrossRef]
19. Zoidis, P.; Papathanasiou, I.; Polyzois, G. The Use of a Modified Poly-Ether-Ether-Ketone (PEEK) as an Alternative Framework Material for Removable Dental Prostheses. A Clinical Report. *J. Prosthodont.* **2016**, *25*, 580–584. [CrossRef]
20. Roehling, S.; Astasov-Frauenhoffer, M.; Hauser-Gerspach, I.; Braissant, O.; Woelfler, H.; Waltimo, T.; Kniha, H.; Gahlert, M. In Vitro Biofilm Formation on Titanium and Zirconia Implant Surfaces. *J. Periodontol.* **2017**, *88*, 298–307. [CrossRef]
21. Hahnel, S.; Wieser, A.; Lang, R.; Rosentritt, M. Biofilm formation on the surface of modern implant abutment materials. *Clin. Oral Implant. Res.* **2015**, *26*, 1297–1301. [CrossRef]
22. Ionescu, A.C.; Hahnel, S.; König, A.; Brambilla, E. Resin composite blocks for dental CAD/CAM applications reduce biofilm formation in vitro. *Dent. Mater.* **2020**, *36*, 603–616. [CrossRef] [PubMed]
23. Habibi, Y.; Dawid, M.T.; Waldecker, M.; Rammelsberg, P.; Bomicke, W. Three-year clinical performance of monolithic and partially veneered zirconia ceramic fixed partial dentures. *J. Esthet. Restor. Dent.* **2020**, *32*, 395–402. [CrossRef] [PubMed]
24. Reissmann, D.R.; Benecke, A.W.; Aarabi, G.; Sierwald, I. Development and validation of the German version of the Orofacial Esthetic Scale. *Clin. Oral Investig.* **2015**, *19*, 1443–1450. [CrossRef] [PubMed]

2

Realization of a Dental Framework by 3D Printing in Material Cobalt-Chromium with Superior Precision and Fitting Accuracy

André Edelmann *, Lisa Riedel and Ralf Hellmann

Applied Laser and Photonics Group, University of Applied Sciences Aschaffenburg, 63743 Aschaffenburg, Germany; s7040@h-ab.de (L.R.); ralf.hellmann@th-ab.de (R.H.)

* Correspondence: andre.edelmann@th-ab.de

Abstract: We report on the generation of a cobalt-chromium dental framework with superior precision and fitting accuracy using selective laser melting. The objective of this study is the reduction of surface roughness and the possibility to manufacture a dental framework with high precision for passive fit with attachments, in particular a round tack. After selective laser melting, the dental framework is thermally post processed at 750 °C, shot-blasted with glass and highly polished. Nominal to actual 3D form deviation is analyzed by stripe light projection, revealing deviations being less than 250 μm, i.e., warpage is as low as to permit dental application and accurate passive fit. In particular, the critical area of the dental framework, the fixture to the implant (overdenture) shows negligible deviations. This superior fitting accuracy is confirmed by joining the bar with a testing stylus.

Keywords: additive manufacturing; dental application; superior accuracy

1. Introduction

Dental implant therapy is since more than 30 years a common practice in the contemporary restorative and surgical dentistry of partially and fully edentulous patients [1–6]. Different polymers and metals were qualified in terms of biocompatibility, with respect to their soft tissue responses and good clinical performance over long periods [7–9]. Among a variety of implant component shapes, one of the most distinguished representatives is the dental implant bar [10,11]. With reference to selective laser melting (SLM), as a beneficial additive manufacturing method for dental technology, titanium and cobalt-chrome alloys are the most prominent and approved metals for dental implant therapy [12–15].

For full anatomical restorations, the dental bar is designed to support partial dentures. Bars are typically employed in a variety of advanced designs with different, complex attachments and retentions (Figure 1 exemplifies details of such a bar), to take into account complex clinical situations and provide maximum comfort for the patient. Dental bars are manufactured in various geometries, such as, e.g., Preci-Horax bars, Dolder bars with joints, abutments and attachments, as well as freely designable bar shapes [10,16]. For a long time, cast bars with welded or soldered prefabricated attachments were the standard in implant-supported restoration of the maxilla and mandible [17,18]. However, these conventional restorations may shrink, expand or have unwanted inclusions as a result of the casting and joining processes [19,20]. During the last decade, precision milling evolved as current the state-of-the-art manufacturing technology to meet the increasing expectations in accuracy and stress-free fit as well as design flexibility [19,21,22].

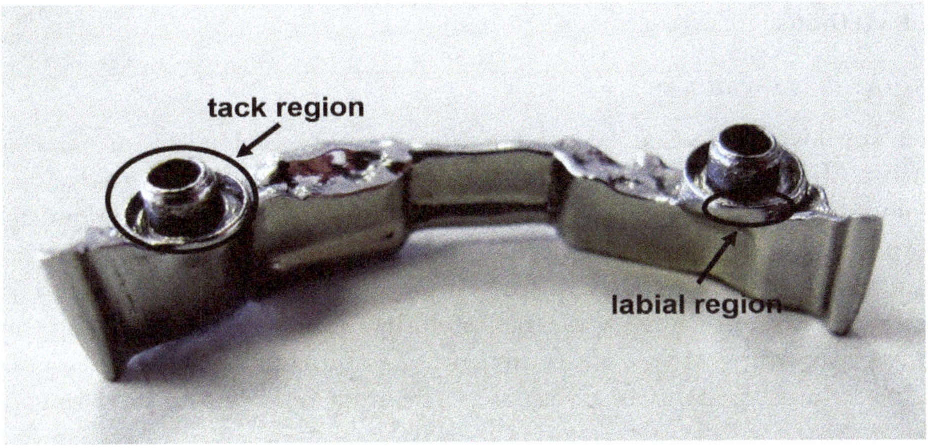

Figure 1. SLM fabricated dental framework.

Proper angulation and positioning of dental implants and the superstructure are essential to achieve acceptable prosthetic outcomes and long term success of implants and implant-supported prostheses, in turn striving superior demands on the fitting accuracy of bars with respect to shape divergence and surface roughness, e.g., in the labial region of the bar as indicated in Figure 1. In addition, surface properties should promote the integration of soft tissue while minimizing plaque and bacterial retention [23].

Therefore, different corrective techniques such as abrasive blasting, precision grinding or electrical discharge machining are employed to improve the surface and accuracy of dental bars. Though a clear definition of acceptable deviations in precision is not yet available [11], it was shown by Romero et al. and others that gaps in the range between 10 µm and 200 µm will be sufficient in meeting the criteria of passive fit between a cast bar superstructure and its interface with an implant abutment [24–27]. This prevents stress in the prosthesis-abutment-screw-implant complex, and, as a consequence, technical complications such as, e.g., fracture of the abutment, prosthesis or implant or biological complications including discomfort or pain to the patient or even bone fracture, respectively [9,28]. In fact, CNC-milled implant superstructures outperform the accuracy of fit that can be achieved with cast metal frameworks [29–31].

As a novel method in prosthodontics and orthodontics, additive manufacturing (AM) combines the advantages of high design flexibility, short manufacturing cycles enabling individual and small series production, high precision and a balanced selection of qualified polymer materials and metals. AM thus has the potential and is indeed already in use, beyond pure rapid prototyping, to replace conventional technologies, shorten process chains and improve dental implant technology [32–34]. Nonetheless, the demanding requirements in terms of precision and passive fit, as well as surface quality still challenge AM.

Against this background, we highlight the potential of SLM by exemplifying a complex shaped bar made of CoCrW. To facilitate the details of the complex design, in particular a thin walled hollow cylinder attachment as part of a full dental framework, which has not been previously reported by SLM, and to improve the surface roughness achievable with SLM, powders with different particle size distributions have been comparatively studied. The reduction of surface roughness is associated with reducing the necessary efforts in post processing, in turn enabling rapid, individualized manufacturing [11]. In addition and detail, achievable density and surface roughness have been optimized by investigating the influence of the applied laser fluence. Smallest shape deviations and high passive fit of highly polished bars lead to good passive fit as demonstrated by a testing stylus, typically used by dental laboratory technicians. In particular, the area of support of the tack that facilitates the connection to the implant is sensitive to roughness and shape deviations hampering precise passive fit.

2. Materials and Methods

2.1. Selective Laser Melting Conditions

For SLM, we employed a Realizer SLM 50 (Realizer GmbH, Bielefeld, Germany) equipped with a $P_L = 100$ W yttrium fiber laser (IPG, YLM-100). Spot size of the laser is set to $d_{spot} = 20$ µm at focus position. The machine processes under argon atmosphere with a 0.1% oxygen level. The build platform was kept at $\vartheta_{plate} = 200$ °C to maintain the machined part at an elevated temperature as to avoid deformation by curling due to residual stress. The input energy density E_d is varied in the range of 52 J/mm^3 to 92 J/mm^3 by varying the hatch distance y_{hatch} and keeping the laser power at $P_L = 55$ W, the exposure time at $t_{exp} = 20$ µm and the point distance at $x_{point} = 6$ µm, and layer thickness $z_{layer} = 50$ µm constant, respectively. The thus resulting energy density is calculated by Equation (1) [13,35].

$$E_d = \frac{P_L\, t_{exp}}{x_{point}\, y_{hatch}\, z_{layer}} \tag{1}$$

2.2. Powder Characterization

In this study, we analyze and process commercially available CoCrW metal powder (Eisenbacher GmbH, Wörth am Main, Germany). The chemical composition of this powder is as listed in Table 1.

Table 1. Chemical composition of CoCrW powder.

wt%	Cobalt	Chromium	Tungsten	Silicon	Manganous	Iron	Others
Powder	62.44	27.50	8.09	1.52	0.2	0.11	<0.1

Important fabrication material parameters for processing metallic powder in AM systems are the flowability and the powder density. If the flowability is too low, a homogenous covering of powder over the build plate in the SLM machine cannot be ensured and, in addition, a low powder density can lead to a higher porosity of the fabricated components [36]. For a more detailed investigation of the build quality regarding the powder characteristics, we divide the powder by sieving into the fraction A32 and A45. The notation refers to the d90 value of the grain size distribution. The fraction in A32 contains powder where 90% of the grain sizes are below $d_g < 32$ µm, whereas 90% of grain sizes in fraction A45 are below $d_g < 45$ µm. For each of these two powder batches we measure the flow time and the powder density. The results are shown in Table 2. The flowability, which influences the coating of the powder bed, is determined by measuring the flow rate using a Hall-Flowmeter according DIN EN ISO 4490. The powder density, influencing the homogeneity and density of the powder bed and thus the accessible relative density of the SLM built part, is measured according DIN ISO 697.

Table 2. Flowability and powder density of powder A32 and A45.

	A 32	A45
flow time (s)	19.1 ± 0.1	14.5 ± 0.3
powder density (g/cm^3)	3.6 ± 0.1	3.1 ± 0.1

Comparing powder sections A32 with A45, a higher flow time is found for A32. For this sieved particle size, the averaged grain sizes are smaller and, as a result, a higher probability of agglomeration by intermolecular interactions such as Van-der-Waals forces and higher contact surfaces of smaller particles come predominantly into play. As a result, higher stiction appears and the flowability is reduced [37,38]. In addition, the lowest powder density is found for A45, as for the A32 powder fraction an increase of finer grain sizes gets relevant and larger particles cannot fill the free spaces [39,40].

The moisture of the powder, which reduces the flow rate and thus the coating of the powder bed and which may also lead to higher gas porosity, is determined by weighting in combination with a drying chamber (PCE-MA 110, PCE Germany GmbH). We determine the moisture of both powder batches being under 0.01% and, therefore, exclude any influence of moisture to the flowability and powder density.

Figure 2 depicts the morphology of the powder and the particle size distribution of the different powder batches A32 and A45. In the powder samples, a spherical characteristic with minor satellites is observed which are free of porosity. The particle size distribution of the powder was analyzed by a Camsizer X2 based on dynamic digital image analysis methods according to ISO 13322-2 (Retsch Technology GmbH). This particle size distribution and morphology allows good flowability and packing density, as was demonstrated in a flowability test conducted using the Hall flowmeter funnel.

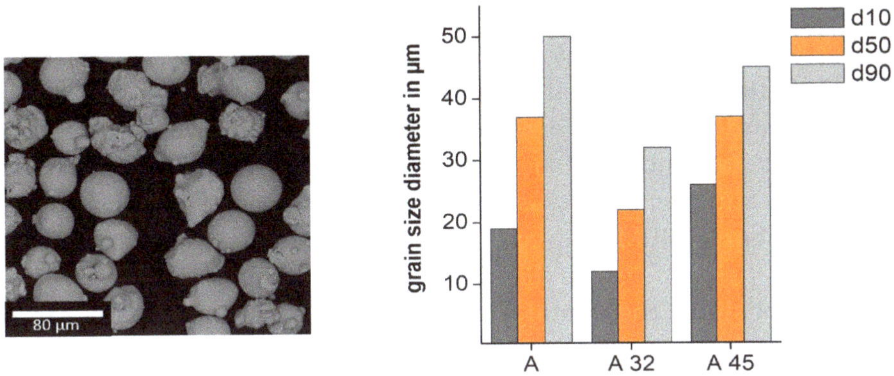

Figure 2. SEM images of Powder A (**left**) and particle size distribution of powder batch A, A32 and A45 (**right**).

2.3. Mechanical Properties

We evaluate the mechanical properties of SLM specimens based on powder batch A and comparing the results with the product specifications of CoCrW-powder (Eisenbacher Dentalwaren, Wörth am Main, Germany) [41]. By using tensile test specimens we measure the tensile strength with $\sigma_m = 365$ MPa, Young's modulus with $E = 170$ GPa, elongation with $\epsilon_b = 18\%$ and yield strength with $\sigma_{ys} = 567$ MPa (AG-Xplus, Shimadzu, Kyoto, Japan). The Vickers hardness HV10/30 on the top surface of test cubes (edge length $a = 10$ mm) results to $h_{vickers} = 365$ HV (Falcon 5000, Innovatest, Maastricht, The Netherlands). For the thermal expansion coefficient we obtain $\Delta l = 14.5 \times 10^{-6}\ K^{-1}$ (DIL 402 Expedis, Netzsch, Selb, Germany) by using cylindrical specimens with a diameter of $d = 6$ mm and a length of $l = 50$ mm and applying a heating rate of $r_{heat} = 5$ K/s up to $\vartheta_{max} = 300$ °C. The mechanical properties are combined in Tables 3 and 4.

Table 3. Tensile strength, Young's modulus, elongation and yield strength of SLM fabricated CoCrW specimens.

	Tensile Strength	Young's Modulus	Elongation	Yield Strength
SLM	969 MPa	170 GPa	18%	567 MPa
reference [41]	1021 MPa	196 GPa	8%	642 MPa

Table 4. Vickers hardness and thermal expansion coefficient of SLM fabricated CoCrW specimens.

	Hardness	Thermal Expansion
SLM	365 HV	$14.5 \times 10^{-6}\ K^{-1}$
reference [41]	356 HV	$14.25 \times 10^{-6}\ K^{-1}$

Additionally we have taken polished cut images of test specimens in combination with SEM and EDX analysis. We have found, in gerneral, homogeneous microstructure with grain boundaries, at which we observe segregations of Wolfram. In Figure 3 the images of the mircostructure is shown.

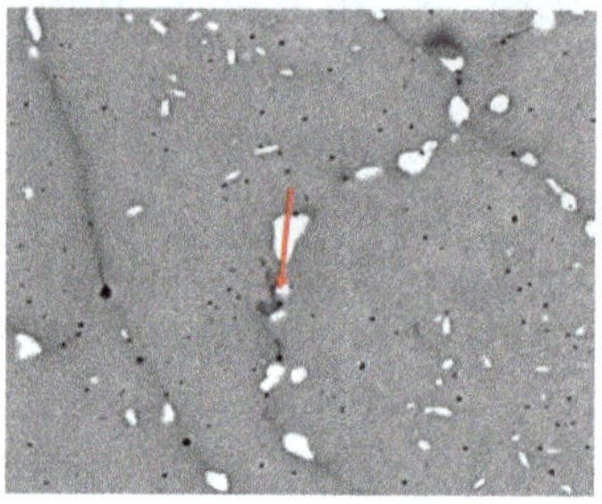

Figure 3. SEM image of CoCrW microstructure.

2.4. *Experimental Flow Chart*

The flow chart of the experimental tasks carried out in this report is shown in Figure 4. Beside the metallurgical and physical examination of powders and test specimen, the generation of the dental framework is conducted as follows. Beginning from digital data, obtained by anonymized patient data and prepared in .stl-data format, we have additively built both specimen for testing and the dental bar by SLM (implant fabrication). Here we focus particularly on the surface roughness by optimizing the particle size distribution of the metal powder. After post processing by thermal treatment and polishing, the dental framework is characterized with particular focus on 3D form deviation and fitting accuracy.

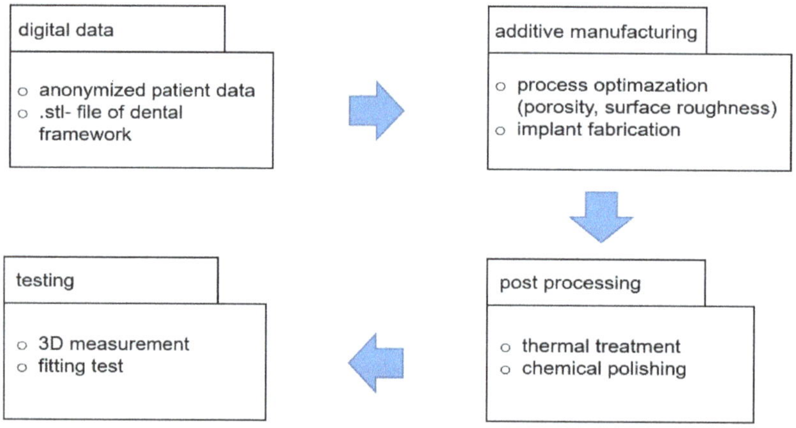

Figure 4. Experimental work flow carried out to fabricate the dental framework.

3. Results and Discussion

3.1. *Optimization of Density and Roughness*

In medical application and in particular in dental restoration, a high quality of the additive manufactured parts is needed. An important quality factor refers to the remaining porosity in the SLM part. By using well defined process parameters, the porosity of SLM parts is, in general accessible, below one percent. As previous, comprehensive studies on selective laser melting have shown, the porosity in the material sensitively depends on the energy density [42–46]. If the energy density is too high, gas porosity appears and if, in contrast, the input of the energy is to low, lack-of-fusion porosity appears [47].

In the following, we compare the processing of the fine powder section A32 and the coarse powder A45, as to evaluate the remaining porosity in the volume of the SLM part. We process both powder batches with the same process parameters, yet varying the applied energy density from $E_d = 52\ \mathrm{J/mm^3}$ to $E_d = 92\ \mathrm{J/mm^3}$. While we keep the laser power P_L, the point distance x_{point}, the exposure time t_{exp} and the layer thickness with z_{layer} constant, respectively, we vary the hatch distance y_{hatch} to accomplish different energy densities (as shown in Section 2.1). For each parameter set we built four cuboids with the dimensions of $V = 4 \times 4 \times 3$ mm^3 and measure the porosity by applying Archimedes method. The results for powder A32 and powder A45 are summarized in Figure 5.

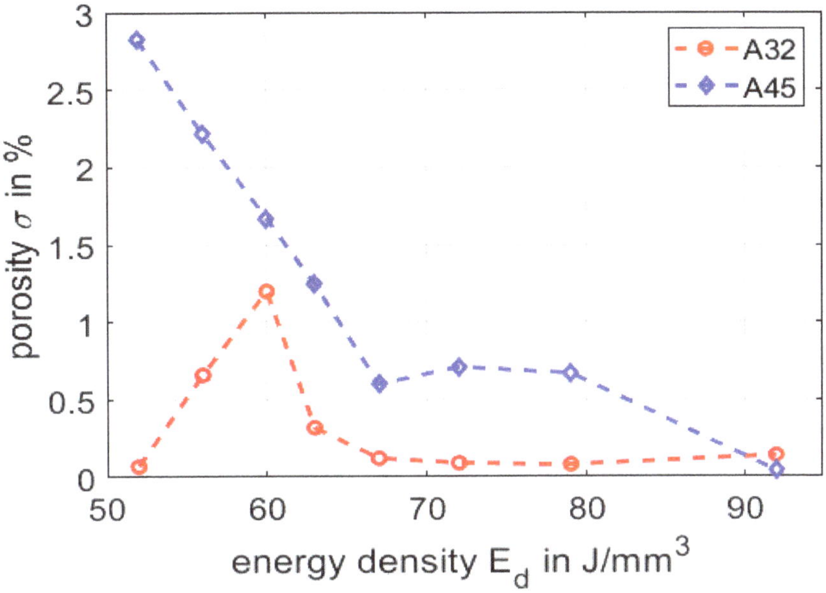

Figure 5. Comparison of the porosity of A32 and A45 in dependency of the energy density.

By processing powder A45 and increasing the energy density, the porosity drops from $\sigma = 2.8\%$ to $\sigma = 0.04\%$. We attribute this decrease to larger particle sizes, leading to lack-of-fusion porosities by lower energy inputs. In contrast, applying the finer powder A32, we find a peak value of the porosity with $\sigma = 1.2\%$ at an energy density of $E_d = 60$ J/mm^3, whereas for energy densities between $E_d = 67$ J/mm^3 and $E_d = 92$ J/mm^3, respectively, we have measured a rather low and stable porosity between $\sigma = 0.1\%$ and $\sigma = 0.2\%$. Here we assume the optimum between the lack-of-fusion and gas porosity. Considering both powder fraction A32 and A45, we find porosities of below one percent at higher energy densities of $E_d = 67$ J/mm^3. Therefore we define the process window for both powder fractions between $E_d = 67$ J/mm^3 and $E_d = 92$ J/mm^3. In this range the porosity is below one percent for both powder fractions, indicating an appropriate build quality.

One of the further limiting factors in the fabrication of high accuracy additive manufactured parts refers to the surface roughness, which we quantify by the common roughness parameter R_z. Deviations in the surface roughness lead to deviations in the accuracy of the part geometry and increase the necessary post processing efforts. Therefore, we discuss the two considered powder batches regarding the accessible surface roughness in dependence of the applied energy input during SLM. Surface roughness was analyzed using a laser scanning microscope (LSM VK-X200, Keyence).

The surface roughness of SLM parts, in general, depends on the grain size distribution of processed powder and used process parameters [48–50]. Furthermore, the surface roughness appears different on top and side surfaces, with respect to the build direction. In Figure 6 the surface roughness R_z is shown for the top and side surfaces for the powder A32 and powder A45 as function of the applied energy density. A suitable process window regarding the porosity is already defined by the porosity between the energy density of $E_d = 63$ J/mm^3 and $E_d = 92$ J/mm^3.

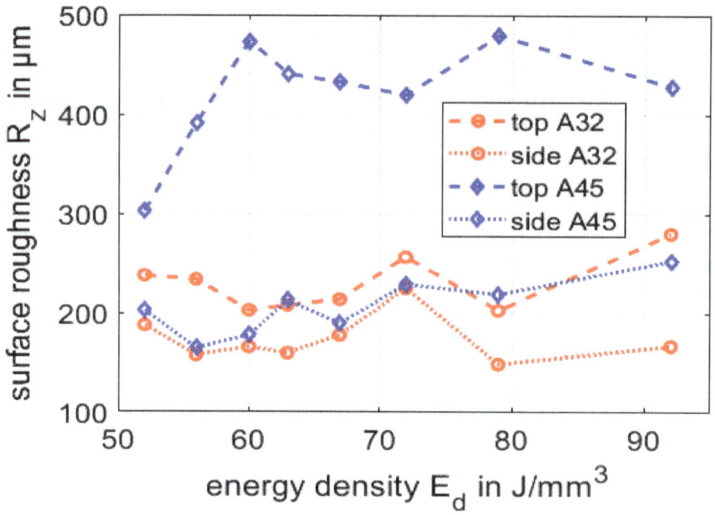

Figure 6. Comparison of surface roughness of the top and side surfaces.

Comparing the surface roughness as given in Figure 6, R_Z of the top surface of powder A45 is highest with $R_Z > 400$ µm, whereas the corresponding values of A32 (top), A32 (side) and A45 (side), respectively, are below $R_Z < 300$ µm. The roughness of the top surfaces of specimen made of A32 and A45 can jointly be explained by the particle size distribution. By processing coarser powder particles a rough surface appears due to sintering of particles on the top surface. The cavities between coarser powder particles cannot be filled with finer powder particles. In contrast, the side surfaces roughness of powder A45 and A32 is rather similar to each other, i.e., the influence of particle size distribution is less pronounced. Here smaller particles of both powder batches are sintered at the side surfaces and the quality of the SLM side surfaces depends mainly on the energy input [50]. As an interim conclusion, best surface roughness for the top and side surfaces is found for powder batch A32 with $R_Z < 300$ µm for the top and $R_Z < 200$ µm for the side. For dental application a low value of the surface roughness is needed allowing the fabrication of geometries with high accuracy and lowest effort in surface finishing of the respective components.

3.2. Fabrication of Dental Framework

To highlight the potential of of CoCrW for dental applications, we exemplify the SLM fabrication by generating a sophisticated dental framework (dental bar with attachements). In Figure 7 the finished dental framework is shown, after post processing with a thermal treatment of up to 750 °C, glass spheres blasting of the surface (grain size of 90–150 µm) and chemical polishing (the polishing step is done by a dental laboratory). Thermal treatment was carried out in a standard oven (Nabertherm) at a temperature of 750 °C (heating phase 45 min), temperature hold for 55 min and natural cooling. The resulting fitting accuracy is tested by a dental testing gauge (stylus) without significant deviation.

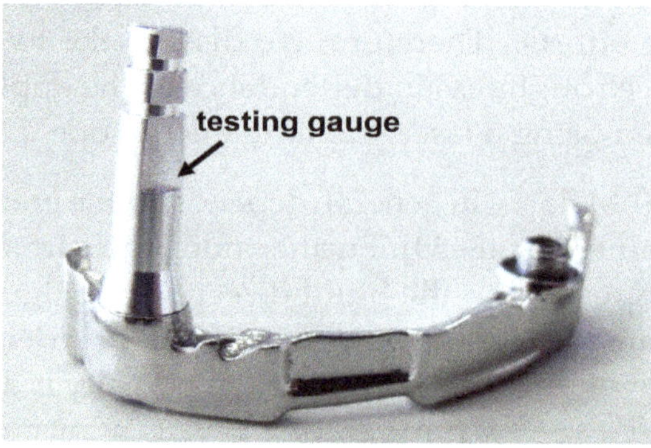

Figure 7. Dental framework with testing gauge.

Verification of the geometrical accuracy of the dental framework is done by 3D inspection (3D scanning) and comparison of the actual values with the nominal values. Shape deviations and shape variance analysis as compared to the original CAD data is provided by stripe line projection using Atos Core and ATOS Professional V8-SR1 software (GOM, Brunswick, Germany). The results are shown in Figure 8 in different orientations. The maximum deviation for the whole dental framework is less than $d_x \leq 0.25$ mm. This fabrication accuracy excludes thermal warpage of the structure and well-defined energy input during the build process. In particular the critical area around the fixture of the dental implant shows very good precision with deviations to the nominal value of less than $d_x \leq 15$ µm.

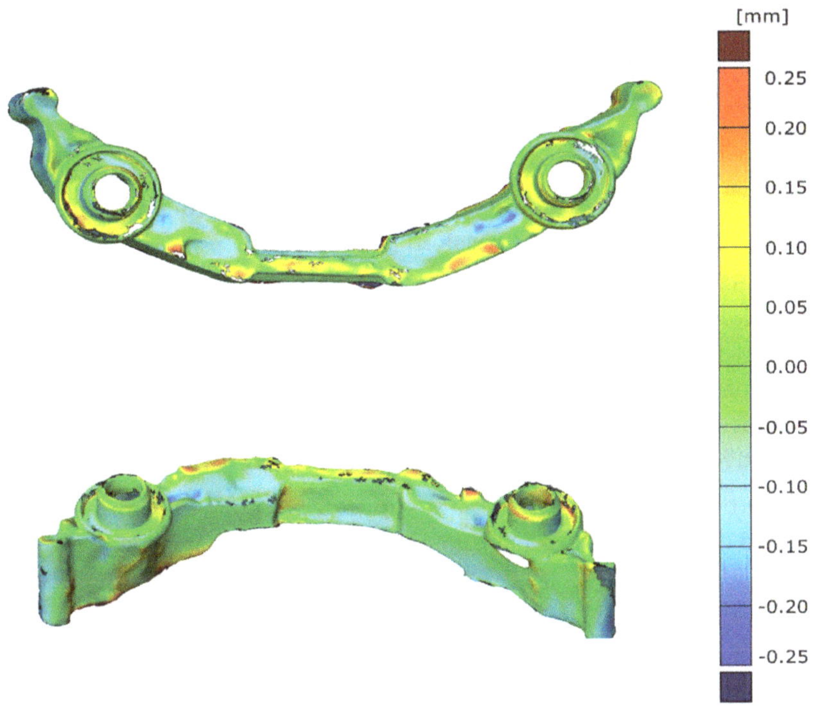

Figure 8. Nominal/actual value comparison of the dental framework—top view (above) and side view (below).

4. Conclusions

We demonstrated additive manufacturing of a dental framework (dental bar) with superior precision and fitting accuracy. In particular, using a fine sized particle distribution leads to significant improvement of the surface roughness fulfilling the recommendations for dental applications. A proper setting of the SLM laser and scanning parameters, in particular the applied laser energy density, leads to a minimized shape deviation and warping of the fabricated dental implant. As a result and to exemplify and highlight the potential of selective laser melting, a CoCrW dental implant components, a dental bar with attachments on the contact area and small sized round tack with thin walls and sufficient roughness, is demonstrated, which is commonly difficult to process with conventional processes.

Author Contributions: Conceptualization, A.E. and R.H.; methodology, A.E.; validation, A.E. and L.R.; formal analysis, A.E. and L.R.; investigation, A.E. and L.R.; data curation, A.E. and L.R.; writing—original draft preparation, A.E. and R.H.; writing—review and editing, A.E. and R.H.; visualization, A.E.; supervision, R.H.; project administration, R.H.; funding acquisition, R.H. All authors have read and agreed to the published version of the manuscript.

Abbreviations

The following abbreviations are used in this manuscript:

SLM selective laser melting
AM additive manufacturing

References

1. Jemt, T. Failures and complications in 391 consecutively inserted fixed prostheses supported by Brånemark implants in edentulous jaws: A study of treatment from the time of prosthesis placement to the first annual checkup. *Int. J. Oral Maxillofac. Implants* **1991**, *6*, 270–276.
2. Wee, A.G.; Aquilino, S.A.; Schneider, R.L. Strategies to achieve fit in implant prosthodontics: A review of the literature. *Int. J. Prosthodont.* **1999**, *12*, 167–178. [PubMed]
3. Kalpana, D.; Sanjana, J.R.; Kumara Raju Kurapati, S.; Joel Koshy, J. Comparative evaluation of one piece and two piece dental implants—A review. *Int. J. Sci. Res.* **2017**, *6*, 49–50.
4. Pjetursson, B.E.; Asgeirsson, A.G.; Zwahlen, M.; Sailer, I. Improvements in implant dentistry over the last decade: Comparison of survival and complication rates in older and newer publications. *Int. J. Oral Maxillofac. Implants* **2014**, *29*, 308–324. [CrossRef] [PubMed]
5. Devaraju, K.; Rao, S.J.; Joseph, J.K.; Kurapati, S.K. Comparison of biomechanical properties of different implant-abutment connections. *Indian J. Dent. Sci.* **2018**, *10*, 180–183.
6. Thalji, G.; McGraw, K.; Cooper, L.F. Maxillary Complete Denture Outcomes: A Systematic Review of Patient-Based Outcomes. *Int. J. Oral Maxillofac. Implants* **2016**, *31*, 169–181. [CrossRef]
7. Örtorp, A.; Jemt, T. CNC-milled titanium frameworks supported by implants in the edentulous jaw: A 10-year comparative clinical study. *Clin. Implant Dent. Relat. Res.* **2012**, *14*, 88–99. [CrossRef]
8. Lowe, L.G.; Shcherbukhin, V.M. An implant-supported, cobalt-chromium milled bar and nonflanged attachment-retained overdenture to rehabilitate the edentulous mandible. *J. Prosthet. Dent.* **2009**, *102*, 46–51. [CrossRef]
9. Kioleoglou, I.; Pissiotis, A.; Konstantinos, M. Accuracy of fit of implant-supported bars favricated on definitive casts made of different dental stones. *J. Clin. Exp. Dent.* **2018**, *10*, 252–263.
10. Rinke, S.; Rasing, H.; Gersdorff, N.; Buergers, R.; Roediger, M. Implant supported over dentures with different bar designs: A retrospective evaluation after 5–19 years of clinical function. *J. Adv. Prosthodont.* **2015**, *7*, 338–343. [CrossRef]
11. Gehrke, P.; Dinkel, J.; Fischer, C.; Schmenger, K.; Sader, R. Surface roughness and necessity of manual refinishing requirements of CAD/CAM-manufatured titanium and cobalt-chrome bars—A pilot study. *Open Dent. J.* **2019**, *13*, 316–326. [CrossRef]
12. Chen, G.; Zeng, X.; Wang, Z.; Guan, K.; Peng, C. Fabrication of removable partial denture framework by selective laser melting. *Adv. Mater. Res.* **2011**, *317–319*, 174–178. [CrossRef]
13. Hong, M.-H.; Ki Min, B.; Kwon, T.-Y. The influence of process parameters on the surface roughness of a 3D-printed CoCr Dental alloy produced via selective laser melting. *Appl. Sci.* **2016**, *6*, 401–411. [CrossRef]
14. Kanazawa, M.; Iwaki, M.; Shunsuke, M.; Naoyuki, N. Fabrication of titanium alloy framework for complete dentures by selective laser melting. *J. Prosthet. Dent.* **2014**, *112*, 1441–1447. [CrossRef] [PubMed]
15. Konieczny, B.; Szczesio-Wlodarczyk, A.; Sokolowski, J.; Bociong, K. Challenges of Co–Cr Alloy Additive Manufacturing Methods in Dentistry—The Current State of Knowledge (Systematic Review). *Materials* **2020**, *13*, 3524. [CrossRef]
16. Weinländer, M.; Piehslinger, E.; Krennmair, G. Removable implant prosthodontic rehabilitation of the edentulous mandible: Five-year results of different prosthetic anchorage concepts. *Int. J. Oral Maxillofac. Implants* **2010**, *25*, 589–597.
17. Mericske-Stern, R. Prosthetic considerations. *Aust. Dent. J.* **2008**, *53*, 49–59. [CrossRef]
18. Waddell, J.N.; Payne, A.G.; Swain, M.V.; Kieser, J.A. Scanning electron microscopy observations of failures of implant overdenture bars: A case series report. *Clin. Implant Dent. Relat. Res.* **2010**, *12*, 26–38. [CrossRef]

19. Abduo, J.; Lyons, K.; Bennani, V.; Waddell, N.; Swain, M. Fit of screwretained fixed implant frameworks fabricated by different methods: A systematic review. *Int. J. Prosthodont.* **2011**, *24*, 207–220.
20. Paniz, G.; Stellini, E.; Meneghello, R.; Cerardi, A.; Gobbato, E.A.; Bressan, E. The precision of fit of cast and milled full-arch implant-supported restorations. *Int. J. Oral Maxillofac. Implants* **2013**, *28*, 687–693. [CrossRef]
21. Katsoulis, J.; Mericske-Stern, R.; Yates, D.M.; Izutani, N.; Enkling, N.; Blatz, M.B. In vitro precision of fit of computer-aided design and computeraided manufacturing titanium and zirconium dioxide bars. *Dent. Mater.* **2013**, *29*, 945–953. [CrossRef] [PubMed]
22. Miyazaki, T.; Hotta, Y.; Kunii, J.; Kuriyama, S.; Tamaki, Y. A review of dental CAD/CAM: Current status and future perspectives from 20 years of experience. *Dent. Mater. J.* **2009**, *28*, 44–56. [CrossRef] [PubMed]
23. Bollen, C.M.; Lambrechts, P.; Quirynen, M. Comparison of surface roughness of oral hard materials to the threshold surface roughness for bacterial plaque retention: A review of the literature. *Dent. Mater.* **1997**, *13*, 258–269. [CrossRef]
24. Romero, G.G.; Engelmeier, R.; Powers, J.M.; Canterbury, A. Accuracy of three corrective techniques for implant bar fabrication. *J. Prosthet. Dent.* **2000**, *84*, 602–607. [CrossRef] [PubMed]
25. Abduo, J.A.; Lyons, K.L. Effect of vertical misfit on strain within screw-retained implant titanium and zirconia frameworks. *J. Prosthodont Res.* **2012**, *56*, 102–109. [CrossRef]
26. Karl, M.; Winter, W.; Taylor, T.D.; Heckmann, S.M. In vitro study on passive fit in implant-supported 5-unit fixed partial dentures. *Int. J. Oral Maxillofac. Implants* **2004**, *19*, 30–37.
27. Hanif, A.; Qureshi, S.; Sheikh, Z.; Rashid, H. Complications in implant dentistry. *Eur. J. Dent.* **2017**, *11*, 135–140. [CrossRef]
28. Clelland, N.L.; Papazoglou, E.; Carr, A.B.; Gilat, A. Comparison of strains transferred to a bone sumulant among implant overdenture bars with various levels of misfir. *J. Prosthodont.* **1995**, *4*, 243–250. [CrossRef]
29. Torsello, F.; di Torresanto, V.M.; Ercoli, C.; Cordaro, L. Evaluation of the marginal precision of one-piece complete arch titanium frameworks fabricated using five different methods for implant-supported restorations. *Clin. Oral Implant. Res.* **2008**, *19*, 772–779. [CrossRef]
30. Takahashi, T.; Gunne, J. Fit of implant frameworks: An in vitro comparison between two fabrication techniques. *J. Prosthet. Dent.* **2003**, *89*, 256–260. [CrossRef]
31. Buzayan, M.M.; Yunus, N.B. Passive fit in screw retained multi-unit implant prosthesis understanding and achieving: A review of the literature. *J. Indian Prosthodont. Soc.* **2014**, *14*, 16–23. [CrossRef] [PubMed]
32. Di Giacomo, A.P.; Cury, P.R.; Airton, D.; DaSilva, M.; DaSilva, V.L.; Sergio, D.; Ajzen, A. A selective laser sintering prototype guide used to fabricate immediate interim fixed complete arch prostheses in flapless dental implant surgery: Technique description and clinical results. *J. Prosthet. Dent.* **2016**, *116*, 874–879. [CrossRef] [PubMed]
33. Jamshidinia, M.; Wang, L.; Tong, W.; Ajlouni, R.; Kovacevic, R. Fatigue properties of a dental implant produced by electron beam melting. *J. Mater. Process. Technol.* **2015**, *226*, 255–263. [CrossRef]
34. Lima, J.; Anami, L.; Araujo, R.; Pavanelli, C. Removable Partial Dentures: Use of Rapid Prototyping. *J. Prosthodont.* **2014**, *23*, 588. [CrossRef]
35. Cherry, J.; Davies, H.; Mehmood, S.; Lavery, N.; Brown, S.; Sienz, J. Investigation into the effect of process parameters on microstructural and physical properties of 316L stainless steel parts by selective laser melting. *Int. J. Adv. Manuf. Technol.* **2015**, *76*, 869–879. [CrossRef]
36. Spierings, A.B.; Levy, G. Comparision of density of stainless steel parts produced with selective laser melting using different powder grades. In Proceedings of the Annual International Solid Freeform Fabrication Symposium, Austin, TX, USA, 3–5 August 2009.
37. Nguyen, Q.B.; Nai, M.L.S.; Zhu, Z.; Sun, C.N.; Wei, J.; Zhou, W. Characteristics of Inconel Powders for Powder-Bed Additive Manufacturing. *Engineering* **2017**, *3*, 695–700. [CrossRef]
38. Clayton, J. Optimising metal powders for additive manufacturing. *Met. Powder Rep.* **2014**, *69*, 14–17. [CrossRef]
39. Lee, Y.S.; Zhang, W. Mesoscopic simulation of heat transfer and fluid flow in laser powder bed additive manufacturing. In Proceedings of the International Solid Free Form Fabrication Symposium, Austin, TX, USA, 12 August 2015.
40. Karapatis, N.P.; Egger, G.; Gygax, P.E.; Glardon, R. Optimization of powder layer density in selective laser sintering. In Proceedings of the 1999 International Solid Freeform Fabrication Symposium, Austin, TX, USA, 25 April 1999.

41. Eisenbacher Dentalwaren ED GmbH. *Product Specification of Kera S-Powder*; Eisenbacher Dentalwaren ED GmbH: Wörth am Main, Germany, 2015
42. Maamoun, A.H.; Xue, Y.F.; Elbestawi, M.A.; Veldhuis, S.C. Effect of Selective Laser Melting Process Parameters on the Quality of Al Alloy Parts: Powder Characterization, Density, Surface Roughness, and Dimensional Accuracy. *Materials* **2018**, *11*, 2343. [CrossRef]
43. Prashanth, K.G.; Scudino, S.; Maity, T.; Das, J.; Eckert, J. Is the energy density a reliable parameter for materials synthesis by selective laser melting? *Mater. Res. Lett.* **2017**, *5*, 386–390. [CrossRef]
44. Aboulkhaira, N.T.; Everitt, N.M.; Ashcroft, I.; Tuck, C. Reducing porosity in AlSi10Mg parts processed by selective laser melting. *Addit. Manuf.* **2014**, *1–4*, 77–86. [CrossRef]
45. Zhang, L.-C.; Attar, H. Selective Laser Melting of Titanium Alloys and Titanium Matrix Composites for Biomedical Applications: A Review. *Adv. Eng. Mater.* **2016**, *18*, 463–475. [CrossRef]
46. Kempen, K.; Thijs, L.; Van Humbeeck, J.; Kruth, J.-P. Mechanical properties of AlSi10Mg produced by Selective Laser Melting. *Phys. Procedia* **2012**, *39*, 439–446. [CrossRef]
47. Pleass, C.; Jothi, S. Influence of powder characteristics and additive manufacturing process parameters on the microstructure and mechanical behaviour of Inconel 625 fabricated by Selective Laser Melting. *Addit. Manuf.* **2018**, *24*, 419–431. [CrossRef]
48. Dadbakhsh, S.; Hao, L.; Jerrard, P.G.E.; Zhang, D.Z. Experimental investigation on selective laser melting behaviour and processing windows of in situ reacted Al/Fe2O3 powder mixture. *Powder Technol.* **2012**, *231*, 112–121. [CrossRef]
49. Calignano, F.; Manfredi, D.; Ambrosio, E.P.; Iuliano, L.; Fino, P. Influence of process parameters on surface roughness of aluminum parts produced by DMLS. *Int. J. Adv. Manuf. Technol.* **2013**, *67*, 2743–2751. [CrossRef]
50. Yang, T.; Liu, T.; Liao, W.; MacDonald, E.; Wei, H.; Chen, X.; Jiang, L. The influence of process parameters on vertical surface roughness of the AlSi10Mg parts fabricated by selective laser melting. *J. Mater. Process. Technol.* **2019**, *266*, 26–36. [CrossRef]

3

Effects of Polyacrylic Acid Pre-Treatment on Bonded-Dentine Interfaces Created with a Modern Bioactive Resin-Modified Glass Ionomer Cement and Subjected to Cycling Mechanical Stress

Salvatore Sauro [1,2,*], Vicente Faus-Matoses [3], Irina Makeeva [2], Juan Manuel Nuñez Martí [1], Raquel Gonzalez Martínez [1], José Antonio García Bautista [1] and Vicente Faus-Llácer [3]

1 Departamento de Odontologia, Facultad de Sciencia de la Salud, Universidad CEU Cardenal Herrera, 46115 Valencia, Spain; juan.nunez@uchceu.es (J.M.N.M.); raquel.gonzalez@uchceu.es (R.G.M.); joseanto@uchceu.es (J.A.G.B.)

2 Department of Therapeutic Dentistry, Sechenov University Russia, 119435 Moscow, Russia; irina_markovina@mail.ru

3 Departamento de Estomatología, Facultad de Medicina y Odontología, Universitat de Valencia, 46010 Valencia, Spain; fausvj@uv.es (V.F.M.); Vicente.J.Faus@uv.es (V.F.L.)

* Correspondence: salvatore.sauro@uchceu.es

Abstract: Objectives: Resin-modified glass ionomer cements (RMGIC) are considered excellent restorative materials with unique therapeutic and anti-cariogenic activity. However, concerns exist regarding the use of polyacrylic acid as a dentine conditioner as it may influence the bonding performance of RMGIC. The aim of this study was to evaluate the effect of different protocols for cycling mechanical stress on the bond durability and interfacial ultramorphology of a modern RMGIC applied to dentine pre-treated with/without polyacrylic acid conditioner (PAA). **Methods:** The RMGIC was applied onto human dentine specimens prepared with silicon-carbide (SiC) abrasive paper with or without the use of a PAA conditioner. The specimens were immersed in deionised water for 24 h then divided in 3 groups. The first group was cut into matchsticks (cross-sectional area of 0.9 mm^2) and tested immediately for microtensile bond strength (MTBS). The second was first subjected to load cycling (250,000 cycles; 3 Hz; 70 N) and then cut into matchsticks and tested for MTBS. The third group was subjected to load cycling (250,000 cycles; 3 Hz; 70 N), cut into matchsticks, and then immersed for 8 months storage in artificial saliva (AS); these were finally tested for MTBS. The results were analysed statistically using two-way ANOVA and the Student–Newman–Keuls test ($\alpha = 0.05$). Fractographic analysis was performed using FE-SEM, while further RMCGIC-bonded dentine specimens were aged as previously described and used for interfacial ultramorphology characterisation (dye nanoleakage) using confocal microscopy. **Results:** The RMGIC applied onto dentine that received no pre-treatment (10% PAA gel) showed no significant reduction in MTBS after load cycling followed by 8 months of storage in AS ($p > 0.05$). The RMGIC–dentine interface created in PAA-conditioned SiC-abraded dentine specimens showed no sign of degradation, but with porosities within the bonding interface both after load cycling and after 8 months of storage in AS. Conversely, the RMGIC–dentine interface of the specimens with no PAA pre-treatment showed no sign of porosity within the interface after any of the aging protocols, although some bonded-dentine interfaces presented cohesive cracks within the cement after prolonged AS storage. However, the specimens of this group showed no significant reduction in bond strength ($p < 0.05$) after 8 months of storage in AS or load cycling ($p > 0.05$). After prolonged AS storage, the bond strength value attained in RMGIC–dentine specimens created in PAA pre-treated dentine were significantly higher than those observed in the specimens created with no PAA pre-treatment in dentine. **Conclusions:** PAA conditioning of dentine prior to application of RMGIC induces no substantial effect on the bond strength after short-term storage, but its use may increase the risk of collagen degradation at the bonding interface after prolonged aging. Modern RMGIC applied without PAA dentine pre-treatment may have greater therapeutic synergy with saliva during cycle occlusal load, thereby enhancing the remineralisation and protection of the bonding interface.

Keywords: adhesion; bioactive; cycling mechanical stress; dentine; longevity; resin-modified glass ionomer cements; polyacrylic acid treatment

---

1. Introduction

Glass ionomer cements (GICs) were introduced for the first time in dentistry by Wilson and Kent in 1969 [1] as an innovative class of dental material able to set via an acid-base reaction after mixing fluoro-aluminosilicate glass particles (FAS) with a polyacrylic acid solution (PAA) [2]. Low viscosity polyacids, such as maleic and itaconic acids were incorporated within the PAA solution to improve the handling and setting of GICs [3–5]. Tartaric acid was also incorporated into the PAA solution to enhance the handling properties and increase the working time [6,7].

It is well known that the initial setting occurs due to a gelation reaction between the fluoro-aluminosilicate glass particles and polyalkenoate acids [8], followed by a proper hardening phase characterised by the cross-linking of the carboxylic groups present in the polymeric chains with calcium and aluminium ions present in the FAS. However, the final chemical reaction for complete setting occurs during the following 48 h [6,7], although the final "maturation" of the cement may take several months due to the slow release of aluminium ions from the glass particles. It is also important to highlight that sodium and fluoride ions are not usually involved in the setting reaction, but rather, these ions remain unreacted within the matrix, and are released gradually into the surrounding environment (e.g., bioactivity) [9,10]. Indeed, for this reason, GICs present unique therapeutic anti-cariogenic activity, which is mainly attributed to the release of fluoride (F^-) ions and to their buffering properties [11–14].

Glass ionomer cements are being used for a wide range of applications in dentistry [2]. These include the restoration of deciduous teeth [15], anterior class III and V restorations [16,17], cementation (luting) of crowns, bridges and orthodontic appliances [18–20], restorations of non-carious teeth with minimal preparation [21,22], and sandwich technique restorations [23,24]. Furthermore, they comprise the main material for atraumatic restorative therapy (ART) [25]. Indeed, subsequent to selective removal of the caries-infected tissues, GICs are applied as therapeutic ion-releasing materials to remineralise the caries-affected tissue left behind inside the dental cavity [26,27]. GICs may also exhibit a number of drawbacks, such as brittleness [28], poor wear resistance, inadequate surface properties [29,30], and sensitivity to high moisture in the oral cavity when newly placed [31].

In order to overcome such drawbacks, several modifications have been introduced to conventional GICs [32–34]. A key modification was the reinforcement of GICs through the incorporation of urethane monomers to produce resin-modified glass ionomer cements (RMGICs) [35,36]. Unlike conventional GICs, RMGICs can be self-activated (self-polymerisation) or light-cured (photo-polymerisation reaction). These "hybrid" materials have been generated to combine the mechanical properties of resin monomers with the anti-carious potential of GICs [37]. Indeed, it has been observed that RMGICs not only release fluoride, but they may also have greater flexural strength and lower solubility compared to conventional GICs [36,37]. RMGICs have a decreased fluoride release and higher creep relative to conventional powder-based ionomers [7]. Although first generation of RMGICs presented slight expansion due to water sorption (from 3.4% up to 11.3%) 24 h after placement [38], modern formulations have overcome this problem [36]. Conventional RMGICs are also characterised by lower mechanical (e.g., Young's modulus and flexural strength) and "inferior" aesthetic properties compared to resin composites [7,38].

A key advance of glass ionomer-based materials is their self-adhesive properties to bind chemically to calcium ions (Ca^{2+}) in the apatite of enamel and dentine through chelation of carboxyl group of acidic polymeric chains [39–41]. However, the self-adhesive mechanism of GIC-based materials to dentine is also due to the micromechanical interlocking achieved by shallow hybridization of the micro-porous collagen network. A 10% solution of PAA is mostly used as an enamel/dentine conditioner to remove the smear layer prior to the application of GIC-based restorative materials. Nevertheless, concerns exist regarding its use, application time, and concentration, as these factors may interfere with the overall bonding performance. Indeed, a high number of adhesive failures between a RMGIC and resin composite have been reported when a polyalkenoic conditioner was used on smear-layer covered dentine [40,41]. Cycling occlusal stress occurring during mastication, swallowing, as well as in cases of parafunctional habits, can affect the integrity of the bonding interface, making it more susceptible to short and long term degradation in the oral environment [42].

The aim of this study was to evaluate the microtensile bond strength (MTBS), after short-term load-cycle aging or after load cycle followed by prolonged aging (8 months) in artificial saliva (AS), of a modern bioactive RMGIC applied to dentine with or without surface pre-conditioning using 10% polyacrylic acid (PAA). Fractographic analysis and interfacial dye-assisted nanoleakage assessment of the bonded interfaces were evaluated using field-emission scanning electron microscopy (FE-SEM) and confocal laser-scanning microscopy (CLSM), respectively.

The tested null hypotheses were that the durability of RMGIC applied with or without the use of a PAA conditioner would be affected by: (i) short-term load-cycle aging; (ii) or load cycle followed by prolonged aging (8 months) in AS.

2. Materials and Methods

2.1. Preparation of Dentine Specimens

Sound human molars were extracted for periodontal or orthodontic reasons and stored in distilled water at 5 °C for no longer than 3 months. The roots were removed 1 mm beneath the cemento–enamel junction using a diamond-embedded blade (high concentration XL 12205; Benetec, London, UK) mounted on a low speed microtome (Remet evolution, REMET, Bologna, Italy). A second parallel cut was made to remove the occlusal enamel and expose mid-coronal dentine.

Two main groups (n = 30 specimens/group) were created based on dentine pre-treatment. Group 1: Specimens were abraded using 320-grit SiC abrasive paper (1 min) under continuous irrigation, followed by a water rinse (20 s), and air-drying (3 s); they were then restored with a light-cured RMGIC (no PAA conditioning). Group 2: Specimens were abraded with 320-grit SiC abrasive paper (1 min), conditioned with 10% PAA gel for 20 s rinsed with water (20 s), dried (3 s), and restored with a light-cured RMGIC (PAA conditioning).

The restorative procedure was performed using the content of two mono-dose capsules of a commercial RMGIC (RIVA light cure HV, Bayswater, VIC, Australia), mixed for 10 s in a trituration unit, and applied in bulk on to the dentine surface and light-cured for 30 s with a light-curing unit (Radii plus, SDI Ltd, Bayswater VIC, Australia) with a LED light source (>1000 mW/cm^2).

The experimental design required that each main group be subsequently subdivided into three sub-groups (n = 10 specimens) based on the aging protocol: (1) CRT: no aging (control, 24 h in deionised water); (2) LC: Load cycling (250,000 cycles in artificial saliva); (3) LC-AS: Load cycling (250,000 cycles in artificial saliva), followed by prolonged water storage (8 months in artificial saliva).

The composition of the artificial saliva was (AS: 0.103 g·L^{-1} of $CaCl_2$, 0.019 g·L^{-1} of $MgCl_2{\cdot}6H_2O$, 0.544 g·L^{-1} of KH_2PO_4, 30 g·L^{-1} of KCl and 4.77 g·L^{-1} HEPES (acid) buffer, pH 7.4). The specimens in the subgroup LC and LC-AS were mounted in plastic rings with acrylic resin for load cycle testing (250,000 cycles; 3 Hz; 70 N). A compressive load was applied to the flat surface of the RMGIC using a 5-mm diameter spherical stainless steel plunger attached to a cyclic loading machine (model S-MMT-250NB; Shimadzu, Tokyo, Japan) while immersed in AS [43].

2.2. Micro-Tensile Bond Strength (MTBS) and Fracture Analysis (FE-SEM)

The specimens were sectioned using a hard-tissue microtome (Remet evolution, REMET, Bologna, Italy) in both the X and Y planes across the dentine-RMGIC interface, obtaining approx. 20 matchstick-shaped specimens from each tooth with cross-sectional areas of 0.9 mm^2. All the specimens were stored at 100% humidity, and were then (i) immediately cut into matchsticks, or (ii) load cycled and then cut into matchsticks, or (iii) load cycled, cut into matchsticks, and then stored for 8 months in AS; specimens were finally subjected to an MTBS test. The latter was performed using a microtensile bond strength device with a stroke length of 50 mm, peak force of 500 N, and a displacement resolution of 0.5 mm. Modes of failure were classified as a percentage of adhesive (A), mixed (M) or cohesive (C) failures when the failed interfaces were examined at 30X magnification by stereoscopic microscopy. Five representative fractured specimens from each sub-group were critical-point dried and mounted on aluminium stubs with carbon cement. The specimens were gold-sputter-coated and imaged using field-emission scanning electron microscopy (FE-SEM S-4100; Hitachi, Wokingham, UK) at 10 kV and a working distance of 15 mm.

Bond strength values in MPa were initially assessed for normality distribution and variances homogeneity using Kolmogorov-Smirnov and Levene's tests, respectively. To analyse if the substrate pre-treatment approaches had an influence on the bond strength, two-way analysis of variance (pre-treatment and substrate condition) was performed. Chi-square analysis was performed to compare the results of failure mode between groups. The significance level was set at $p \leq 0.05$. SPSS V16 for Windows (SPSS Inc., Chicago, IL, USA) was used.

2.3. Ultramorphology of the Bonded-Dentine Interfaces: Confocal Microscopy Evaluation

One dentine-bonded matchstick sample (Ø 0.9 mm^2) was selected from the centre of each tooth in every experimental sub-group. These were coated with a fast-setting nail varnish, applied 1 mm from the bonded interface. They were immersed in a Rhodamine B (Merck KGaA, Darmstadt, Germany) water solution (0.1 wt.%) for 24 h. Subsequently, the specimens were ultrasonicated in distilled water for 5 min and then polished for 30 s each side with a 2400-grit SiC paper. The specimens were finally ultrasonicated again in distilled water for 5 min and submitted for confocal microscopy analysis. Using a confocal scanning microscope (Olympus FV1000, Olympus Corp., Tokyo, Japan) equipped with a 63X/1.4 NA oil-immersion lens and a 543 nm LED illumination, reflection and fluorescence images were obtained with a 1-μm z-step to optically section the specimens to a depth of up to 20 μm below the surface. The z-axis scan of the interface surface was pseudo-coloured arbitrarily for improved exposure and compiled into both single and topographic projections using the CLSM image-processing software (Fluoview Viewer, Olympus Corp., Tokyo, Japan). The configuration of the system was standardised and used at constant settings for the entire investigation [43]. Each dentine interface was investigated completely, and then five optical images were randomly captured. Micrographs representing the most common morphological features observed along the bonded interfaces were captured and recorded.

3. Results

3.1. Micro-Tensile Bond Strength (MTBS) and Failure Mode Analysis

Microtensile bond strength means and standard deviation are expressed in MPa in Table 1. Dentine surface treatments and aging in AS (8 months) had no significant influence on the MTBS results ($p > 0.01$). Interactions between factors were not significant ($p > 0.05$). The MTBS performed at 24 h with the non-load-cycled specimens showed that the use of PAA dentine conditioning induced no significant increase in bond strength ($p > 0.05$), compared to the specimens created by applying the RMGIC on smear layer-covered dentine (no PAA-treatment).

Table 1. The results show the mean ± SD of the MTBS (MPa) to dentine when resin-modified glass ionomer cement was applied after different dentine pre-treatments.

Main Groups Dentine Etching (10% PAA gel)	24 h AS (CTR)	Load Cycling in AS (LC)	Load Cycling and 8-Month in AS (LC-AS)
No PAA (95/5)	16.3 ± 5.9 (A1) (5/25/70)	16.4 ± 4.1 (A1) (2/10/88)	13.1 ± 4.6 (A1) (10 */55 */35 *)
Yes PAA (100/0)	21.5 ± 4.8 (A1) (0/15/85)	21.1 ± 5.5 (A1) (3/17/80)	14.2 ± 5.2 (A2) (13 */65 */22 *)

Percentage (%) of total number of beams (intact sticks/pre-failed sticks) in the dentine treatment groups and percentage of failure modes (adhesive/mix/cohesive). The same letter indicates no differences in columns with different dentine treatments maintained in the same aging conditions. The same number indicates differences in rows for the same dentine treatment but different aging conditions ($p > 0.05$). The symbol (*) indicates significant differences in the mode of failure in the same treatment group after different aging conditions.

Likewise, after load cycling, the specimens created in dentine pre-treated using PAA showed a bond strength comparable ($p > 0.05$) to that obtained with the specimens created with the RMGIC applied onto dentine surfaces that received no PAA conditioning.

The specimens created in dentine pre-treated with PAA and those without PAA conditioning showed no significant difference ($p > 0.05$) after LC-AS aging compared to the specimens in the control group (24 h) or those in the group where the specimens where subjected to load cycling only. The only significant difference ($p < 0.05$) in terms of bond strength was observed after LC-AS aging; this occurred between the specimens created in dentine pre-treated with PAA and those without PAA conditioning.

3.2. Failure and Fractographic FE-SEM Analysis

Most of the specimens from all groups failed predominantly in cohesive mode within RMGIC (range: 70–88%) and in mixed mode (10–25%) after 24 h and load cycling aging (Table 1), while most of the specimens tested after LC-AS aging failed prevalently in mixed mode (range: 55–65%) compared to those tested after 24 h or load cycling only ($p < 0.05$). The percentage of adhesive failures after LC-AS aging was significantly higher ($p < 0.05$) (range: 10–13%) in the specimens in both PAA and no- PAA groups compared to those tested after 24 h or load cycling (range 2–5%).

The SEM fractographic results at 24 h and after load cycling aging are shown in Figure 1. In short, the specimens created without PAA pre-treatment that failed during a microtensile bong strength test mainly in cohesive mode after 24 h of storage in water (Figure 1A) showed a surface covered by residual RMGIC (Figure 2B,C). The specimens created with the use of PAA re-treatment applied on dentine that failed in mixed mode after 24 h storage showed some areas with the presence of unprotected dentinal tubules, which were totally exposed and characterised by the presence of partially demineralised collagen fibrils (Figure 1F,1-F1). Also, the specimens created with the use of no PAA and then subjected to load cycling prevalently showed a surface covered by RMGIC with no exposure of the dentinal tubules (Figure 1G). The specimens created with the use of PAA applied on dentine showed after load cycling only the presence of totally exposed unprotected dentinal tubules (Figure 1F); at higher magnification, it was possible to observe the presence of partially-demineralised collagen fibrils (Figure 1H-1).

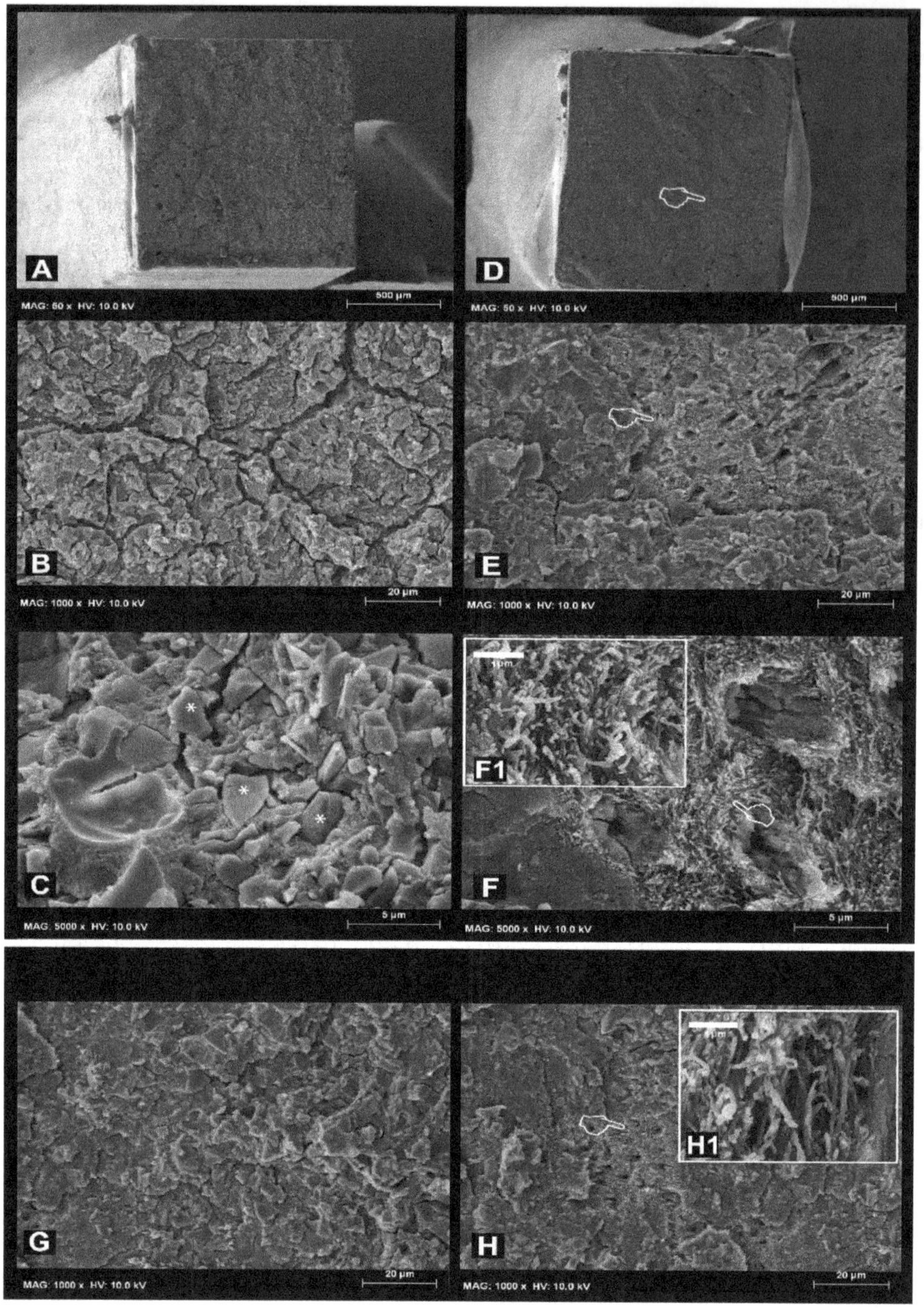

Figure 1. (**A**) Representative SEM micrograph of a specimen created with the use of no PAA applied on dentine that failed during the microtensile bong strength test in cohesive mode after 24 h of storage in water. At higher magnification, it is possible to note a surface covered by residual RMGIC (**B**) characterized by the presence of particles (*) of fluoroaluminosilicate glass (**C**). (**D**) Representative SEM fractographic analysis of specimens created with the use of PAA applied on dentine that failed in mixed mode after 24 h storage. At higher magnification, it is possible to see the presence of totally exposed unprotected dentinal tubules (pointer), and the presence of some partially demineralised residual collagen fibrils (pointer) (**E**,**F**,**F**-1). (**G**) Representative SEM micrograph of specimen created with the use of no PAA applied on dentine that failed during microtensile bond strength test in cohesive mode after load cycling aging. Also, in this case it is possible to note a surface covered by RMGIC with no dentine exposure. (**H**): Representative SEM fractographic analysis of specimens created with the use of PAA applied on dentine that failed in mixed mode after load cycling aging. It is possible to see the presence of totally exposed unprotected dentinal tubules (pointer), and, at a higher magnification, it is possible to note the presence of partially demineralised collagen fibrils (**H**-1).

The SEM fractographic results after LC-AS aging are depicted in Figure 2. A residual presence of RMGIC (Figure 2B) and a dentine surface devoid of exposed tubules was observed in the specimens created with the use of no PAA mode (Figure 2A); the dentine surface devoid of exposed tubules was still covered by smear layer (Figure 2C). On the other hand, the specimens created with the use of PAA applied on dentine that failed in mixed mode after load cycling and 8 months of storage in AS were characterised by the presence of residual RMGIC and some exposed dentine (Figure 2D). At higher magnification, tubules which were still occluded by residual RMGI were detected, but with no presence of exposed collagen fibrils was observed; these probably degraded over time during the prolonged aging in AS.

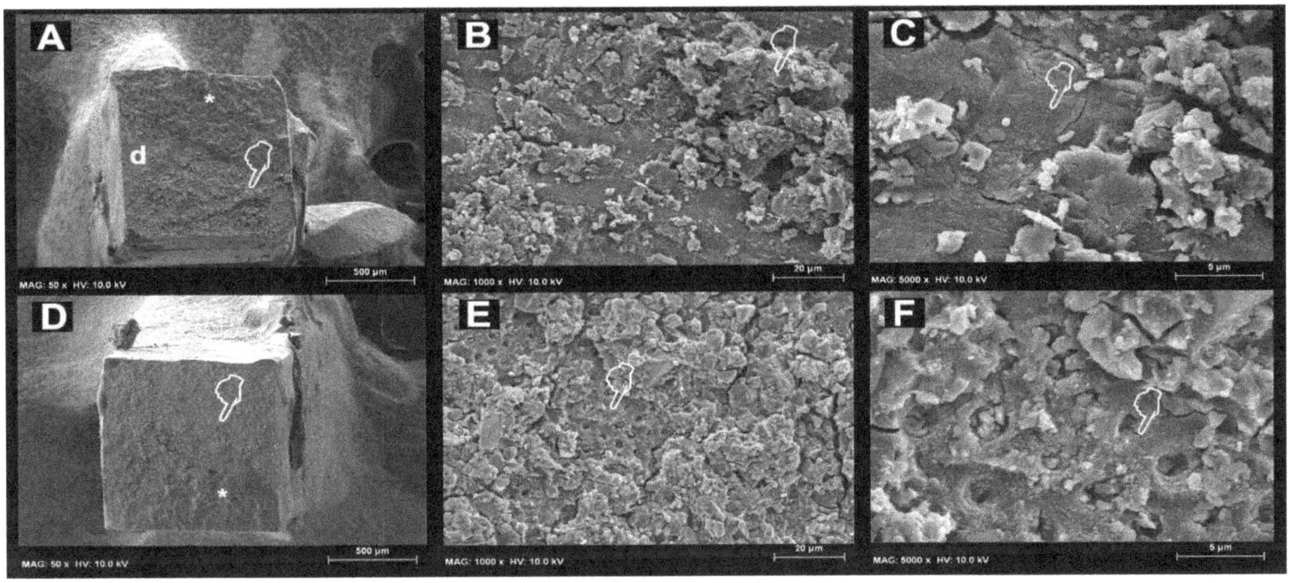

Figure 2. SEM micrographs obtained after load cycle followed by prolonged AS storage. (**A**) Representative SEM micrograph of specimen created with the use of no PAA applied on dentine that failed during microtensile bong strength test in mixed mode, where it is possible to see residual RMGIC (pointer), compact residual RMGIC (*) and some exposed dentine (d). (**B**) At higher magnification, it is possible to note a surface covered by residual RMGIC [pointer] and a dentine surface (pointer) with no exposed tubules but still covered by smear layer (**C**), (**D**); Representative SEM fractographic analysis of specimens created with the use of PAA applied on dentine that failed in mixed mode after 8 months of storage in AS which is characterised by the presence of residual RMGIC (*) and dentine (pointer). (**E**) At higher magnification, it is possible to observe the presence of exposed dentinal tubules (pointer) surrounded by residual RMGIC particles. (**F**) At even higher magnification it is possible to note the tubules are still occluded, but with no presence of exposed collagen fibrils, which probably degraded over time during prolonged aging in AS.

3.3. Ultramorphology of the Bonded-Dentine Interfaces: Confocal Microscopy Evaluation

The results of the ultramorphology and nanoleakage analysis of the RMGIC-dentine interfaces performed through dye-assisted confocal microscopy at 24 h and after load cycling only are shown in Figure 3. In short, at 24 h, the RMGIC applied onto dentine without PAA pre-treatment presented a gap-free interface characterised by a thin interdiffusion layer, which absorbed the fluorescent solution (Rhodamine B) through the dentinal tubules (Figure 3A). Conversely, the RMGIC applied onto the dentine pre-treated with PAA presented a thicker and more porous interdiffusion layer (Figure 3B). The RMGIC-dentine specimens created by applying the RMGIC onto the dentine pre-treated with no PAA and subjected to short-term load-cycle, showed an interdiffusion layer which was slightly thinner compared to that of the control specimens (24 h), (Figure 3C). This morphological features were also observed in the specimens bonded using RMGIC onto dentine pre-treated with 10% PAA and then subjected to load cycling. Indeed, such an aging protocol had no effect on the overall morphology of the interface, but the interdiffusion layer clearly appeared thinner than that observed in the specimens at 24 h (Figure 3C).

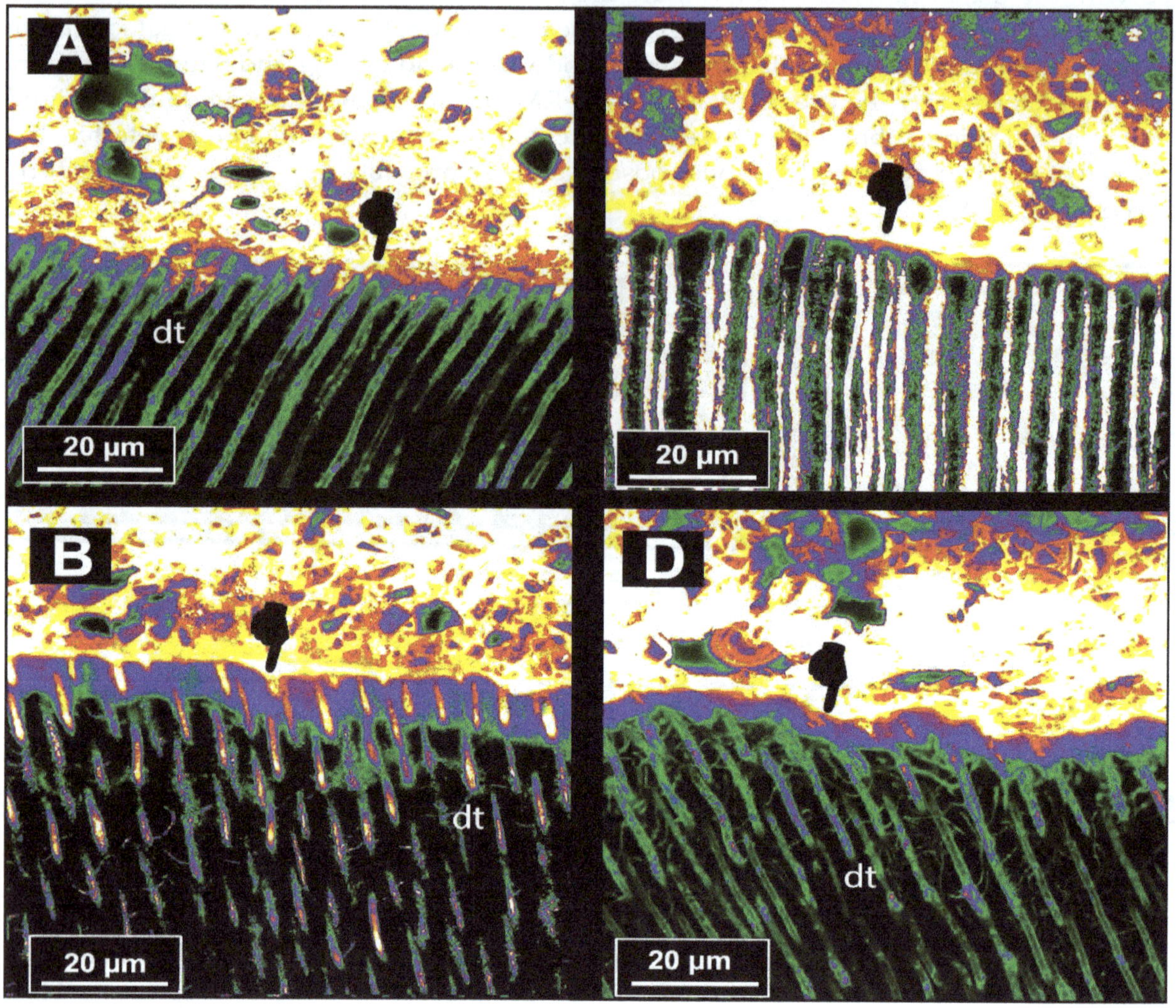

Figure 3. Confocal images of interfaces at 24 h or after short-term cycle load aging. (**A**) CLSM projection image exemplifies the interfacial characteristics at 24 h of the bond–dentine interface created by application of the resin-modified glass ionomer cement (RMGIC) onto dentine without PAA pre-treatment. It is possible to see a permeable gap-free interface that absorbed the fluorescein solution through the dentinal tubules (dt). In particular, this highlighted the existence of a thin interdiffusion layer (pointer). (**B**) CLSM projection at 24 of a representative bond-dentine interfaces created by RMGIC applied onto dentine pre-treated with PAA. In this case, it is possible to appreciate a thicker interdiffusion layer that absorbed the fluorescein solution through the dentinal tubules (dt) (**C**) A representative CLSM projection of a RMGIC-dentine interface created by applying the RMGIC onto a dentine pre-treated with no PAA and subjected to load cycling. It is possible to observe that such an aging protocol had no effect on the overall morphology of the interface, although the interdiffusion layer appears slightly thinner (pointer) than that observed in picture (**A**). (**D**) A representative CLSM projection of a RMGIC-dentine interface created by applying the RMGIC onto a dentine pre-treated with 10% PAA and subjected to load cycling. Also, in this case, it is possible to observe that such an aging protocol had no effect on the overall morphology of the interface, but the interdiffusion layer appears clearly thinner (pointer) than that observed in picture (**B**), which represents the same specimens subjected to no load-cycle aging.

The results of the ultramorphology and nanoleakage analysis of the RMGIC-dentine interfaces after LC-AS aging are shown in Figure 4. In this case, it was noted that the RMGIC-dentine interface of the RMGIC applied onto the dentine surface pre-treated with no PAA often presented cohesive fractures within the RMGIC layer; these were probably created during specimen preparation due to the brittle characteristics of such a material (Figure 4A). Conversely, the RMGIC-dentine interface created by applying the RMGIC onto a dentine pre-treated with PAA and then subjected to prolonged AS storage showed a remaining thin permeable interdiffusion layer, which may indicate the presence of porosities causing collagen degradation during subsequent prolonged water storage (Figure 4B).

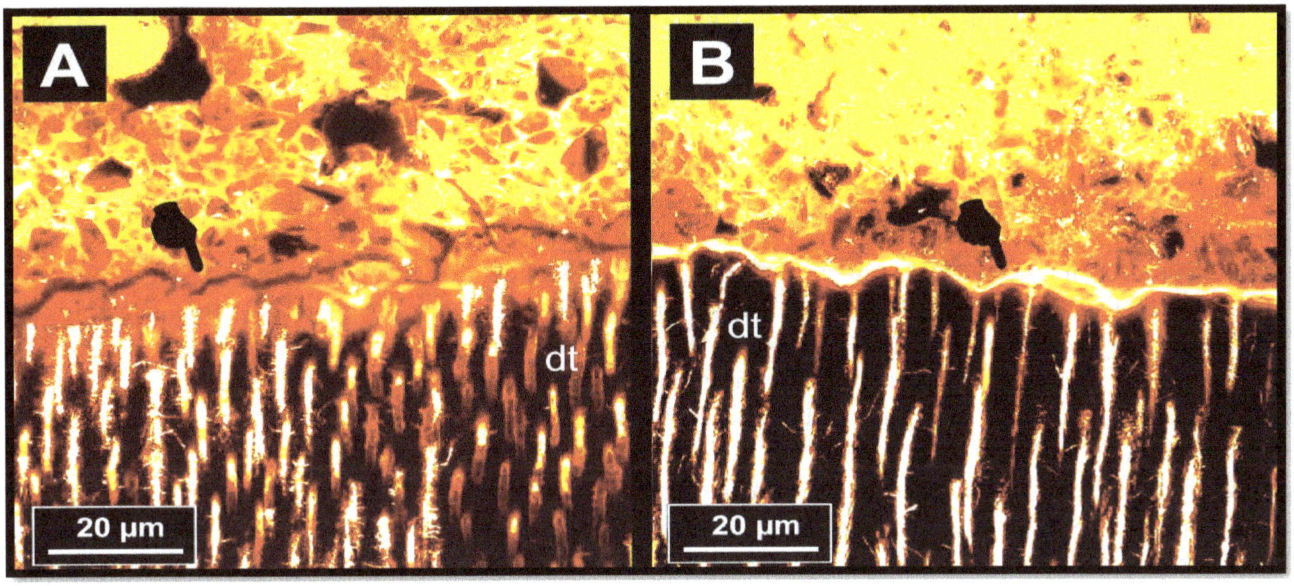

Figure 4. Confocal images of interfaces after cycle load aging and prolonged AS aging. (**A**) A representative CLSM projection of a RMGIC-dentine interface created by applying the RMGIC onto a dentine pre-treated with no PAA and subjected to prolonged AS storage. It is possible to observe the presence of a cohesive fracture within the RMGIC layer (pointer), probably created during specimen preparation (polishing) due to the brittle characteristics of such a material. This observation is supported by the absence of a permeable interfusion layer at RMGIC-dentine interface due to the maturation of the latter after prolonged storage in AS. Conversely, the RMGIC-dentine interface created by applying the RMGIC onto a dentine pre-treated with PAA and then subjected to prolonged AS storage (**B**) shows a remaining thin permeable interdiffusion layer (pointer), which indicates the presence of porosities created subsequent to collagen degradation during prolonged water storage.

4. Discussion

Therapeutic minimally invasive dentistry encompasses the philosophy of preservation of reparable dental tissues, along with the use of remineralising approaches to re-establish as much as possible of the mechanical properties of such tissues [44]. Glass-ionomer materials can be considered the main self-adhesives [45,46] and ion-releasing restorative materials available in clinics nowadays which are able to achieve such a target. However, it is believed that the overall bonding performance of such materials may be maximised if the dental substrates are pre-treated with a diluted polyacrylic acid conditioner (PAA 10%) [47,48]. Indeed, PAA conditioners remove the smear layer from dentine and enamel surfaces, consequently making the HAp directly accessible to interact with glass ionomer cements. Moreover, a slight dentine demineralisation occurs subsequent to PAA application, and a submicron interdiffusion layer is formed, which provides micromechanical retention [47–49]; the residual HAp within the demineralised collagen fibrils may also serve as receptors for additional chemical interaction [44–48]. The use of PAA as a dentine conditioner is still a theme of debate with modern resin-modified GIC [40,41], especially when considering its effect on the durability and remineralisation of dentine-bonded interfaces [43]. Furthermore, it has been recently demonstrated [50] that with conventional RMGICs such as Vitrebond Plus (3M ESPE), due to a great level energy accumulation at the dentine bonding interface during cycle load, there was evident fluorescent permeability associated with a lack of hermetic sealing.

The results of our study are in accordance those of Toledano at al. [50], as all the specimens applied in dentine pre-treated with or without PAA showed remining permeability at the bonding interface. Indeed, our current results demonstrated that the RMGIC tested in this study after the application on dentine without PAA pre-treatment presented a thin gap-free interface characterised by a thin layer of Rhodamine B absorbed through dentinal tubules (Figure 3A). In contrast, the interface of the RMGIC applied onto the dentine pre-treated with PAA was characterised by more Rhodamine B accumulation, which was due to a lack of sealing of dentinal tubules (Figure 3B), as well as a thicker layer of PAA-demineralised dentine, which remained non-infiltrated by the RMGIC [43,50].

However, after short-term load-cycle aging, the RMGIC-dentine specimens created using the RMGIC in dentine without PAA pre-treatment showed only a very thin interdiffusion layer characterised by slight fluorescence signal at the interface. As described by Toledano at al. [50], such a reduction in porosities at the bonding interface may have been due to apatite-like precipitation and remineralisation induced at the interface during mechanical cycling stress. Conversely, the specimens created with the RMGIC applied after PAA dentine pre-treatment also showed that the thickness fluorescent signal at the interface was reduced compared to the same specimens at 24 h (Figure 3C), although such a porous layer was thicker than that observed when using no PAA dentine pre-treatment. In this case, it is possible that the level of mineral precipitation was not so suitable for remineralising all the porosities within the interdiffusion layer, especially at its bottom. Indeed, Kim at al. [51] recently shown that GIC-based materials fail to completely remineralise apatite-depleted dentine due to a lack of nucleation of new apatite, even when biomimetic remineralising analogues were employed during the aging period [52].

It is important to highlight that such short-term load cycle aging was not able to induce any significant change in the microtensile bond strength, and no difference in the mode of failure in both groups of specimens (PAA vs. PAA dentine pre-treatment) was observed, compared to the control specimens at 24 h. Conversely, the results of this study showed that the specimens created with the representative RMGIC applied in dentine pre-treated with PAA showed a significant reduction in bond strength after LC-AS aging compared to specimens tested after 24 h or after short-term load cycle aging. Moreover, the LC-AS aging protocol induce also a significant change in the mode of failure; RMGIC applied in dentine pre-treated with or without PAA presented more adhesive qualities compared to all the other groups. Therefore, while the first null hypothesis is totally rejected, the second one that the durability of RMGIC applied with or without the use of PAA conditioner would be affected by load cycle followed by prolonged aging (8 months) in AS tested must be partially rejected.

Some of the current results are in accordance with those reported by Inoue et al. [45], who showed that the use of PAA conditioner before application of GIC-based materials offered no significant increase of the MTBS to dentine. Similar results were also recently reported by Sauro et al. [43], who showed that RMGIC applied onto dentine pre-treated with PAA showed significant μTBS reduction after 6 months of AS storage alone or in combination with load cycling ($p > 0.05$). Moreover, they also showed that for the RMGIC-dentine interface, specimens were affected by degradation/nanoleakage after aging, unlike the interfaces created without the use of PAA conditioning, which showed signs of remineralisation/maturation of the bonding interface.

The fractographic SEM analysis performed in this study showed that pre-treating the dentine with PAA could, in some cases, cause clear exposure of the collagen fibrils both before and after prolonged AS storage. Moreover, such fibrils were less abundant after prolonged AS storage compared to those observed in the specimens aged in AS for 24 h (Figure 2F). These specimens also showed a significant increase in the number of adhesive failures. In accordance with previously-published results [40,41,43], current fractographic SEM results showed that the specimens created with the use of no dentine PAA conditioner that failed in adhesive mode presented with dentine still covered by residual RMGIC, as the fracture occurred just above the dentine surface (Figure 2C).

It is hypothesised that such a result could be attributed to hydrolytic degradation processes that occurs over time within the collagen. Indeed, the use of PAA to pre-treat the dentine tissue may have demineralised the dentine collagen and activated endogenous matrix collagenolytic (MMP 1, MMP 8 and MMP 13) and gelatinolytic (MMP 2 and MMP 9) metalloproteinases [53]. It was also demonstrated [54] that high concentration of carboxylic groups in PAA acid conditioner may cause the formation a PAA-based polymeric gel layer within the bonding interface, which induces more water sorption at the interface. The RMGIC itself may also have degraded and become more porous over time in AS, thereby facilitating diffusion of water towards the glass-ionomer–dentine interface and causing an acceleration of the degradation processes [55].

The results of the ultramorphology and nanoleakage analysis of the RMGIC-dentine interfaces after prolonged AS storage showed that when RMGIC were applied onto the dentine surface, pre-treated with no PAA, and then subjected to prolonged AS storage, a thin permeable interdiffusion layer remained. This outcome may support the hypothesis that a bonding interface is usually characterised by the presence of porosities created subsequent to collagen degradation during prolonged water storage (Figure 4B). Conversely, the specimens created with the use of no PAA dentine conditioning showed that the absorbing layer at the interface seen at 24 h examination (Figure 3A) disappeared after prolonged AS storage (Figure 4A) due to the maturation of such areas [55], and possible remineralisation [43,56]. Indeed, the therapeutic properties (e.g., ion releasing) of RMGIC may have induced the growth of mineral crystals and remineralisation within the bonded-dentine interface, which interfered with the proteolytic action of endogenous dentine metalloproteinases [56,57].

This latter hypothesis is in accordance with previous studies that demonstrated the fluoride might inhibit both pro- and active forms of MMP 2 and MMP 9 [58]. Moreover, Makowski & Ramsby [59] reported that mineral precipitation, as well as apatite formation, may inhibit MMP activity through the formation of [Ca-PO/MMP] complexes. Sauro et al. [43] have recently reported that such a remineralising potential of RMGIC may increase if they are applied onto dentine pre-treated with bioactive glass in air-abrasion systems, and then conditioned with or without the use of a PAA conditioning gel.

In conclusion, within the limitations of this in vitro study, it is possible to affirm that the clinical decision of using a PAA conditioner should be based upon the histological features of the dentine retained after cavity preparation (e.g., sound or caries-affected dentine). However, modern RMGICs may be used for dentine restorations with or without the use of PAA pre-treatment, but it is important to consider that such a type of acid etching procedure might increase the risk of degradation at the bonding interface after prolonged service in oral cavity under mechanical cycling stress and prolonged saliva immersion. Conversely, in cases of no PAA dentine pre-treatment, it might be possible to have a synergic combination between GIC-based materials, saliva, and cycle occlusal load, which may enhance the therapeutic properties of RMGIC to induce mineralisation and protection of the bonding interface, thereby achieving more long-lasting restorations.

Author Contributions: For research articles with several authors, a short paragraph specifying their individual contributions must be provided. The following statements should be used "Conceptualization, S.S. and I.M..; Methodology, V.F.M., J.M.N.M.; Validation, S.S., V.F.L.; Formal Analysis, R.G.M., J.A.G.B.; Investigation, S.S., I.M., V.F.M., X.X.; Resources, V.F.L., I.M.; Data Curation, X.X.; Writing-Original Draft Preparation, S.S.; Writing-Review & Editing, S.S..; Supervision, V.F.L, S.S., I.M.; Project Administration, S.S., V.F.L., I.M.; Funding Acquisition, V.F.L, I.M.", please turn to the CRediT taxonomy for the term explanation. Authorship must be limited to those who have contributed substantially to the work reported.

Acknowledgments: We declare that we have no proprietary, financial, professional or other personal interest of any nature or kind in any product, service, and/or company that could be construed as influencing the position presented in, or the review of this manuscript. The authors of this article would like to thank SDI (Australia) for donating us the RMGIC (RIVA LC) and the PAA conditioner used in this study.

References

1. Wilson, A.D.; Kent, B.E. The glass-ionomer cement, a new translucent dental filling material. *J. Appl. Chem. Biotechnol.* **1971**, *21*, 313. [CrossRef]
2. Wilson, A.D.; Nicholson, J.W. *Acid-Base Cements: Their Biomedical and Industrial Applications*; Cambridge University Press: Cambridge, UK, July 2005; Volume 3.
3. Prosser, H.J.; Powis, D.R.; Wilson, A.D. Glass-ionomer cements of improved flexural strength. *J. Dent. Res.* **1986**, *65*, 146–148. [CrossRef] [PubMed]
4. Alhalawani, A.M.; Curran, D.J.; Boyd, D.; Towler, M.R. The role of poly(acrylic acid) in conventional glass polyalkenoate cements. *J. Polym. Eng.* **2016**, *36*, 221–237. [CrossRef]
5. Guggenberger, R.; May, R.; Stefan, K.P. New trends in glass-ionomer chemistry. *Biomaterials* **1998**, *19*, 479–483. [CrossRef]
6. McCabe, J.F.; Walls, A.W. (Eds.) *Applied Dental Materials*; John Wiley & Sons: Hoboken, NJ, USA, May 2013.
7. Anusavice, K.J.; Shen, C.; Rawls, H.R. *Phillips' Science of Dental Materials*; Elsevier Health Sciences: Amsterdam, The Netherlands, 2013.
8. Wilson, A.D. The chemistry of dental cements. *Chem. Soc. Rev.* **1978**, *7*, 265–296. [CrossRef]
9. Nicholson, J.W. Chemistry of glass-ionomer cements: A review. *Biomaterials* **1998**, *19*, 485–494. [CrossRef]
10. Zainuddin, N.; Karpukhina, N.; Hill, R.G.; Law, R.V. A long-term study on the setting reaction of glass ionomer cements by 27 Al MAS-NMR spectroscopy. *Dent. Mater.* **2009**, *25*, 290–295. [CrossRef] [PubMed]
11. Preston, A.J.; Higham, S.M.; Agalamanyi, E.A.; Mair, L.H. Fluoride recharge of aesthetic dental materials. *J. Oral Rehabil.* **1999**, *26*, 936–940. [CrossRef] [PubMed]
12. Forsten, L. Resin-modified glass ionomer cements: Fluoride release and uptake. *Acta Odontol. Scand.* **1995**, *53*, 222–225. [CrossRef] [PubMed]
13. Forss, H.; Jokinen, J.; Spets-Happonen, S.; Seppä, L.; Luoma, H. Fluoride and mutans streptococci in plaque grown on glass ionomer and composite. *Caries Res.* **1991**, *25*, 454–458. [CrossRef] [PubMed]
14. Preston, A.J.; Mair, L.H.; Agalamanyi, E.A.; Higham, S.M. Fluoride release from aesthetic dental materials. *J. Oral Rehabil.* **1999**, *26*, 123–129. [CrossRef] [PubMed]
15. De Amorim, R.G.; Leal, S.C.; Frencken, J.E. Survival of atraumatic restorative treatment (ART) sealants and restorations: A meta-analysis. *Clin. Oral Investig.* **2012**, *16*, 429–441. [CrossRef] [PubMed]
16. Van Dijken, J.W. 3-Year clinical evaluation of a compomer, a resin-modified glass ionomer and a resin composite in class III restorations. *Am. J. Dent.* **1996**, *9*, 195–198. [PubMed]
17. Abdalla, A.I.; Alhadainy, H.A.; Garcia-Godoy, F. Clinical evaluation of glass ionomers and compomers in class V carious lesions. *Am. J. Dent.* **1997**, *10*, 18–20. [PubMed]
18. Leevailoj, C.; Platt, J.A.; Cochran, M.A.; Moore, B.K. In vitro study of fracture incidence and compressive fracture load of all-ceramic crowns cemented with resin-modified glass ionomer and other luting agents. *J. Prosthet. Dent.* **1998**, *80*, 699–707. [CrossRef]
19. Pascotto, R.C.; de Lima Navarro, M.F.; Capelozza Filho, L.; Cury, J.A. In vivo effect of a resin-modified glass ionomer cement on enamel demineralization around orthodontic brackets. *Am. J. Orthod. Dentofac.* **2004**, *125*, 36–41. [CrossRef]
20. Jokstad, A.; Mjör, I.A. Ten years' clinical evaluation of three luting cements. *J. Dent.* **1996**, *24*, 309–315. [CrossRef]
21. Murdoch-Kinch, C.A.; McLean, M.E. Minimally invasive dentistry. *J. Am. Dent. Assoc.* **2003**, *134*, 87–95. [CrossRef] [PubMed]
22. Peumans, M.; de Munck, J.; Mine, A.; van Meerbeek, B. Clinical effectiveness of contemporary adhesives for the restoration of non-carious cervical lesions. A systematic review. *Dent. Mater.* **2014**, *30*, 1089–1103. [CrossRef] [PubMed]
23. Terata, R.; Nakashima, K.; Kubota, M. Effect of temporary materials on bond strength of resin-modified glass-ionomer luting cements to teeth. *Am. J. Dent.* **2000**, *13*, 209–211. [PubMed]
24. McLean, J.W.; Powis, D.R.; Prosser, H.J.; Wilson, A.D. The use of glass-ionomer cements in bonding composite resins to dentine. *Br. Dent. J.* **1985**, *158*, 410–414. [CrossRef] [PubMed]
25. Andersson-Wenckert, I.E.; Kieri, C. Durability of extensive class II open-sandwich restorations with a resin-modified glass ionomer cement after 6 years. *Am. J. Dent.* **2004**, *17*, 43–50. [PubMed]

26. Yamaga, R.; Nishino, M.; Yoshida, S.; Yokomizo, I. Diammine silver fluoride and its clinical application. *J. Osaka Univ. Dent. Sch.* **1972**, *12*, 1–20. [PubMed]
27. Sauro, S.; Osorio, R.; Watson, T.F.; Toledano, M. Influence of phosphoproteins' biomimetic analogs on remineralization of mineral-depleted resin–dentin interfaces created with ion-releasing resin-based systems. *Dent. Mater.* **2015**, *31*, 759–777. [CrossRef] [PubMed]
28. Xie, D.; Brantley, W.A.; Culbertson, B.M.; Wang, G. Mechanical properties and microstructures of glass-ionomer cements. *Dent. Mater.* **2000**, *16*, 129–138. [CrossRef]
29. Peutzfeldt, A.; Garcia-Godoy, F.; Asmussen, E. Surface hardness and wear of glass ionomers and compomers. *Am. J. Dent.* **1997**, *10*, 15–17. [PubMed]
30. Ahmed, N.; Zafar, M.S. Effects of wear on hardness and stiffness of restorative dental materials. *Life Sci. J.* **2014**, *11*, 11–18.
31. Um, C.M.; Øilo, G. The effect of early water contact on glass-ionomer cements. *Quintessence Int.* **1992**, *1*, 23.
32. Moshaverinia, A.; Roohpour, N.; Chee, W.W.L.; Schricker, S.R. A review of powder modifications in conventional glass-ionomer dental cements. *J. Mater. Chem.* **2011**, *21*, 1319–1328. [CrossRef]
33. Moshaverinia, A.; Ansari, S.; Moshaverinia, M.; Roohpour, N.; Darr, J.A.; Rehman, I. Effects of incorporation of hydroxyapatite and fluoroapatite nanobioceramics into conventional glass ionomer cements (GIC). *Acta Biomater.* **2008**, *4*, 432–440. [CrossRef] [PubMed]
34. Moshaverinia, A.; Ansari, S.; Movasaghi, Z.; Billington, R.W.; Darr, J.A.; Rehman, I.U. Modification of conventional glass-ionomer cements with N-vinylpyrrolidone containing polyacids, nano-hydroxy and fluorapatite to improve mechanical properties. *Dent. Mater.* **2008**, *24*, 1381–1390. [CrossRef] [PubMed]
35. Wilson, A.D. Resin-modified glass-ionomer cements. *Int. J. Prosthodont.* **1989**, *3*, 425–429.
36. Soncini, J.A.; Maserejian, N.N.; Trachtenberg, F.; Tavares, M.; Hayes, C. The Longevity of amalgam versus compomer/composite restorations in posterior primary and permanent teeth: Findings from the new england children's amalgam trial. *J. Am. Dent. Assoc.* **2007**, *138*, 763–772. [CrossRef] [PubMed]
37. McCabe, J.F. Resin-modified glass-ionomers. *Biomaterials* **1998**, *19*, 521–527. [CrossRef]
38. Sauro, S.; Pashley, D. Strategies to stabilise dentine-bonded interfaces through remineralising operative approaches - State of The Art. *Int. J. Adhes. Adhes.* **2016**, *69*, 39–57. [CrossRef]
39. Tyas, M.J.; Burrow, M.F. Adhesive restorative materials: A review. *Aust. Dent. J.* **2004**, *49*, 112–121. [CrossRef] [PubMed]
40. Inoue, S.; Abe, Y.; Yoshida, Y.; De Munck, J.; Sano, H.; Suzuki, K.; Lambrechts, P.; Van Meerbeek, B. Effect of conditioner on bond strength of glass-ionomer adhesive to dentin/enamel with and without smear layer interposition. *Oper. Dent.* **2004**, *29*, 685–692. [PubMed]
41. De Munck, J.; Van Meerbeek, B.; Yoshida, Y.; Inoue, S.; Suzuki, K.; Lambrechts, P. Four-year water degradation of a resin-modified glass-ionomer adhesive bonded to dentin. *Eur. J. Oral Sci.* **2004**, *112*, 73–83. [CrossRef] [PubMed]
42. Toledano, M.; Cabello, I.; Aguilera, F.S.; Osorio, E.; Osorio, R. Effect of in vitrochewing and bruxism events on remineralization, at the resin-dentin interface. *J. Biomech.* **2015**, *48*, 14–21. [CrossRef] [PubMed]
43. Sauro, S.; Watson, T.; Moscardó, A.P.; Luzi, A.; Feitosa, V.P.; Banerjee, A. The effect of dentine pre-treatment using bioglass and/or polyacrylic acid on the interfacial characteristics of resin-modified glass ionomer cements. *J. Dent.* **2018**, *73*, 32–39. [CrossRef] [PubMed]
44. Watson, T.F.; Atmeh, A.R.; Sajini, S.; Cook, R.J.; Festy, F. Present and future of glass ionomersand calcium-silicate cements as bioactive materials in dentistry: biophotonics-based interfacial analyses in health and disease. *Dent. Mater.* **2014**, *30*, 50–61. [CrossRef] [PubMed]
45. Inoue, S.; Van Meerbeek, B.; Abe, Y.; Yoshida, Y.; Lambrechts, P.; Vanherle, G.; Sano, H. Effect of remaining dentin thickness and the use of conditioner on micro-tensile bond strength of a glass-ionomer adhesive. *Dent. Mater.* **2001**, *17*, 445–455. [CrossRef]
46. Yoshida, Y.; Van Meerbeek, B.; Nakayama, Y.; Snauwaert, J.; Hellemans, L.; Lambrechts, P.; Vanherle, G.; Wakasa, K. Evidence of chemical bonding at biomaterial–hard tissue interfaces. *J. Dent. Res.* **2000**, *79*, 709–714. [CrossRef] [PubMed]
47. Van Meerbeek, B.; Vargas, M.; Inoue, S.; Yoshida, Y.; Peumans, M.; Lambrechts, P.; Vanherle, G. Adhesives and cements topromote preservation dentistry. *Oper. Dent.* **2001**, *26*, 119–144.

48. Van Meerbeek, B.; Inoue, S.; Perdigao, J.; Lambrechts, P.; Vanherle, G. *Enamel and Dentin Adhesion*; Summitt, J.B., Robbins, J.W., Schwartz, R.S, Eds.; Quintessence Publishing Co.: Chicago, IL, USA, 2001; pp. 178–235.
49. Lin, A.; McIntyre, N.; Davidson, R. Studies on the adhesion of glass ionomer cements to dentin. *J. Dent. Res.* **1992**, *71*, 1836–1841. [CrossRef] [PubMed]
50. Toledano, M.; Osorio, R.; Osorio, E.; Cabello, I.; Toledano-Osorio, M.; Aguilera, F.S. In vitro mechanical stimulation facilitates stress dissipation and sealing ability at the conventional glass ionomer cement-dentin interface. *J. Dent.* **2018**, *73*, 61–69. [CrossRef] [PubMed]
51. Kim, Y.K.; Yiu, C.K.; Kim, J.R.; Gu, L.; Kim, S.K.; Weller, R.N.; Pashley, D.H.; Tay, F.R. Failureof a glass ionomer to remineralise apatite-depleted dentin. *J. Dent. Res.* **2010**, *89*, 230–235. [CrossRef] [PubMed]
52. Gu, L.S.; Kim, J.; Kim, Y.K.; Liu, Y.; Dickens, S.H.; Pashley, D.H.; Ling, J.Q.; Tay, F.R. Achemical phosphorylation-inspired design for Type I collagen biomimeticremineralization. *Dent. Mater.* **2010**, *26*, 1077–1089. [CrossRef] [PubMed]
53. Nishitani, Y.; Yoshiyama, M.; Wadgaonkar, B.; Breschi, L.; Mannello, F.; Mazzoni, A.; Carvalho, R.M.; Tjäderhane, L.; Tay, F.R.; Pashley, D.H. Activation of gelatinolytic/collagenolytic activity in dentin by self-etching adhesives. *Eur. J. Oral Sci.* **2006**, *114*, 160–166. [CrossRef] [PubMed]
54. Es-Souni, M.; Fischer-Brandies, H.; Zaporojshenko, V.; Es-Souni, M. On the interactionof polyacrylic acid as a conditionning agent with bovine enamel. *Biomaterials* **2002**, *23*, 2871–2878. [CrossRef]
55. Sidhu, S.K.; Watson, T.F. Interfacial characteristics of resin-modified glass-ionomermaterials: A study on fluid permeability using confocal fluorescence microscopy. *J. Dent. Res.* **1998**, *77*, 1749–1759. [CrossRef] [PubMed]
56. Sauro, S.; Watson, T.F.; Thompson, I.; Toledano, M.; Nucci, C.; Banerjee, A. Influence of air-abrasion executed with PAA-bioglass 45S5 on the bonding performance of a resin-modified glass ionomer cement. *Eur. J. Oral Sci.* **2012**, *120*, 168–177. [CrossRef] [PubMed]
57. Brackett, M.G.; Agee, K.A.; Brackett, W.W.; Key, W.O.; Sabatini, C.; Kato, M.T.; Buzalaf, M.A.; Tjäderhane, L.; Pashley, D.H. Effect of sodium fluoride on theendogenous MMP activity of dentin matrices. *J. Nat. Sci.* **2015**, *1*, e118. [PubMed]
58. Tezvergil-Mutluay, A.; Seseogullari-Dirihan, R.; Feitosa, V.P.; Cama, G.; Brauer, D.S.; Sauro, S. Effects of Composites Containing Bioactive Glasses on Demineralized Dentin. *J. Dent. Res.* **2017**, *96*, 999–1005. [CrossRef] [PubMed]
59. Makowski, G.S.; Ramsby, M.L. Differential effect of calcium phosphate andcalcium pyrophosphate on binding of matrix metalloproteinases to fibrin: comparison to a fibrin-binding protease from inflammatory joint fluids. *Clin. Exp. Immunol.* **2004**, *136*, 176–187. [CrossRef] [PubMed]

4

Studies on the Curing Efficiency and Mechanical Properties of Bis-GMA and TEGDMA Nanocomposites Containing Silver Nanoparticles

Izabela Barszczewska-Rybarek [1,*] and Grzegorz Chladek [2]

[1] Department of Physical Chemistry and Technology of Polymers, Silesian University of Technology, 44-100 Gliwice, Poland

[2] Institute of Engineering Materials and Biomaterials, Silesian University of Technology, 44-100 Gliwice, Poland; Grzegorz.Chladek@polsl.pl

* Correspondence: Izabela.Barszczewska-Rybarek@polsl.pl

Abstract: Bioactive dimethacrylate composites filled with silver nanoparticles (AgNP) might be used in medical applications, such as dental restorations and bone cements. The composition of bisphenol A glycerolate dimethacrylate (Bis-GMA) and triethylene glycol dimethacrylate (TEGDMA) mixed in a 60/40 wt% ratio was filled from 25 to 5000 ppm of AgNP. An exponential increase in resin viscosity was observed with an increase in AgNP concentration. Curing was performed by way of photopolymerization, room temperature polymerization, and thermal polymerization. The results showed that the polymerization mode determines the degree of conversion (*DC*), which governs the ultimate mechanical properties of nanocomposites. Thermal polymerization resulted in a higher *DC* than photo- and room temperature polymerizations. The *DC* always decreased as AgNP content increased. Flexural strength, flexural modulus, hardness, and impact strength initially increased, as AgNP concentration increased, and then decreased at higher AgNP loadings. This turning point usually occurred when the *DC* dropped below 65% and moved toward higher AgNP concentrations, according to the following order of polymerization methods: photopolymerization < room temperature polymerization < thermal polymerization. Water sorption (WS) was also determined. Nanocomposites revealed an average decrease of 16% in *WS* with respect to the neat polymer. AgNP concentration did not significantly affect WS.

Keywords: silver nanocomposite; dimethacrylate; molecular structure; flexural properties; water sorption

---

1. Introduction

Recently, polymeric biomaterials with microbiological activity have increasingly gained attention in the potential treatment of various types of inflammation or infection [1]. In dentistry and orthopedy, biomaterials based on dimethacrylates have a superior status, serving as restorative dental materials [2] and bone cements [3–5]. The most commonly used monomers of this type are: 2,2′-bis-[4-(2-hydroxy-3-methacryloyloxy propoxy)phenyl]propane (Bis-GMA) and triethylene glycol dimethacrylate (TEGDMA)—a diluting monomer (Scheme 1) [2–5]. Their polymerization results in a highly crosslinked composite matrix [6,7]. One of the negative consequences of this process is polymerization shrinkage, which causes interfacial gap formation. This phenomenon is responsible for the microleakage and accumulation of bacteria beneath and around the reconstruction, causing tissue inflammation and recurrent caries [8–10].

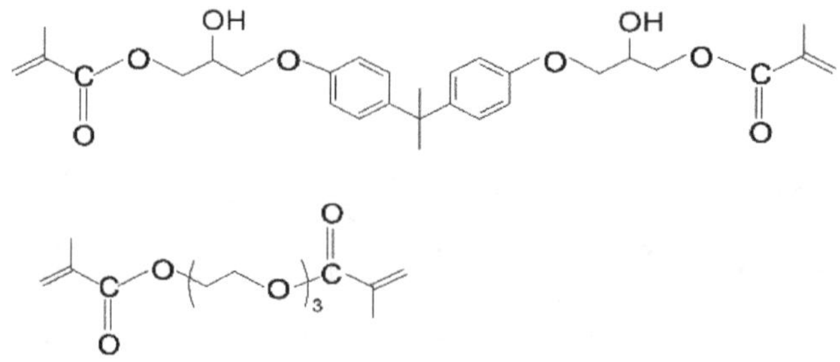

Scheme 1. The Bis-GMA and TEGDMA chemical structure.

It is widely recognized that the interaction of a restorative material with microorganisms is important for its longevity and effectiveness [9]. It might be improved by the incorporation of antimicrobial substances into tooth reconstruction or bone cement [10–12]. The group of *Streptococcus mutans* has been described as the most important bacteria related to the formation of dental caries [10,13,14]. Complications of bone replacements are, in turn, primarily caused by staphylococci, in particular, *Staphylococcus aureus* [15]. Faced with such problems, the need to further develop dental restorative materials, adhesives, and bone cements containing antimicrobial agents has arisen.

A variety of nanoparticles are currently under investigation in order to improve the antibacterial properties of biomaterials. Polymeric nanocomposites filled with nanoparticles, such as calcium phosphate [16,17], zinc oxide [13,18,19], titanium dioxide [20], gold [21,22], and silver (AgNP) [13,16,23–28] have shown promising capabilities in reducing bacterial proliferation, thereby preventing the degradation of tissue and restoration.

AgNP advantages, such as a wide spectrum and long-term antibacterial activity, low toxicity, and good biocompatibility with human cells have led to its application in medical products, such as wound dressings, catheters, and prostheses [28]. AgNP has also been applied in several areas of dentistry [24–29] and orthopedy [15,23,26]. Literature provides much evidence for the antibacterial action of AgNP-containing dental materials against oral streptococci [13,26–28]. On the other hand, bone cements filled with AgNP exhibited antimicrobial activity against staphylococci, such as *Staphylococcus aureus*, *Staphylococcus epidermidis*, and *Acinetobacter baumannii* [23,26]. The decrease in the development of recurrent caries and formation of bacterial biofilm on tooth restoration [16,27,30] and bone cementation [23] was achieved by the introduction of AgNP at the concentration of 500 to 5000 ppm.

Despite evident benefits of nanocomposites with microbiological activity, their potential is limited by the nanofiller agglomeration process at a high nanofiller volume fraction. If the nanofiller content exceeds a critical value, the polymerization extent decreases, which leads to a decrease in polymer network homogeneity [31]. The number of pendant groups, pendant chains, or even free monomer molecules within the poly(dimethacrylate) matrix increases. Consequently, macroscopic properties of the composite are negatively influenced [32]. Additionally, the elution of unreacted monomer from a reconstruction may negatively influence the biological compatibility of the applied biomaterial. The literature has revealed that the greater the content of nanoparticles in the composite, the greater the amount of monomers in the eluate [29].

In view of the above, knowledge regarding structure-property relationships within nanocomposites represents a crucial aspect. The literature, dealing with dimethacrylate systems filled with AgNP, is still lacking a thorough study on this issue.

The purpose of this study was to characterize polymer nanocomposites obtained by photochemical, room temperature, and thermal polymerizations of Bis-GMA/TEGDMA 60/40 wt% composition enriched with silver nanoparticles (AgNP). The AgNP content was increased from 25 to 5000 ppm. The work focused on differences induced by the polymerization initiation methods and AgNP content on the degree of conversion, mechanical properties, and water sorption. Mechanical examination of nanocomposites included the determination of the modulus of elasticity, flexural strength, hardness, and impact resistance.

2. Results

In the present study, the mixture of Bis-GMA and TEGDMA at 60/40 wt% ratio was loaded with AgNP in the quantity of 25 to 5000 ppm. As shown in Table 1, eight Bis-GMA/TEGDMA/AgNP resin compositions were produced using the solvent casting method. n-Hexane was used as a solvent.

Table 1. The AgNP concentrations in Bis-GMA/TEGDMA/AgNP compositions, AgNP concentrations in AgNP/hexane colloids, and colloid amounts used in nanocomposite manufacturing.

AgNP Concentration in Bis-GMA/TEGDMA/AgNP Compositions (ppm)	AgNP Concentration in hexane Colloid (ppm)	The Amount of AgNP/hexane Colloid (g)
25	100	25.0
50	100	50.0
100	100	100.0
150	100	150.0
250	100	250.0
500	100	500.0
1500	500	300.4
5000	1000	502.5

Before polymerization, Bis-GMA/TEGDMA/AgNP compositions, as well as the neat Bis-GMA/TEGDMA mixture, were tested for viscosity. An exponential increase in viscosity with AgNP concentration was observed (Figure 1).

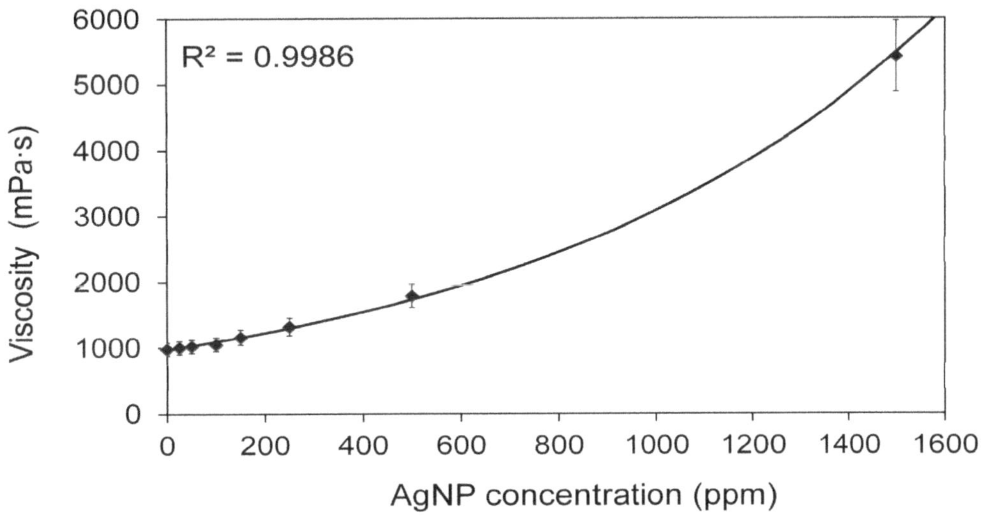

Figure 1. The relationship between viscosity and AgNP concentration in Bis-GMA/TEGDMA/AgNP compositions. All results were statistically significant ($p < 0.05$).

As shown in Figure 1, by increasing the AgNP concentration from 0 to 1500 ppm, the viscosity increased from 980 to 5420 mPa·s. Above 1500 ppm of AgNP, the viscosity increased dramatically, which necessitated the use of another torque in further studies. Consequently, 98 mPa·s was determined for the sample filled with 5000 ppm of AgNP. This value could not be compared with the previous results, found using the torque designed for lower viscosities. Thus, this value was not taken into account when the correlation between viscosity and AgNP concentration was constructed.

The monomer mixtures were then activated for polymerization in three ways:

1. Photopolymerization—by the addition of CQ (camphorquinone) 0.4 wt.% and DMAEMA (N,N-dimethylaminoethyl methacrylate) 1 wt.%;

2. Room temperature polymerization—by the addition of BPO (benzoyl peroxide) 0.5 wt% and DMPT (N,N-dimethyl-p-toluidine) 0.05 wt%;
3. Thermal polymerization—by the addition of BPO 1 wt%.

Macroscopic observations led to the first conclusion that the polymerization initiation mechanism restricts the AgNP capacity in the nanocomposite.

Photopolymerization was limited by 250 ppm of AgNP. A higher AgNP content resulted in a poor sample quality, which was mechanically weak and brittle. The absorption of UV-VIS radiation was suspected as the key factor responsible for this limitation. To check this hypothesis, UV-VIS analysis was performed on the neat Bis-GMA/TEGDMA composition, as well as its AgNP loaded modifications. As shown in Figure 2, all samples were likely to absorb UV-VIS radiation within the range of 190 to 300 nm, with the maximum at around 215 nm. However, the absorption intensity of nanocomposites was higher than the absorption intensity of the neat network. The higher the AgNP quantity, the higher the absorption intensity. This region corresponds to the CQ absorption in the UV region [33]. Additionally, CQ absorbs electromagnetic radiation in the VIS region from 400 to 550 nm, with the maximum absorption intensity at 467 nm [33]. This part of the spectra remained free from absorption bands of Bis-GMA/TEGDMA/AgNP (Figure 2b).

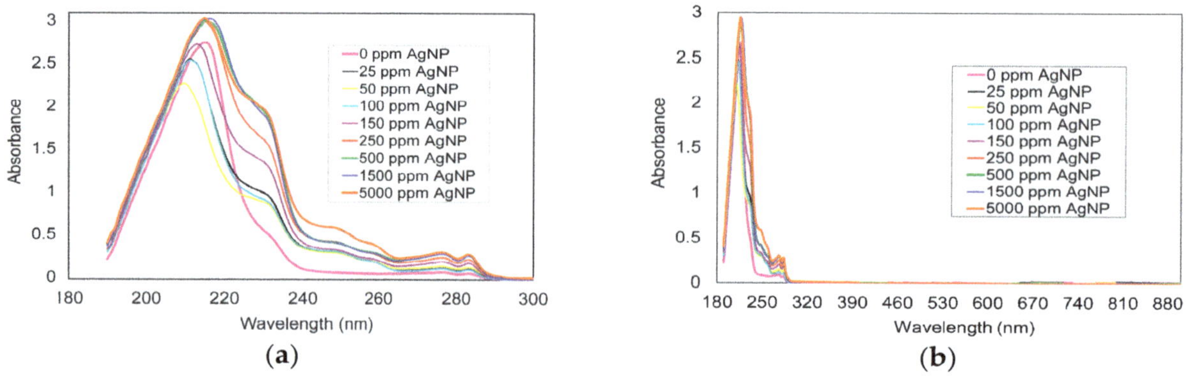

Figure 2. UV/VIS spectra of the pristine Bis-GMA/TEGDMA and its AgNP loaded modifications in the range of: (**a**) 190–300 nm; (**b**) 190–900 nm.

In the case of room temperature polymerization, 1500 ppm of AgNP was the maximum concentration that could be employed to maintain a good visual quality of the sample. The introduction of 5000 ppm of AgNP caused an enormous increase in the viscosity of the resinous system. This prevented the escape of air bubbles before the polymer was hardened. Consequently, a significant weakening of the nanocomposite was observed.

Thermal initiation was successfully adopted to produce nanocomposites of a high quality and durability over the whole AgNP concentration range.

Following the initial sample quality assessment, the AgNP concentration range was narrowed individually for each group of nanocomposites according to the polymerization technique. Thus, the following maximum AgNP concentrations were set up in a sample preparation for further studies: 250 ppm—photopolymerization, 1500 ppm—room temperature polymerization, and 5000 ppm—thermal polymerization. The list of tested samples and their names are presented in Table 2.

Table 2. The Bis-GMA/TEGDMA/AgNP nanocomposite samples studied and their names: Ph (photopolymerization), RT (room temperature polymerization), T (thermal polymerization).

AgNP Concentration in Nanocomposite (ppm)	Sample Name		
	Photopolymerization	Room Temperature Polymerization	Thermal Polymerization
0	Ph0	RT0	T0
25	Ph25	RT25	T25
50	Ph50	RT50	T50
100	Ph100	RT100	T100
150	Ph150	RT150	T150
250	Ph250	RT250	T250
500	-	RT500	T500
1500	-	RT1500	T1500
5000	-	-	T5000

In Table 3, the results for the degree of conversion (*DC*) and polymerization shrinkage (*S*) are summarized.

Table 3. The polymerization shrinkage and degree of conversion in studied Bis-GMA/TEGDMA/AgNP nanocomposites.

Sample	Polymerization Shrinkage (%)	Degree of Conversion (%)
Ph0	8.37 ± 0.58 [1]	69.8 ± 6.0 [31,32]
Ph25	8.22 ± 0.60 [2,6]	67.2 ± 7.0 [33]
Ph50	8.01 ± 0.70 [3,7]	64.8 ± 4.6 [34,35,f]
Ph100	7.41 ± 0.62 [4,6]	60.2 ± 4.2 [g]
Ph150	6.95 ± 0.96 [5,7,a,b]	54.8 ± 5.6 [31,34,h]
Ph250	5.44 ± 0.53 [1–5,c,d]	50.2 ± 7.5 [32,33,35,i,j]
RT0	8.39 ± 0.60 [8,9]	69.6 ± 5.4 [36,39,k]
RT25	8.13 ± 0.70 [10]	68.0 ± 4.9 [37,40]
RT50	7.99 ± 0.62 [11]	66.8 ± 4.7 [41,l]
RT100	7.84 ± 0.44 [12]	65.4 ± 7.2 [38,42]
RT150	7.77 ± 0.78 [13,a]	61.4 ± 7.2 [m]
RT250	7.66 ± 0.73 [14,c]	60.2 ± 6.3 [j,n]
RT500	7.41 ± 0.62 [8,15]	56.2 ± 7.7 [36–38,o]
RT1500	5.34 ± 0,59 [9–15,e]	52.0 ± 9.0 [39–42,p]
T0	8.50 ± 0.50 [16,23]	78.2 ± 5.5 [43,k]
T25	8.37 ± 0.43 [17,24]	78.0 ± 5.7 [44]
T50	8.28 ± 0.57 [18,25]	78.2 ± 5.4 [45,f,l]
T100	8.19 ± 0.48 [19,26]	77.4 ± 7.0 [46,g]
T150	8.13 ± 0.69 [20,27,b]	76.8 ± 7.0 [47,h,m]
T250	8.11 ± 0.51 [21,28,d]	76.6 ± 7.2 [48,i,n]
T500	8.01 ± 0.70 [22,29]	73.8 ± 4.9 [49,o]
T1500	7.15 ± 0.74 [16–22,30,e]	70.4 ± 7.4 [50,p]
T5000	5.01 ± 0.99 [23–30]	43.6 ± 7.8 [43–50]

[1–50] $p < 0.05$—statistically significant results within the nanocomposite series. [a–p] $p < 0.05$—statistically significant results between nanocomposites, having the same AgNP content, but obtained in different polymerization modes.

The *DC* in the neat networks produced by photo- and room temperature polymerizations was almost the same and equaled 70%. The *DC* in the thermally polymerized neat network was higher and equaled 78%. However, a statistically significant difference was only found for the RT0 and T0 couple. The average polymerization shrinkage of the neat networks was 8.4% and there was no statistically significant difference between the Ph0, RT0, and T0 samples.

The analysis of results for nanocomposites showed that the introduction of AgNP into the Bis-GMA/TEGDMA matrix resulted in a decrease of the *DC* and *S* (polymerization shrinkage).

The higher the AgNP concentration, the lower the *DC* and *S*. It is worth noting that the *DC* in T5000 did not achieve a satisfactory degree of conversion, which was 43.6%. Statistically significant decreases in the *DC*, with respect to the neat networks, were found, beginning from the following AgNP concentrations: 150 ppm—for photopolymerization, 500 ppm—for room temperature polymerization, and 5000 ppm—for thermal polymerization. An analogous analysis of the results for *S* allowed for the specification of the following AgNP concentrations, which resulted in statistically significant decreases in *S*, with respect to the neat networks, respectively: 250 ppm, 500 ppm, and 1500 ppm.

A detailed analysis of the *DC* and *S* led to the conclusion that both parameters increased by the initiation mechanism according to the following order: photopolymerization < room temperature polymerization < thermal polymerization. The *DC* in nanocomposites obtained by thermal polymerization was usually statistically significantly higher than the *DC* in nanocomposites obtained by photopolymerization and room temperature polymerization.

In Table 4, the results for flexural properties are summarized. It may be seen that the flexural strength (σ) and flexural modulus (E) depend on the AgNP concentration.

Table 4. The flexural properties of studied Bis-GMA/TEGDMA/AgNP nanocomposites.

Sample	Flexural Strength (MPa)	Flexural Modulus (MPa)
Ph0	88.6 ± 9.1 [1,5]	3819.4 ± 255.8 [40]
Ph25	92.4 ± 11.7 [2,6,a]	3848.5 ± 210.5 [41,45]
Ph50	98.3 ± 11.7 [3,7,b]	4039.2 ± 361.9 [42,46]
Ph100	97.4 ± 8.7 [4,8,c]	3897.2 ± 314.3 [43,47]
Ph150	74.4 ± 7.7 [1–4,9,d,f]	3179.6 ± 343.6 [44,45–47,p]
Ph250	57.6 ± 6.8 [5–9,e,g]	1808.2 ± 254.9 [40–44,q,r]
RT0	79.8 ± 10.2 [10,h]	3610.5 ± 316.0 [48,54]
RT25	88.2 ± 9.8 [11,16,i]	3665.6 ± 248.6 [49,55]
RT50	95.5 ± 9.0 [12,17,j]	3822.3 ± 292.7 [50,56,61]
RT100	98.5 ± 10.4 [13,18,k]	4001.6 ± 442.3 [51,57,62]
RT150	96.7 ± 10.8 [10,14,19,a,f,l]	3746.8 ± 290.3 [52,58]
RT250	89.6 ± 5.9 [15, 20,c,g,m]	3336.5 ± 307.4 [53,59,61,62,q,s]
RT500	73.1 ± 7.8 [11–15,n]	2676.8 ± 227.8 [47–53,60,t]
RT1500	68.1 ± 7.1 [16–20,o]	1905.9 ± 289.8 [54–60,u]
T0	100.3 ± 6.8 [21,25,h]	3872.5 ± 297.9
T25	109.0 ± 11.0 [26,27,33,a,i]	4034.0 ± 437.6
T50	112.0 ± 12.5 [28,34,b,j]	4066.4 ± 415.0
T100	120.16 ± 8.4 [21,29,35,c,k]	4044.4 ± 272.6 [61]
T150	124.8 ± 6.3 [22,30,36,d,l]	4066.5 ± 407.3 [p]
T250	129.3 ± 15.8 [23,26,31,37,e,m]	4153.5 ± 303.4 [62,r,s]
T500	129.2 ± 11.2 [24,32,38,n]	4210.6 ± 396.6 [63,t]
T1500	96.6 ± 7.2 [27–32,39,o]	4596.1 ± 590.6 [64,u]
T5000	58.7 ± 6.0 [25,33–39]	3368.9 ± 479.4 [61–64]

[1–64] $p < 0.05$—statistically significant results within the nanocomposite series. [a–u] $p < 0.05$—statistically significant results between nanocomposites, having the same AgNP content, but obtained in different polymerization modes.

The flexural strength of the neat networks derived from room temperature polymerization (79.8 MPa) and photopolymerization (88.6 MPa) was lower than that from thermal polymerization (100.3 MPa). The results for only the RT0 and T0 couple were statistically significant. The elasticity of the pristine networks was similar ($p \geq 0.05$) and it was characterized by the average E value of 3767.5 MPa. By filling Bis-GMA/TEGDMA with AgNP, increases in both elastic properties were observed. The flexural strength of nanocomposites produced by photopolymerization increased by 11%, whereas the modulus increased by 6%. σ of samples produced by room temperature polymerization increased by 23%, whereas E increased by 11%. Thermally activated polymerizations resulted in the greatest increases in σ and E, which correspond, respectively, to 29 and 19%. The detailed analysis of results for σ and E within particular series, led to the observation that their values increased with an increasing AgNP content at the beginning (low AgNP concentrations), but then decreased with an increasing AgNP content at high AgNP concentrations. The maximum values of σ were noted for the following nanocomposites: Ph50, RT100, and T250, whereas the maximum values for E were found for: Ph50, RT100, and T1500. Statistically significant drops in σ with respect to the pristine networks were recorded for the first time for Ph150 and T5000. σ of none of the chemically cured nanocomposites revealed statistically significant decreases with respect to RT0. The first statistically significant drop in E, with respect to Ph0, was recorded for Ph250, whereas with respect to RT0, it was recorded for RT1500. None of the thermally cured samples showed statistically significant decreases in E with respect T0. This result may be due to the fact that in thermally activated samples, the DC was relatively high (in most cases it was higher than 70%) compared to Ph or RT samples.

When comparing the elastic properties of nanocomposites by the polymerization method, the following order of increasing σ and E might be constructed: photopolymerization < room temperature polymerization < thermal polymerization. Statistical analysis showed that thermally polymerized materials had a significantly higher bending strength than products of photo- and room temperature polymerizations. The same tendency could be found by comparing results for modulus; however, they did not usually show statistical significance.

The decreases in σ and E, observed with increasing AgNP concentration in nanocomposites, coincide with the decreasing DC. The comprehensive analysis of changes in the DC, σ, and E led to the conclusion that AgNP in the Bis-GMA/TEGDMA/AgNP nanocomposites can play a reinforcing role, by increasing σ and E, when the DC is at a minimum of about 65%.

In Table 5, the results for the hardness and impact strength of studied materials are summarized.

Table 5. Hardness and impact resistance of studied Bis-GMA/TEGDMA/AgNP nanocomposites.

Sample	Hardness (N/mm^2)	Impact Resistance (kJ/m^2)
Ph0	115.1 ± 9.5^{1}	$4.57 \pm 0.35^{26,30}$
Ph25	117.9 ± 6.1^{2}	$4.77 \pm 0.36^{27,31}$
Ph50	$123.3 \pm 16.4^{3,6}$	$4.82 \pm 0.47^{28,32}$
Ph100	$122.8 \pm 10.6^{4,7}$	$4.21 \pm 0.45^{29,33,g}$
Ph150	$100.9 \pm 12.1^{5,6,7,a,b}$	$3.41 \pm 0.35^{26–29,34,h}$
Ph250	$81.4 \pm 7.3^{1–5,c,d}$	$2.48 \pm 0.31^{30–34,i,j}$
RT0	$110.2 \pm 7.6^{8,9}$	$4.07 \pm 0.37^{35,40,k}$
RT25	117.7 ± 4.2^{10}	$4.24 \pm 0.44^{36,41,l}$
RT50	121.3 ± 6.5^{11}	$4.25 \pm 0.42^{37,42,m}$
RT100	128.5 ± 13.1^{12}	$4.27 \pm 0.49^{38,43,n}$
RT150	$130.2 \pm 15.1^{8,13,16,a}$	$4.03 \pm 0.44^{39,44,o}$
RT250	$122.7 \pm 14.5^{14,c}$	$3.67 \pm 0.36^{45,j,p}$
RT500	$113.1 \pm 11.6^{15,16,e}$	$3.34 \pm 0.28^{35–39,46,q}$
RT1500	$83.94 \pm 6.7^{9–15,f}$	$2.26 \pm 0.15^{40–46,r}$
T0	$121.8 \pm 11.6^{17,19,22}$	$5.20 \pm 0.28^{47,50,56,k}$
T25	$126.4 \pm 12.1^{18,20,23}$	$5.38 \pm 0.51^{51,57,l}$
T50	$130.5 \pm 15.5^{21,24}$	$5.47 \pm 0.56^{48,52,58,m}$
T100	139.2 ± 18.3	$5.54 \pm 0.44^{49,53,59,64,f,n}$
T150	143.2 ± 21.7^{b}	$5.30 \pm 0.45^{54,60,h,o}$
T250	$142.8 \pm 20.8^{25,d}$	$4.73 \pm 0.45^{55,61,64,i,p}$
T500	$148.5 \pm 13.0^{17,18,e}$	$4.42 \pm 0.50^{47–49,62,q}$
T1500	$149.1 \pm 7.1^{19–21,f}$	$4.06 \pm 0.41^{50–55,63,r}$
T5000	$158.9 \pm 13.5^{22–25}$	$2.26 \pm 0.15^{56–63}$

$^{1–64}$ $p < 0.05$—statistically significant results within the nanocomposite series. $^{a–r}$ $p < 0.05$—statistically significant results between nanocomposites, having the same AgNP content, but obtained in different polymerization modes.

The hardness (H) of pristine networks did not differ significantly and the average value equaled 115.7 N/mm^2. In the composite series, the values of H increased to a certain AgNP limiting content and afterwards, they decreased. Thus, the following nanocomposites were characterized by the highest hardness in the series: Ph50, RT150, and T5000, which correspond to the following percentage increases, respectively: 7%, 18%, and 30%. Statistically significant decreases in H, with respect to pristine polymers, were found for Ph250 and RT1500, i.e., for nanocomposites with the highest AgNP loadings in the photo- and room temperature polymerized series. The hardness of the thermally polymerized samples increased over the whole concentration range. Moreover, the T5000 nanocomposite was characterized by the highest hardness noted in this study.

When comparing the hardness of nanocomposites according to the initiation mechanism, the following increasing order can be constructed: photopolymerization < room temperature polymerization < thermal polymerization. However, these results were usually not statistically significant.

When comparing the impact strength of pristine polymers by the polymerization technique, the values might be ordered accordingly: room temperature polymerization (4.07 kJ/m^2) < photopolymerization (4.57 kJ/m^2) < thermal polymerization (5.20 kJ/m^2). Statistically significant results were produced for the RT0 and T0 couple. The same order of polymerization techniques might be constructed if a_n of nanocomposites was analyzed. The results for nanocomposites obtained by thermal polymerization were statistically significantly higher compared to results for their counterpart samples produced in photo- or chemically initiated processes.

By comparing results in the nanocomposite series, it can be seen that the impact strength increased as the AgNP content increased up to a certain limit and then decreased, with a further increase of AgNP concentration. The impact resistance of photopolymerized samples reached the maximum in Ph50, which corresponded to 5.5% income with respect to Ph0. The impact resistance (a_n) of samples polymerized on the chemical route increased by 4.9%, which was recorded for RT100. Thermal polymerization resulted in a 6.5% increase in a_n, which was achieved for T100. All these increases were statistically insignificant with respect to the pristine polymers. Statistically significant drops in a_n of nanocomposites, with respect to the pristine polymers, were noted for Ph250, RT500, and T500.

In Figure 3, the results for water sorption (WS) are shown. It may be seen that AgNP incorporation caused the decrease in the values by around 16.5%. The average WS of nanocomposites was 33.2 μg/mm^3, whereas the WS of pristine polymers equaled 37.7 μg/mm^3. The polymerization technique did not significantly influence WS ($p \geq 0.05$).

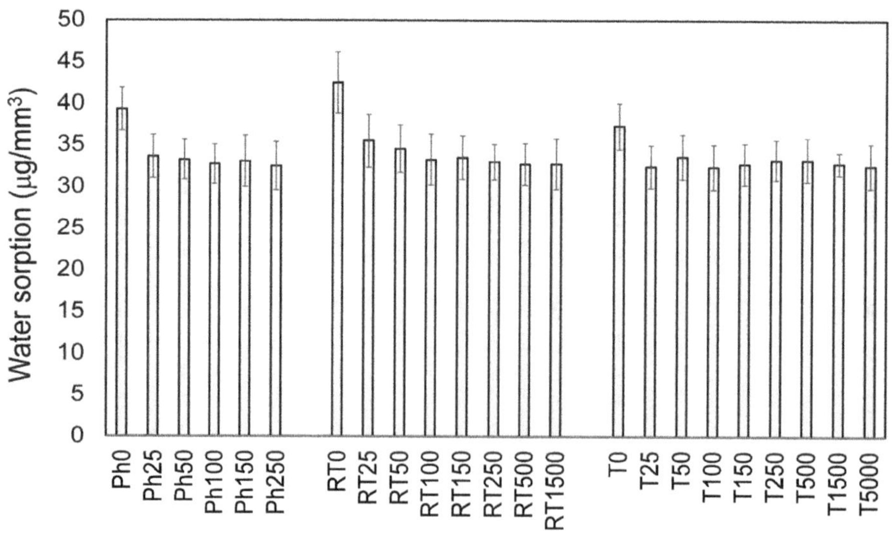

Figure 3. Water sorption of Bis-GMA/TEGDMA/AgNP nanocomposites. The statistically significant results were obtained between pristine polymers and nanocomposites in each series ($p < 0.05$).

3. Discussion

The present paper describes research regarding the effect of AgNP concentration in the Bis-GMA/TEGDMA 60/40 wt% on the viscosity of its liquid form, as well as structural, physical, and mechanical properties of hardened materials.

The results showed that AgNP concentration influences Bis-GMA/TEGDMA/AgNP resin viscosity, which increases as the AgNP content increases. An exponential increase in viscosity resulted in the enormously limited flowability of the mixture filled with 5000 ppm of AgNP. This means that the concentration of AgNP in the Bis-GMA/TEGDMA/AgNP mixture should not be higher than 1500 ppm. A higher AgNP concentration may considerably restrict resin flowability, which gives rise to air bubble trapping and can exclude the possibility of introducing other fillers, typically used in dental composites and bone cements to improve their mechanical characteristics.

The structure-property relationships were tested for Bis-GMA/TEGDMA/AgNP nanocomposites obtained by radical polymerization of the dimethacrylate matrix, which was initiated according to three mechanisms:

1. Photopolymerization—commonly used for direct curing of dental restorations [2];
2. Room temperature chemical polymerization—commonly used in bone cementation [3];
3. Thermal polymerization—commonly used in industrial processes for the manufacturing of thick parts [34].

The neat networks were characterized by the *DC* from 70 to 78%, which is in agreement with the literature data. The polymerization of dimethacrylates is never complete. A considerable fraction of the double bonds remains unreacted because of immobilization, caused by a set of certain complex features, such as autoacceleration, autodeceleration, steric isolation, and vitrification [6,7,35–38]. This has been demonstrated in many studies on the photopolymerization [35,36], room temperature polymerization [37], and thermal polymerization [38] of Bis-GMA/TEGDMA systems. The *DC* of 78% was the highest measured in this study and corresponded to the thermally polymerized sample. It can be explained by the effects of temperature on the polymerization kinetics. It is well-known that the higher polymerization temperature, the higher the final conversion in the dimethacrylate network. Heating provides the energy to improve the segmental mobility of the polymer chain and makes more residual unsaturation sites accessible for polymerization [35,36]. Additionally, the thermodynamic miscibility of Bis-GMA and TEGDMA monomers is greater at elevated temperatures. They can undergo phase separation at room temperature, which can result in the formation of more heterogeneous networks [36]. In the early stage of the thermal polymerization process, the temperature was kept at 40 °C for 1 h. At this temperature, the BPO decomposition rate was slow enough that the system nearly did not polymerize [39] and the viscosity decreased sufficiently enough to allow air bubbles to escape. Due to the preheating of liquid samples, high macroscopic homogeneity of the cured materials was maintained, despite the increase in viscosity. Gradually raising the temperature to 100 °C, in combination with a 24 h total polymerization time, resulted in materials of the highest structural homogeneity and best mechanical performance. The temperature of 100 °C was higher than the glass temperature of the Bis-GMA/TEGDMA polymer network [36]. It was chosen to intensify segmental mobility during post-curing.

The results for the *DC* in nanocomposites showed that it depends on the AgNP concentration, as well as the polymerization initiation mechanism.

The decrease in *DC* with the increase of AgNP concentration is likely caused by the increasing distance between double bonds. The free volume in the nanocomposite is occupied by the AgNP agglomerates. The higher the AgNP concentration, the higher the tendency of forming larger agglomerates [31]. As the dimensions of agglomerates and their number increase, the reactive groups drift further apart and thus become less available and less reactive.

The following general order of increasing *DC* according to polymerization methods: photopolymerization < room temperature polymerization < thermal polymerization, results from a variety of factors. The poorest curing efficiency of photopolymerization might be explained by the presence of partially overlapping absorption of Bis-GMA/TEGDMA/AgNP and CQ in the UV region. Even though the UV/VIS spectrum was free from any absorption bands from Bis-GMA/TEGDMA/AgNP in the VIS region, where CQ absorbs in the 400–550 nm range, the curing efficiency in nanocomposites produced by photopolymerization was insufficient when AgNP content exceeded 250 ppm. The effectiveness of room temperature polymerization was most likely restricted by the excessive high viscosity of the resin system, which causes the trapping of air bubbles. The highest *DC* of nanocomposites manufactured by thermal polymerization can be explained by the same kinetic factors as mentioned above. However, it has to be noted that the T5000 nanocomposite was characterized by the *DC* of 44%. Since the *DC* lower than 50% gives the information of free monomer occurrence in the system, 1500 ppm might be proposed as a maximum AgNP concentration in possible potential applications of studied nanocomposites [40].

Since *S* is the consequence of the *DC*, as predicted, the same trend in *S* values was observed with increasing AgNP content and polymerization technique.

The results also showed that mechanical properties of Bis-GMA/TEGDMA/AgNP nanocomposites mainly depend on the *DC* in the dimethacrylate polymer matrix, which is governed by the initiation mechanism (Figure 4).

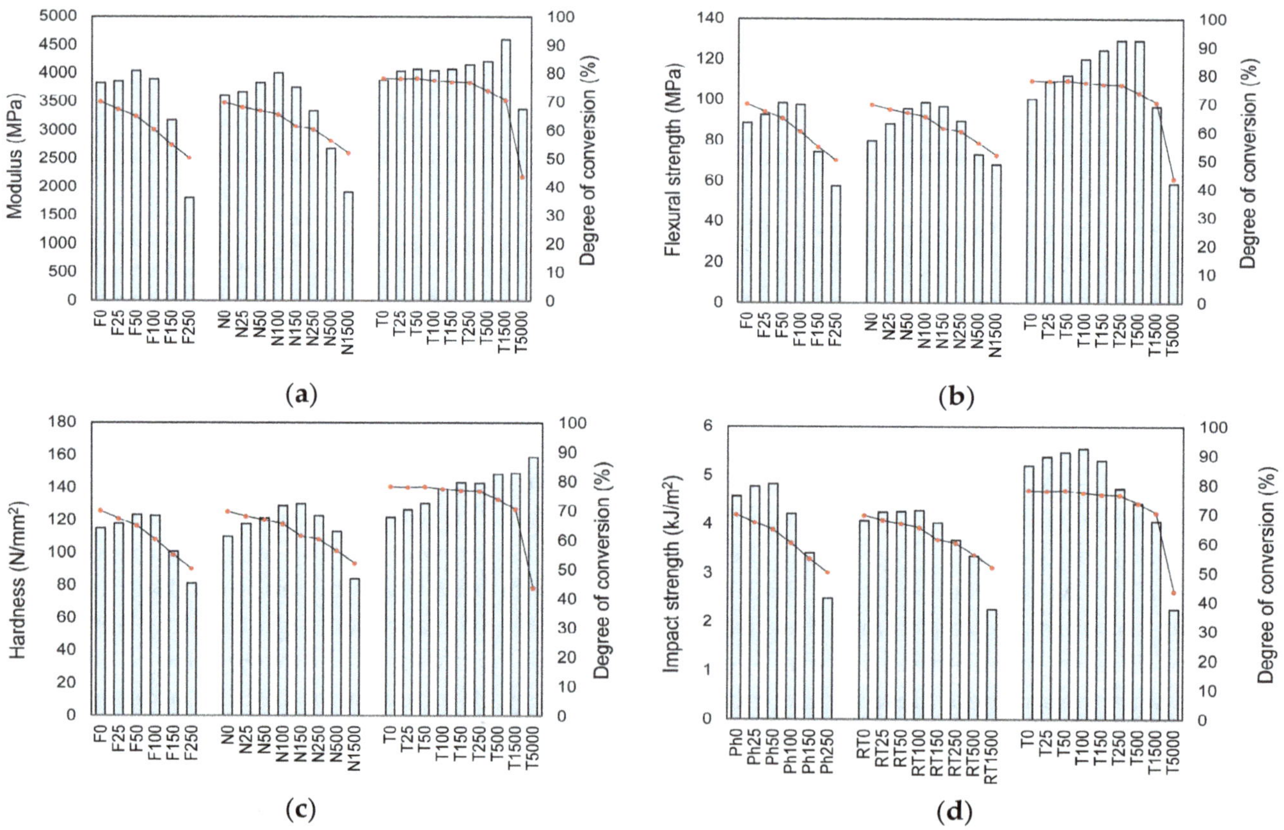

Figure 4. The comparison of mechanical properties with the degree of conversion: (**a**) modulus; (**b**) flexural strength; (**c**) hardness; (**d**) impact resistance. Bar charts correspond to mechanical properties, whereas line charts correspond to the *DC*.

Thermal polymerization resulted in a higher flexural strength, modulus, and hardness than photopolymerization and room temperature polymerization. Impact strength increased accordingly: room temperature polymerization < photopolymerization < thermal polymerization. The top position of thermally polymerized nanocomposites in these arrangements might be attributed to their maximum *DC* and the best sample quality. The lowest a_n of chemically polymerized nanocomposites might be attributed to lower *DC* and a larger number of air bubbles trapped in the sample. Since the room temperature polymerization begins just after mixing the components of the initiation system, the resin viscosity increases radically in a short time and perfect trapped air removal is unattainable. For this reason, bone cements typically display an overall porosity ranging from 2 to 18% [41,42]. This means that the latter property may be considerably deteriorated by air trapped bubbles, which are specific for room temperature polymerization.

As can be seen from Figure 4, mechanical properties usually increased at the beginning, at lower AgNP concentrations, and then decreased, when AgNP concentrations exceeded a certain level. The decreases in σ, E, H, and a_n, which were observed with increasing AgNP concentration in nanocomposites, coincide with the decreasing *DC*. This result coincides with previous findings, which show that the modulus, mechanical strength, and hardness decrease as the degree of conversion decreases [6,7]. The detailed analysis of changes in the *DC*, σ, and E leads to the conclusion that AgNP in the Bis-GMA/TEGDMA/AgNP nanocomposites can play a reinforcing role on the condition that the *DC* is at a minimum of 65%. In the series of nanocomposites obtained by thermal polymerization, hardness increased throughout the series, regardless of the degree of conversion. Therefore, hardness might be considered as the least sensitive to the *DC* property.

Taking the above considerations into account, the following AgNP concentrations might be recommended as the upper limits for manufacturing Bis-GMA/TEGDMA/AgNP nanocomposites with a satisfactory physico-mechanical performance: 250 ppm—for photopolymerization and 1500 ppm—for room temperature and thermal polymerizations.

The water sorption of the nanocomposites studied decreases with the mere addition of AgNP by an average of 16% and an increase in its concentration does not significantly influence the WS behavior. This result might be attributed to the hydrophobic character of AgNP [43].

4. Materials and Methods

4.1. Materials

The dimethacrylate resins: Bis-GMA and TEGDMA, components of the initiation systems: CQ (camphorquinone), DMAEMA (*N*,*N*-dimethylaminoethyl methacrylate), and DMPT (*N*,*N*-dimethyl-*p*-toluidine) were purchased from Sigma-Aldrich (St. Louis, MO, USA) and used as received. The BPO initiator—(benzoyl peroxide) came from POCh (Gliwice, Poland) and it was purified by dissolving in chloroform (POCh, Gliwice, Poland) and precipitated by adding methanol (POCh, Gliwice, Poland). n-Hexane was purchased from POCh (Gliwice, Poland) and was used as received.

AgNP colloid in hexane of the 1000 ppm concentration was purchased from AMEPOX Co. Ltd. (Lodz, Poland). The AgNP/hexane colloid was used as received or diluted with n-hexane to the concentrations of 500 and 100 ppm (Table 1). The mean particle size was 22.8 nm, as measured in a previous study [44].

4.2. Preparation of AgNP-Loaded Resin Compositions

The monomer blend consisted of Bis-GMA and TEGDMA in a 60/40 wt% ratio. It was loaded with AgNP. Eight concentrations of AgNP: 25, 50, 100, 150, 250, 500, 1500, and 5000 ppm, were prepared by solvent casting, with the use of n-hexane as a solvent.

First, 40 g of TEGDMA was dissolved in 100 mL of n-hexane. Next, the precisely measured amount of AgNP/hexane colloid was added to the TEGDMA solution in n-hexane (Table 1). Mixing was performed in an Erlenmayer flask on a magnetic stirrer for 10 min. Hexane was evaporated from the TEGDMA/AgNP/hexane dispersion in a rotary evaporator (IKA RV-10, Staufen, Germany) for 20 min, under the pressure of 50 mbar and then for 20 min, under the pressure of 5 mbar. The effectiveness of the evaporation procedure was confirmed in the ^{1}H NMR experiments (UNITY INOVA, Varian, 300 MHz, Palo Alto, CA, USA), which did not show the presence of peaks corresponding to n-hexane on

1H NMR spectra. TEGDMA loaded with AgNP was then blended with 60 g of Bis-GMA. Mixing was performed in a glass vessel with a mechanical stirrer at 40 °C for 20 min.

4.3. Curing Procedure

Polymerizations were carried out in 12 cm diameter Petri dishes and 10 mm diameter Teflon O-rings placed on a glass surface. The polymer amounted to the obtained thicknesses of 2 and 1 mm, respectively.

4.3.1. Photopolymerization

Bis-GMA/TEGDMA/AgNP liquid compositions, loaded with AgNP in the concentration specified in Table 1 were mixed with 0.4 wt.% of CQ (initiator) and 1 wt.% of DMAEMA (reducer) and poured into molds. Before irradiation, the sample surface was covered with a PET (poly(ethylene terephtalate)) film in order to avoid the oxygen inhibition effect. The mixtures were irradiated with a mercury UV/VIS lamp (FAMED-1, Zywiec, Poland, power 375 W) set at a distance of 10 cm for 15 min.

4.3.2. Room Temperature Polymerization (Chemical Polymerization)

Bis-GMA/TEGDMA/AgNP liquid compositions, loaded with AgNP in the concentration specified in Table 1, were divided into two equimass portions. One of them was mixed with 0.5 wt% of BPO (radical polymerization initiator) and the other with 0.05 wt% of DMPT (redox activator for BPO). To perform curing, both components were thoroughly mixed for 60 s. After stirring, the mixtures were poured into molds, covered with PET film, and left for 24 h.

4.3.3. Thermal Polymerization

Bis-GMA/TEGDMA/AgNP liquid compositions, loaded with AgNP in the concentration specified in Table 1, were mixed with 1 wt% of BPO, poured into molds, and polymerized in a drying oven under nitrogen—reducing oxygen inhibition, by raising the temperature gradually from 40 to 100 °C over 24 h [40]. First, the polymerizing mixture was reheated at 40 °C for 1 h; next, the temperature was increased to 70 °C and maintained at that temperature overnight; and finally, the temperature was increased to 100 °C and maintained for 2 h.

4.4. UV/VIS Spectroscopy

The UV/VIS spectra of pristine Bis-GMA/TEGDMA monomer composition, as well as its modifications with AgNP, were recorded over a wavelength ranging from 190 to 500 nm, utilizing a UV/VIS spectrometer (UV 2600, Shimadzu Co., Kyoto, Japan) with a 10-cm path-length quartz cuvette.

4.5. Viscosity

The viscosity (η, mPa·s) of liquid Bis-GMA/TEGDMA and its compositions with AgNP was measured by means of a rotating spindle viscometer (Brookfield Fungilab Viscometer, Visco Star Plus L, Barcelona, Spain) at 25 °C, according to PN-ISO 2555 (Plastics—Resins in the liquid state or as emulsions or dispersions—Determination of apparent viscosity by the Brookfield method). Viscosity was measured using the appropriate spindle, which allowed for recording viscosity values between 10% and 90% torque. Compositions containing 0 to 1500 ppm AgNP were tested utilizing the same spindle of the designation "1". The composition containing 5000 ppm was characterized by a significantly higher viscosity, which required the use of a spindle with the designation of "3".

4.6. Polymerization Shrinkage

The density of resinous compositions (d_m) was measured utilizing a liquid pyknometer at 25 °C according to ISO 1675 (Plastics—Liquid resins—Determination of density by the pyknometer method). Their cured forms were tested for density (d_p) according to Archimedes' principle, on the Mettler

Toledo XP Balance with a 0.01 mg accuracy (Greifensee, Switzerland) with the density determination kit at 25 °C. Water was used as the immersing liquid. The volumetric shrinkage (S) was determined by the following equation:

$$S(\%) = \frac{d_p - d_m}{d_p} \times 100 \tag{1}$$

4.7. Degree of Conversion

The degree of conversion (DC) in the polymer matrix of studied nanocomposites was determined by using an FTIR spectrophotometer (Bio-Rad Laboratories, FTS 175C, Hercules, CA, USA). The spectra of the monomers and their polymers were recorded with 128 scans at a resolution of 1 cm^{-1}. The monomer samples were tested as very thin films on KBr pellets. The cured samples were pulverized into fine powder with a particle diameter of less than 24 μm and analyzed as KBr pellets. The DC was calculated from the decrease of the absorption band at 1637cm^{-1}, referring to the C=C stretching vibration ($A_{C=C}$), in relation to the peak at 1609 cm^{-1} assigned to aromatic stretching vibrations (A_{Ar}) [45]:

$$DC(\%) = \left(1 - \frac{(A_{C=C}/A_{Ar})_{polymer}}{(A_{C=C}/A_{Ar})_{monomer}}\right) \times 100 \tag{2}$$

4.8. Mechanical Properties

4.8.1. Flexural Properties

The flexural modulus (E) and flexural strength (σ) were determined in accordance with ISO 178 (Plastics—Determination of flexural properties) in three-point bending tests, using a universal testing machine (Zwick Z020, Ulm, Germany). The rectangular samples (length × width × thickness: 40 mm × 10 mm × 2 mm) were tested. E and σ were calculated according to the following equations:

$$E\ (\mathrm{MPa}) = \frac{P_1 l^3}{4bd^3\delta} \tag{3}$$

$$\sigma\ (\mathrm{MPa}) = \frac{3Pl}{2bd^2} \tag{4}$$

where, P is the maximum load, P_1 is the load at a selected point of the elastic region of the stress–strain plot, l is the distance between supports, b is the specimen width, d is the specimen thickness, and δ is the deflection of the specimen at P_1.

4.8.2. Hardness

The ball indentation hardness (H) was determined according to ISO 2039-1 (Plastics—Determination of hardness—Part 1: Ball indentation method) on the VEB Werkstoffprüfmaschinen apparatus (Leipzig, Germany). The 4 mm-thick disc-like samples were prepared by stacking two 2 mm layers. H was calculated according to the following equation:

$$H\ (\mathrm{MPa}) = \frac{F_m\left(\frac{0.21}{h-h_r+0.21}\right)}{\pi d h_r} \tag{5}$$

where, h_r is the reduced depth of impression (h_r = 0.25 mm), d is the diameter of the ball indenter (d = 5 mm), F_m is the test load on the indenter, and h is the depth of impression.

4.8.3. Impact Strength

The impact strength (a_n) was determined in accordance with DIN 53435 (Testing of plastics. Bending test and impact test on Dynstat test pieces) using VEB Werkstoffprüfmaschinen Dynstat apparatus on rectangular unnotched specimens (length × width × thickness: 15 mm × 10 mm × 2 mm). The following formula was applied to calculate a_n:

$$a_n \left(\frac{\mathrm{kJ}}{\mathrm{m}^2}\right) = \frac{A_n}{bd} \quad (6)$$

where, A_n is the impact energy required to cause a material to fracture, and b and d are the width and thickness of the specimen, respectively.

4.9. Water Sorption

Water sorption was measured according to ISO 4049 (Dentistry—Polymer-based restorative materials). Disc-like specimens (diameter × thickness: 10 mm × 1 mm) of each nanocomposite were dried in a pre-conditioning oven at 37 °C until their weight was constant. This result was recorded as m_0 (Mettler Toledo XP Balance with 0.01 mg accuracy, Greifensee, Switzerland). The specimens were then immersed in distilled water and maintained at 37 °C for a week. After this time, the samples were removed, blotted dry, and weighed (m_1). Water sorption (WS) was calculated using the following formula:

$$\mathrm{WS}\left(\frac{\mu\mathrm{g}}{\mathrm{mm}^3}\right) = \frac{m_1 - m_0}{V_0} \quad (7)$$

where, m_0 is the initial sample weight, V_0 – the initial volume of the sample.

4.10. Statistical Analysis

The experimental results were analyzed using one-way analysis of variance (ANOVA). The pair-wise comparisons were conducted by means of the Student's t-test with a significance level (p) of 0.05. For each physical property, a set of five samples was tested. The results of measurements were expressed as mean values with associated standard deviations.

5. Conclusions

This study explained the AgNP influence on the degree of conversion and mechanical properties of Bis-GMA/TEGDMA/AgNP nanocomposites. It was shown that the higher the AgNP concentration, the lower the *DC*. Among the polymerization methods used, the thermal polymerization resulted in the highest level of curing.

Further analysis showed that AgNP can have a strengthening effect on mechanical properties. However, their values increased at the beginning, at lower AgNP concentrations, and then decreased, as AgNP concentrations exceeded a certain level, which was varied and dependent on the property. Hardness showed the least sensitivity to the *DC*, followed by the modulus, bending strength, and impact resistance, in that order. The latter property, besides possessing the highest sensitivity to the *DC*, was most likely deteriorated by air trapped bubbles, which are specific for chemical polymerization.

Author Contributions: Conceptualization, I.M.B.-R.; methodology and investigation, I.M.B.-R. and G.C.; writing—original draft preparation, review, and editing, I.M.B.-R.; funding acquisition, I.M.B.-R.

Abbreviations

AgNP	Silver nanoparticles
Bis-GMA	2,2′-bis-[4-(2-hydroxy-3-methacryloyloxy propoxy)phenyl]propane
BPO	Benzoyl peroxide

RT	Room temperature polymerization
CQ	Camphorquinone
DC	Degree of conversion
DMPT	*N,N*-dimethyl-*p*-toluidine
DMAEMA	*N,N*-dimethylaminoethyl methacrylate
E	Flexural modulus
H	Hardness
TEGDMA	Triethylene glycol dimethacrylate
Ph	Photopolymerization
S	Polymerization shrinkage
T	Thermal polymerization
WS	Water sorption

References

1. Francolini, I.; Vuotto, C.; Piozzi, A.; Donelli, G. Antifouling and antimicrobial biomaterials: An overview. *APMIS* **2017**, *125*, 392–417. [CrossRef] [PubMed]
2. Powers, J.M.; Sakaguchi, R.L. Restorative materials—Composites and polymers. In *Craig's Restorative Dental Materials*, 13th ed.; Mosby: St. Louis, MI, USA, 2013; ISBN 9780323081085.
3. Khader, B.A.; Towler, M.R. Materials and techniques used in cranioplasty fixation: A review. *Mater. Sci. Eng. C* **2016**, *66*, 315–322. [CrossRef] [PubMed]
4. Vallo, C.I.; Schroeder, W.F. Properties of acrylic bone cements formulated with Bis-GMA. *J. Biomed. Mater. Res.* **2005**, *74B*, 676–685. [CrossRef] [PubMed]
5. Otsuka, M.; Sawada, M.; Matsuda, Y.; Nakamura, T.; Kokubo, T. Antibiotic delivery system using bioactive bone cement consisting of Bis-GMA/TEGDMA resin and bioactive glass ceramics. *Biomaterials* **1997**, *18*, 1559–1564. [CrossRef]
6. Barszczewska-Rybarek, I.; Jurczyk, S. Comparative study of structure-property relationships in polymer networks based on Bis-GMA, TEGDMA and various urethane-dimethacrylates. *Materials* **2015**, *8*, 1230–1248. [CrossRef] [PubMed]
7. Barszczewska-Rybarek, I. Structure-property relationships in dimethacrylate networks based on Bis-GMA, UDMA and TEGDMA. *Dent. Mater.* **2009**, *25*, 1082–1089. [CrossRef] [PubMed]
8. Irie, M.; Suzuki, K.; Watts, D.C. Marginal gap formation of light-activated restorative materials: Effects of immediate setting shrinkage and bond strength. *Dent. Mater.* **2002**, *18*, 203–210. [CrossRef]
9. Mishra, S.K.; Chowdhary, R.; Kumari, S. Microleakage at the Different Implant Abutment Interface: A Systematic Review. *J. Clin. Diagn. Res.* **2017**, *11*, ZE10–ZE15. [CrossRef]
10. Hamouda, I.M. Current perspectives of nanoparticles in medical and dental biomaterials. *J. Biomed. Res.* **2012**, *26*, 143–151. [CrossRef]
11. Ástvaldsdóttir, Á.; Dagerhamn, J.; van Dijken, J.W.V.; Naimi-Akbar, A.; Sandborgh-Englund, G.; Tranæus, S.; Nilsson, M. Longevity of posterior resin composite restorations in adults—A systematic review. *J. Dent.* **2015**, *43*, 934–954. [CrossRef]
12. Karthikeyan, S.; Wagar, A. Nanotechnology and its applications in dentistry. In *Emerging Nanotechnologies in Dentistry*, 2nd ed.; Karthikeyan, S., Wagar, A., Eds.; William Andrew (Elsevier): Norwich, NY, USA, 2017; pp. 1–15, ISBN 9780128122914.
13. Kasraei, S.; Sami, L.; Hendi, S.; AliKhani, M.-Y.; Rezaei-Soufi, L.; Khamverdi, Z. Antibacterial properties of composite resins incorporating silver and zinc oxide nanoparticles on *Streptococcus mutans* and Lactobacillus. *Restor. Dent. Endod.* **2014**, *39*, 109–114. [CrossRef] [PubMed]

14. Beyth, N.; Yudovin-Farber, I.; Bahir, R.; Domb, A.J.; Weiss, E.I. Antibacterial activity of dental composites containing quaternary ammonium polyethylenimine nanoparticles against Streptococcus mutans. *Biomaterials* **2006**, *27*, 3995–4002. [CrossRef] [PubMed]
15. Tunney, M.; Dunne, N.; Einarsson, G.; McDowell, A.; Kerr, A.; Patrick, S. Biofilm formation by bacteria isolated from retrieved failed prosthetic hip implants in an in vitro model of hip arthroplasty antibiotic prophylaxis. *J. Orthop. Res.* **2007**, *25*, 2–10. [CrossRef] [PubMed]
16. Melo, M.A.; Cheng, L.; Zhang, K.; Weir, M.D.; Rodrigues, L.K.; Xu, H.H. Novel dental adhesives containing nanoparticles of silver and amorphous calcium phosphate. *Dent. Mater.* **2013**, *29*, 199–210. [CrossRef] [PubMed]
17. Xu, H.H.K.; Moreau, J.L.; Sun, L.; Chow, L.C. Nanocomposite containing amorphous calcium phosphate nanoparticles for caries inhibition. *Dent. Mater.* **2011**, *27*, 762–769. [CrossRef] [PubMed]
18. Aydin Sevinç, B.; Hanley, L. Antibacterial activity of dental composites containing zinc oxide nanoparticles. *J. Biomed. Mater. Res. B Appl. Biomater.* **2010**, *94*, 22–31. [CrossRef] [PubMed]
19. Tavassoli Hojati, S.; Alaghemand, H.; Hamze, F.; Babaki, F.A.; Rajab-Nia, R.; Rezvani, M.B.; Kaviani, M.; Atai, M. Antibacterial, physical and mechanical properties of flowable resin composites containing zinc oxide nanoparticles. *Dent. Mater.* **2013**, *29*, 495–505. [CrossRef]
20. Poosti, M.; Ramazanzadeh, B.A.; Zebarjad, M.; Javadzadeh, P.; Naderinasab, M.; Shakeri, M.T. Shear bond strength and antibacterial effects of orthodontic composite containing TiO_2 nanoparticles. *Eur. J. Orthod.* **2013**, *35*, 676–679. [CrossRef]
21. Russo, T.; Gloria, A.; De Santis, R.; Amora, U.D.; Balato, G.; Vollaro, A.; Oliviero, O.; Improta, G.; Triassi, M.; Ambrosio, L. Preliminary focus on the mechanical and antibacterial activity of a PMMA-based bone cement loaded with gold nanoparticles. *Bioact. Mater.* **2017**, *2*, 156–161. [CrossRef]
22. Chamundeeswari, M.; Sobhana, S.S.; Jacob, J.P.; Kumar, M.G.; Devi, M.P.; Sastry, T.P.; Mandal, A.B. Preparation, characterization and evaluation of a biopolymeric gold nanocomposite with antimicrobial activity. *Biotechnol. Appl. Biochem.* **2010**, *55*, 29–35. [CrossRef]
23. Prokopovich, P.; Köbrick, M.; Brousseau, E.; Perni, S. Potent antimicrobial activity of bone cement encapsulating silver nanoparticles capped with oleic acid. *J. Biomed. Mater. Res. B Appl. Biomater.* **2015**, *103*, 273–281. [CrossRef] [PubMed]
24. Fatemeh, K.; Mohammad Javad, M.; Samaneh, K. The effect of silver nanoparticles on composite shear bond strength to dentin with different adhesion protocols. *J. Appl. Oral Sci.* **2017**, *25*, 367–373. [CrossRef] [PubMed]
25. Chladek, G.; Kasperski, J.; Barszczewska-Rybarek, I.; Żmudzki, J. Sorption, Solubility, Bond Strength and Hardness of Denture Soft Lining Incorporated with Silver Nanoparticles. *Int. J. Mol. Sci.* **2013**, *14*, 563–574. [CrossRef] [PubMed]
26. Burdușel, A.-C.; Gherasim, O.; Grumezescu, A.M.; Mogoantă, L.; Ficai, A.; Andronescu, E. Biomedical Applications of Silver Nanoparticles: An Up-to-Date Overview. *Nanomaterials* **2018**, *8*, 681. [CrossRef] [PubMed]
27. Kassaee, M.Z.; Akhavan, A.; Sheikh, N.; Sodagar, A. Antibacterial effects of a new dental acrylic resin containing silver nanoparticles. *J. Appl. Polym. Sci.* **2008**, *110*, 1699–1703. [CrossRef]
28. Corrêa, J.M.; Mori, M.; Sanches, H.L.; da Cruz, A.D.; Poiate, I.A.V.P. Silver Nanoparticles in Dental Biomaterials. *Int. J. Biomater.* **2015**, 485275. [CrossRef]
29. Durner, J.; Stojanovic, M.; Urcan, E.; Hickel, R.; Reichl, F.X. Influence of silver nano-particles on monomer elution from light-cured composites. *Dent. Mater.* **2011**, *27*, 631–636. [CrossRef]
30. Nam, K.-Y. In vitro antimicrobial effect of the tissue conditioner containing silver nanoparticles. *J. Adv. Prosthodont.* **2011**, *3*, 20–24. [CrossRef]
31. Shubnikov, A.V. Nanomaterials. In *Advances in Nanotechnology Research and Application*, 2012 ed.; Acton, A.Q., Ed.; ScholarlyEditions™ eBook: Atlanta, GR, USA, 2012; Volume 86, pp. 4339–4579. ISBN 978-1-4649-046-5.
32. Pfeifer, C.S.; Shelton, Z.R.; Braga, R.R.; Windmoller, D.; Machado, J.C.; Stansbury, J.W. Characterization of dimethacrylate polymeric networks: A study of the crosslinked structure formed by monomers used in dental composites. *Eur. Polym. J.* **2011**, *47*, 162–170. [CrossRef]
33. Kamoun, E.A.; Winkel, A.; Eisenburger, M.; Menzel, H. Carboxylated camphorquinone as visible-light photoinitiator for biomedical application: Synthesis, characterization, and application. *Arab. J. Chem.* **2016**, *9*, 745–754. [CrossRef]

34. Abliz, D.; Duan, Y.; Steuernagel, L.; Xie, L.; Li, D.; Ziegmann, G. Curing Methods for Advanced Polymer Composites—A Review. *Polym. Polym. Compos.* **2018**, *21*, 341–348. [CrossRef]
35. Andrzejewska, E. Photopolymerization kinetics of multifunctional monomers. *Prog. Polym. Sci.* **2001**, *26*, 605–665. [CrossRef]
36. Stansbury, J.W. Dimethacrylate network formation and polymer property evolution as determined by the selection of monomers and curing conditions. *Dent. Mater.* **2012**, *28*, 13–22. [CrossRef] [PubMed]
37. Pomrink, G.J.; DiCicco, M.P.; Clineff, T.D.; Erbe, E.M. Evaluation of the reaction kinetics of CORTOSS, a thermoset cortical bone void filler. *Biomaterials* **2003**, *24*, 1023–1031. [CrossRef]
38. Jancar, J.; Wang, W.; DiBenedetto, A.T. On the heterogeneous structure of thermally cured bis-GMA/ TEGDMA resins. *J. Mater. Sci. Mater. Med.* **2000**, *11*, 675–682. [CrossRef] [PubMed]
39. Newcomb, M. Small Radical Chemistry. In *Handbook of Radical Polymerization*, 1st ed.; Matyjaszewski, K., Davis, T., Eds.; John Wiley & Sons: Hoboken, NJ, USA, 2002; Volume 2, pp. 77–116. ISBN 978-0-471-39274-3.
40. Barszczewska-Rybarek, I.; Korytkowska, A.; Gibas, M. Investigations on the structure of poly(dimethacrylate)s. *Des. Monomers Polym.* **2001**, *4*, 301–314. [CrossRef]
41. Bercier, A.; Gonçalves, S.; Lignon, O.; Fitremann, J. Calcium Phosphate Bone Cements Including Sugar Surfactants: Part One—Porosity, Setting Times and Compressive Strength. *Materials* **2010**, *3*, 4695–4709. [CrossRef] [PubMed]
42. Mau, H.; Schelling, K.; Heisel, C.; Wang, J.S.; Breusch, S.J. Comparison of various vacuum mixing systems and bone cements as regards reliability, porosity and bending strength. *Acta Orthop. Scand.* **2004**, *75*, 160–172. [CrossRef] [PubMed]
43. Guo, R.; Peng, L.; Lan, J.; Jiang, S.; Yan, W. Microstructure and hydrophobic properties of silver nanoparticles on amino-functionalised cotton fabric. *Mater. Technol.* **2016**, *31*, 139–144. [CrossRef]
44. Chladek, G.; Mertas, A.; Barszczewska-Rybarek, I.; Nalewajek, T.; Żmudzki, J.; Król, W.; Łukaszczyk, J. Antifungal Activity of Denture Soft Lining Material Modified by Silver Nanoparticles—A Pilot Study. *Int. J. Mol. Sci.* **2011**, *12*, 4735–4744. [CrossRef] [PubMed]
45. Barszczewska-Rybarek, I.M. Quantitative determination of degree of conversion in photocured poly(urethane-dimethacrylate)s by FTIR spectroscopy. *J. Appl. Polym. Sci.* **2012**, *123*, 1604–1611. [CrossRef]

5

Graphene-Induced Osteogenic Differentiation is Mediated by the Integrin/FAK Axis

Han Xie [1], Tong Cao [1], Alfredo Franco-Obregón [2,3] and Vinicius Rosa [1,4,5,*]

1. Faculty of Dentistry, National University of Singapore, 9 Lower Kent Ridge Road, Singapore 119085, Singapore; xiehan512@foxmail.com (H.X.); dencaot@nus.edu.sg (T.C.)
2. Department of Surgery, Yong Loo Lin School of Medicine, National University of Singapore, NUHS Tower Block, Level 8, IE Kent Ridge Road, Singapore 119228, Singapore; suraf@nus.edu.sg
3. BioIonic Currents Electromagnetic Pulsing Systems Laboratory, BICEPS, National University of Singapore, MD6, 14 medical Drive, #14-01, Singapore 117599, Singapore
4. Department of Materials Science and Engineering, National University of Singapore, Blk EA, #03-09 9 Engineering Drive 1, Singapore 117575, Singapore
5. Centre for Advanced 2D Materials and Graphene Research Centre, National University of Singapore, 6 Science Drive 2, Singapore 117546, Singapore

* Correspondence: denvr@nus.edu.sg

Abstract: Graphene is capable of promoting osteogenesis without chemical induction. Nevertheless, the underlying mechanism(s) remain largely unknown. The objectives here were: (i) to assess whether graphene scaffolds are capable of supporting osteogenesis in vivo and; (ii) to ascertain the participation of the integrin/FAK mechanotransduction axis during the osteogenic differentiation induced by graphene. MSC-impregnated graphene scaffolds (n = 6) were implanted into immunocompromised mice (28 days). Alternatively, MSCs were seeded onto PDMS substrates (modulus of elasticity = 130, 830 and 1300 kPa) coated with a single monomolecular layer of graphene and cultured in basal medium (10 days). The ensuing expressions of FAK-p397, integrin, ROCK1, F-actin, Smad p1/5, RUNX2, OCN and OPN were evaluated by Western blot (n = 3). As controls, MSCs were plated onto uncoated PDMS in the presence of mechanotransduction inhibitors (echistatin, Y27632 and DMH1). MSC-impregnated graphene scaffolds exhibited positive immunoexpression of bone-related markers (RUNX2 and OPN) without the assistance of osteogenic inducers. In vitro, regardless of the stiffness of the underlying PDMS substrate, MSCs seeded onto graphene-coated PDMS substrates demonstrated higher expressions of all tested osteogenic and integrin/FAK proteins tested compared to MSCs seeded onto PDMS alone. Hence, graphene promotes osteogenesis via the activation of the mechanosensitive integrin/FAK axis.

Keywords: tissue engineering; differentiation; focal adhesion kinase; bone; nanomaterials; osteoblast; mechanical

---

1. Introduction

Graphene consists of a single sheet of carbon atoms arranged into a tightly packed two-dimensional (2D) honeycomb lattice. Graphene sheets have proven quite amenable to molecular chemical vapor deposition functionalization as well as present high specific surface area and ultrahigh mechanical strength. Graphene can also be produced by (CVD) that is a scalable method to produce high quality graphene substrates in two and three-dimensions [1].

The demonstrated ability of CVD-grown graphene to induce osteogenic differentiation in vitro has rendered this method as a promising platform for cell-based bone tissue engineering and regeneration [2–9]. Notably, stem cells cultured on graphene films with basal growth medium demonstrated elevated expression of osteogenic proteins including Runt-related transcription factor 2 (RUNX2), osteocalcin (OCN), alkaline phosphatase (ALP), and osteopontin (OPN) [2,4,8]. Similarly, three-dimensional graphene substrates (scaffolds and hydrogels) increased the expression of bone-related genes and proteins such as RUNX2, collagen I (COL-1), and OCN [4,10,11]. Graphene film has also been shown to augment the mineralization potential of different somatic and stem cell classes [2,3,7]. Remarkably, MG-63 cells cultured on graphene coated titanium exhibited higher amounts of calcium nodules after 7 days compared to the uncoated controls (12 vs. 8 Ca/ng of DNA) [7]. The osteogenic differentiation achieved with CVD-grown graphene in the absence of osteogenic inductors is highly advantageous for bone tissue engineering as these chemicals and biomolecules present the following shortcomings: (a) dexamethasone is relatively non-specific promoting both osteogenesis as well as adipogenesis in the long-term; (b) bone morphogenetic proteins (BMPs) are expensive and plagued by concerns over their safety and; (c) the systematic administration of glucocorticoids can paradoxically result in bone loss [12–14].

Although graphene has been shown to induce osteogenic differentiation in vitro the intracellular events involved in this phenomenon remain largely unresolved. The physical characteristic of graphene (elastic properties and superficial topographical features such as wrinkles and ripples) may facilitate cell anchorage and thereby, promote stem cell differentiation [2,8]. Previous studies have shown that mesenchymal stem cells (MSCs) undergoing osteogenic differentiation on graphene in the absence of osteogenic inductors, exhibiting an upregulation in the basal expression of collagen I, RUNX2, OCN and OPN as well as other osteogenic genes [2,4,6,10,15]. Graphene activates physiologically-relevant mechanotransduction pathways, stimulating the expression of transcripts for bone morphogenetic protein 2 (BMP-2) and myosin heavy chain [4,6] and supported by findings that myosin heavy-chain mRNA and protein are upregulated by mechanical loading [16]. NIH-3T3 fibroblasts cultured on graphene coated substrates (glass, silicone or polydimethylsiloxane) exhibited enhanced adhesion and spreading and higher expression of F-actin and vinculin. Moreover, fibroblasts grown on graphene exhibited more elaborated stress fiber cytoarchitecture than those fibroblasts grown on uncoated substrates [17]. Cells grown on graphene films or scaffolds exhibited greater activation of focal adhesion kinase (FAK) [17,18], a key component of focal adhesion-mediated mechanotransduction regulating proliferation, differentiation and apoptosis, and other key processes in cellular physiology [19]. Finally, FAK is an essential component of the signal transduction machinery controlling osteogenesis, whereby its suppression disrupts bone formation [20].

Stem cell lineage commitment is modulated by the elastic characteristics of their microenvironments [21]. For instance, MSCs cultured in a rigid hydrogel ($G' = 3600$ Pa) exhibited higher mineralization potential than those cultured in hydrogels with elastic modulus of $G' \leq 1570$ Pa [22]. Similarly, stem cells from human exfoliated deciduous teeth (SHED) exhibit greater potential for osteogenic differentiation with increasing substrate rigidity [23]. Substrate matrix stiffness influences osteogenic differentiation of MSC via mechanosensing pathways conveyed through α-integrins, Rho-associated protein kinase (ROCK) and focal adhesion kinase (FAK) [24,25]. Indeed, an increase in the substrate stiffness enhances osteoblastic differentiation through the α2-integrin-ROCK-FAK-ERK1/2 axis [26]. As graphene has a very high elastic modulus (>1.0 TPa [27]), high in-plane stiffness [3] and remarkable flexibility for out-of-plane deformation [8], it is reasonable to assume that the osteogenic differentiation promoted by this material is similarly triggered and mediated by the activation of the mechanotransduction integrin-FAK axis. Unveiling the intracellular cascade(s) evoked by graphene and governing osteogenic differentiation is thus critical for the effective clinical translation of this carbonaceous and versatile material.

The objectives of this study were: (i) to assess the ability of a graphene scaffold to promote osteogenic differentiation of human MSCs in vivo and; (ii) to test the hypothesis that the osteogenic differentiation of MSCs on graphene is mediated via the activation of the integrin-FAK axis.

2. Results

2.1. Graphene Scaffold Induced Osteogenic Differentiation In Vivo

To evaluate whether graphene was capable of inducing osteogenesis in vivo we seeded MSCs onto a graphene scaffold (red arrows in H&E) before transplantation into the subcutaneous space of SCID mice for four weeks (Figure 1). The histological sections obtained from the scaffolds revealed the formation of bony-like structures resembling primary bone (white arrows in H&E). Immunohistochemical characterization showed that the tissues presented positive expression of the bone-related markers RUNX2 and OPN (green arrows) and for specific human mitochondria antibody (blue arrows).

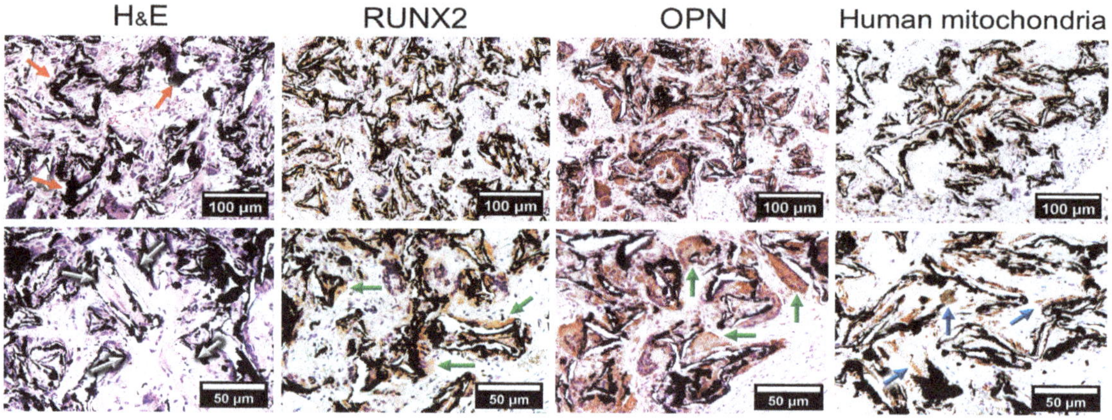

Figure 1. Graphene scaffold induce osteogenic differentiation in vivo. MSCs were seeded onto graphene scaffolds and transplanted into subcutaneous pockets of SCID mice. After four weeks, there was the formation of bony-like structures on the surface of the graphene scaffold (H&E, white arrows) that presented positive expression for the markers of osteogenic differentiation Runt-related transcription factor 2 (RUNX2) and osteopontin (OPN) (green arrows). The positive staining for specific for human mitochondria confirmed that the tissues formed were populated by human cells (blue arrows).

2.2. Activation of Integrin-FAK Axis during Graphene-Mediated Osteogenic Differentiation

To determine whether graphene promotes osteogenic differentiation via the actions of mechanosensitive pathways, we analyzed the expression of key proteins involved in the integrin-FAK axis in response to substrates of diverse mechanical properties. MSCs were seeded onto PDMS substrates with tuned elastic moduli (PDMS) or graphene-coated PDMS (Gp) in the presence or absence of inhibitors. The expression of the proteins was evaluated after 10 days in vitro.

The effective concentrations of inhibitors were ascertained by their ability to suppress proliferation. MSCs were administered different concentrations of echistatin (a Disintegrin), Y-27632 (p160ROCK inhibitor) or DMH1 (Activin receptor-like kinase 2 inhibitor) and their growth monitored for seven days. A decrease in cell proliferation of approximately 30% compared to the control was set as the threshold for effective inhibition. Echistatin significantly inhibited proliferation as early as 1 day ($p < 0.05$) at all concentrations used. However, at 10 nM proliferation was reduced by approximately 30% after seven days (Figure 2A). Effective proliferation inhibition was obtained at a concentration of 50 µM for both Y27632 and DMH1 (Figure 2B,C).

Next, we evaluated whether the integrin-FAK axis was activated during graphene-induced osteogenic differentiation. MSCs were cultured on PDMS substrates of varying stiffness that had been coated with a single monomolecular layer of graphene (Gp), or not. After 10 days, MSCs grown on Gp presented higher expression levels of FAK-p397, as well as all downstream proteins recruited in this axis compared to those seeded on PDMS alone. Highest expressions were observed on graphene-coated substrates (Gp) regardless of the stiffness of the underlying PDMS substrate. The expression of all mechanotransductory-related proteins was decreased by the presence of Echistatin (10 nM), strongly implicating the integrin-FAK axis in the osteogenic differentiation triggered by graphene (Figure 3A,B). The quantification of relative expressions showed that cells grown on Gp exhibited higher protein expression than cells cultured on PDMS alone of similar modulus of elasticity (Figure 3B).

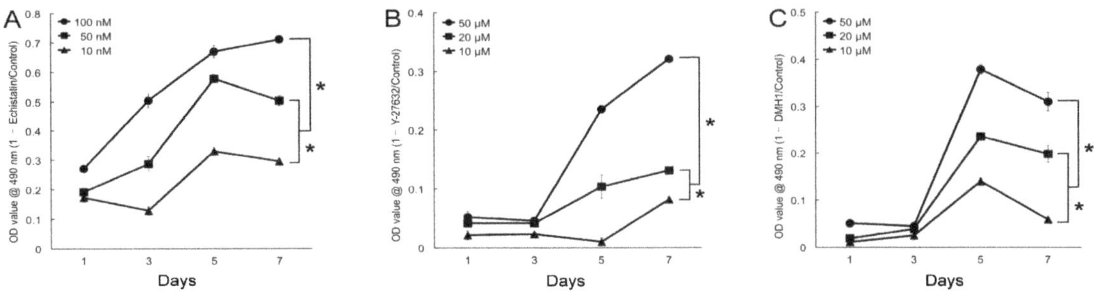

Figure 2. Effects of mechanotransduction inhibitors on cell proliferation. All inhibitors concentrations decreased cell proliferation at all time points compared to controls. After seven days, the proliferation decreased by approximately 30%, when cells were treated with 10 nM of echistatin (**A**) and 50 μM of Y27632 and DMH1 (**B**,**C**) comparing to the untreated control. (* denotes statistical difference between the groups, $p < 0.05$. For the sake of clarity, only the statistical significances at day seven are depicted).

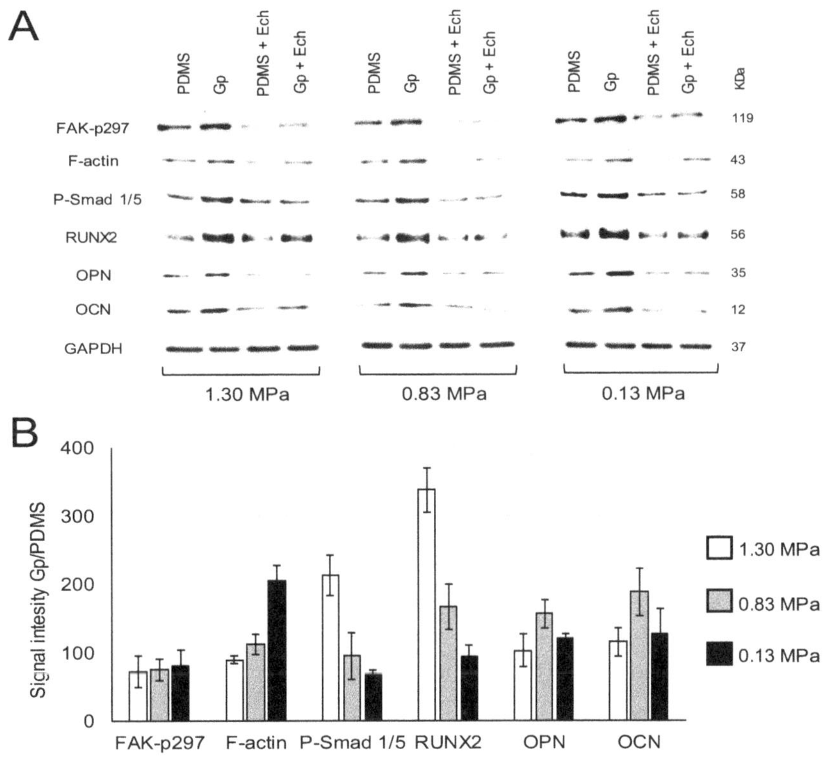

Figure 3. (**A**) Absolute and (**B**) relative expression levels of indicated proteins derived from MSCs grown on PDMS of different stiffnesses (determined by ratio of Sylgard 184 and 527) and graphene-coated PDMS (Gp). Regardless of the stiffness of the underlying substrates, MSC on Gp presented higher expression of physical stimuli-related proteins (FAK-p397, Smad p1/5 and F-actin) and bone-related markers (RUNX2, osteopontin (OPN) and osteocalcin (OCN)) compared to cells cultured on PDMS alone. OPN and OCN expression increased on Gp relative to PDMS (Gp/PDMS) for all stiffnesses tested. (**B**) relative quantification of all groups in the absence of inhibitors. Signal intensity is in arbitrary units. The presence of 10 nM echistatin attenuated the expression of all proteins examined. GAPDH represents housekeeping gene.

Y27632 (50 μM) was used to confirm a downstream role of ROCK1 in the osteogenic differentiation induced by graphene. As previously, regardless of the stiffness of the underlying polymer, MSCs on graphene-coated PDMS exhibited higher expression levels of ROCK1 in conjunction with its downstream affiliated transforming growth factor β modulating protein, Smad 1/5, and bone-related proteins (RUNX2, OPN and OCN), whose expressions were attenuated by the administration of Y27632 (Figure 4A,B).

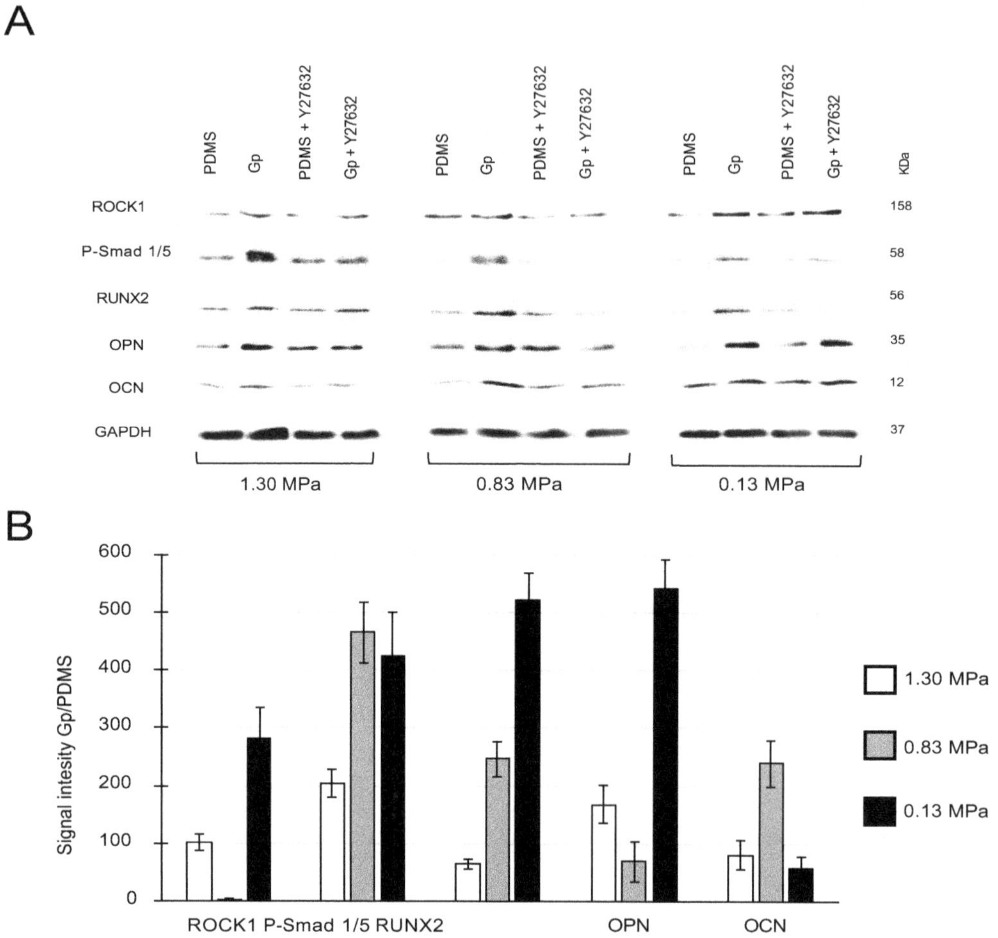

Figure 4. (**A**) Regardless of the stiffness of the underlying substrate (PDMS), Gp upregulated the expression levels of ROCK1, Smad p1/5 and F-actin and bone-related proteins. With the exception of ROCK1/0.83 MPa, Gp increased the expression of all proteins by >50%. (**B**) Relative quantification of all groups in the absence of inhibitors. Signal intensity is in arbitrary units.

Finally, we checked the expression levels of the selected proteins before and after inhibiting Smad p1/5 in response to treatment with DMH1 (50 μM). The expressions of Smad p1/5 and of the downstream bone-related proteins (RUNX2, OPN and OCN) were higher on Gp compared to all PDMS conditions tested. The presence of DMH1 suppressed the expression of all proteins confirming that the osteogenic differentiation on graphene is regulated by the activation of Smad p1/5 (Figure 5A). The quantification of protein expression showed that cells on Gp exhibited increased compared to PDMS for all modulus of elasticities studied (Figure 5B).

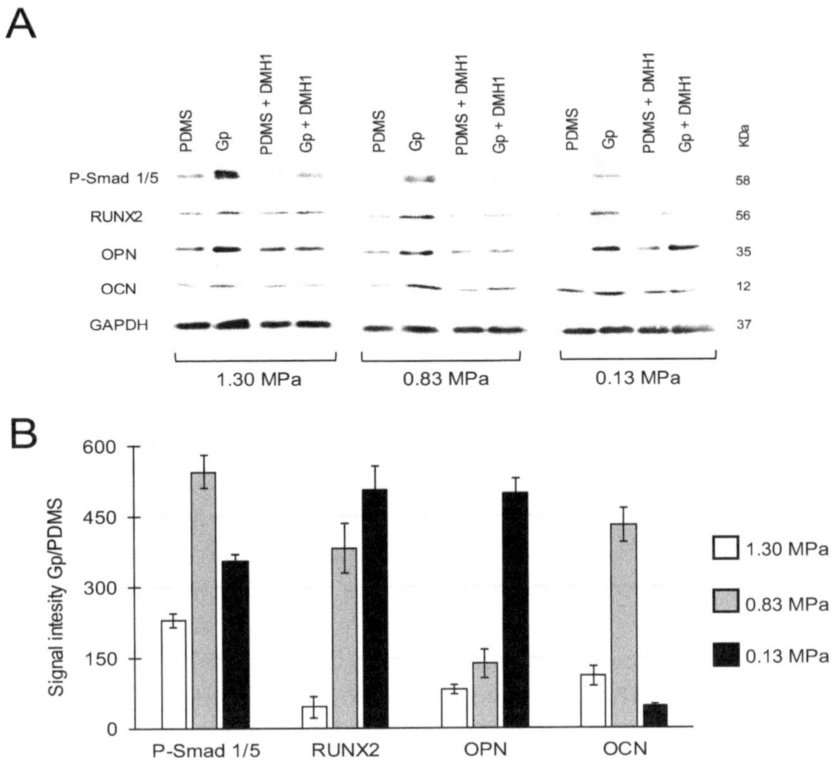

Figure 5. (**A**) MSCs grown on Gp exhibited greater increases of Smad p1/5 and of the classical markers for osteogenic differentiation, RUNX2, OPN and OCN. The expressions of p-SMAD increased by >180% on Gp compared to PDMS alone. The treatment 50 μM of DMHI decreased the expression of all protein studies. (**B**) Relative quantification of all groups in the absence of inhibitors. Signal intensity is in arbitrary units.

3. Discussion

CVD-grown graphene has emerged as a promising platform with which to enhance osteogenic outcome [5,6,8,9,23]. The osteogenic capabilities of CVD-grown graphene have been attributed to its molecular structure, whereby the potential for π–π stacking between the aromatic rings of given osteogenic inducers (e.g., dexamethasone, β-glycerophosphate) and the graphene has been hypothesized. This would act to effectively absorb and immobilize said biomolecules to its surface for more effective cell delivery and enhanced differentiation [3,24]. Seemingly at odds with the previous studies, several other publications have attested to the osteogenic potential of graphene films, scaffolds and hydrogels even in the absence of chemical inductors [2,4,6,8,12]. A resolution to these seemingly disparate discoveries may come with the recent finding that unstimulated paracrine cells plated onto graphene enhance their release of signaling molecules and proteins that are capable of promoting osteogenic differentiation of MCSc cultured onto inert glass substrate [2]. Hence, it is feasible that graphene both promotes the paracrine release of pro-osteogenic biomolecules in the immediate microenvironment as well as enhances their delivery to support osteogenic differentiation [2,4,8,11]. However, the potential of CVD-grown graphene promote osteogenesis in vivo and the cellular mechanisms evoked to allow differentiation remain largely unknown. In this report, the graphene scaffold induced the differentiation of human MSC in vivo (Figure 1). After four weeks from implantation, the histological analysis with H&E revealed the presence of bony-like tissues within the scaffolds resembling primary bone. Notably, the imunnohistochemical analysis of the tissues formed showed positive expression of the transcription factor RUNX2 and OPN. The first is essential for osteoblastic differentiation and skeletal morphogenesis, while OPN is an important bone matrix protein synthesized by osteoblastic cells [25,26]. Positive immunoreactivity to an antibody specific for human mitochondria indicated that the tissues formed was of human origin and confirmed that the cells remained viable for 28 days as well as that they underwent osteogenic differentiation in vivo.

Evidence exists for integrin-mediated mechanical signaling regulating stem cell paracrine factor production and release [10]. We investigated the role of the integrin-FAK-axis in the graphene-induced osteogenic differentiation. The FAK activity is related to alterations in the actin and microtubule filaments. As cells experience changes in forces through integrin contacts that link the extracellular matrix with the cytoskeleton, the FAK is activated modulating corrective cell responses to environmental stimuli [18,27]. Both integrins and FAK proteins are sensitive to physical stimuli and elastic properties of the substrates [28]. Accordingly, the high modulus of elasticity (up to 2.4 TPa) and high flexibility to out-of-plane deformation of graphene [8,22] could modulate the expression of these proteins and trigger a mechano-stimulated osteogenic differentiation. To test this hypothesis, MSC were cultured on PDMS substrates with modulus of elasticity ranging from 130 to 1.3 MPa with or without a coating of graphene. After 10 days, the expressions of the proteins involved in the integrin-FAK axis were evaluated by Western blot.

The expression of FAK-p397 was higher in all graphene-coated PDMS substrates (Gp) compared to PDMS alone (Figure 3). Similar enhancement in FAK expression was observed in fibroblasts cultured on stiff fibronectin gel (66 kPa) compared with a softer one (1050 Pa) [29]. Besides regulating cell adhesion, FAK-p397 is necessary for osteogenic differentiation, as its inhibition decreases RUNX2 expression by ~50% and mineralized matrix deposition by 30% [30].

Additionally, we observed that MSCs on Gp presented higher F-actin expression compared MSCs on uncoated PDMS (Figure 3). F-actin controls the cytoskeleton tension, promotes the phosphorylation of Smad and upregulates the downstream of osteogenic regulatory proteins [31]. The higher expression of RUNX2, OCN and OPN observed in this study may be related to greater substrate-mediated contractile forces reflected by increased F-actin stress fibers that enhances osteoblastic differentiation [18]. In addition, regardless of the stiffness of the underlying PDMS and presence of graphene, cells treated with the integrin inhibitor (echistatin) presented low expression of all proteins analyzed. This inhibitor binds to integrin $\alpha_V\beta_3$ receptor in a nondissociable manner [32] decreasing the expression of FAK, actin cytoskeleton and RhoA, hence, compromising the integrin-FAK signaling [33]. A similar trend ca be observed in Figure 3, confirming that the integrin-FAK complex is triggered by graphene, inducing osteogenic differentiation.

Contractile and mechanical forces associated by stiffer substrates activate RhoA/Rho-associated protein kinase (ROCK) that is essential for the formation of stress fibers and for the activation of Smad signaling imperative for osteogenesis [34,35]. MSCs on Gp exhibited higher expression of ROCK1, Smad p1/5 and both OCN and OPN compared to MSCs seeded onto PDMS alone (Figure 4). The latter are well-recognized signature proteins for the presence and function of mature osteoblasts [2,4]. Conversely, treatment with Y27632 decreased the expressions of ROCK1, Smad p1/5 and bone-related markers. Moreover, periodontal ligament cells treated with Y27632 also showed significant reductions in the expression of osteogenic genes (e.g., fibronectin 1, collagen type I and III, and biglycan) [36]. Together, these findings confirm that the graphene-induced osteogenic differentiation of MSC is mediated by the expression of ROCK1.

Finally, we checked the role of Smad (Figure 5), which is a sensitive regulatory protein that mediates the osteogenic differentiation in MSCs [37]. A single layer graphene increased the expression of Smad p1/5 independently of the stiffness of the underlying PDMS substrate. It is known that the phosphorylated Smad protein complex (e.g., Smad p1/5/8) can translocate into the cell nucleus and directly induce an upstream activator of RUNX2 [37,38], while the suppression of phosphorylation and nuclear translocation of Smad 1/5/8 inhibits the expression of osteogenic genes in MSCs [39]. Smad functions with RUNX2 through direct binding in a transcriptional activator complex during the osteogenic induction [40]. Accordingly, MSCs grown on Gp revealed the increased expression of Smad p1/5 and RUNX2 culminating in higher expressions of OCN and OPN proteins. The expressions decreased by the presence of DMH1 inhibitor confirming that the graphene-induced osteogenic differentiation is regulated by the upstream of Smad proteins.

Despite our provocative findings showing osteogenic induction by CVD-grown graphene in vivo and elucidating an underlying mechanotransduction-related signaling cascade, this work has limitations. For instance, PDMS with tunable properties has been shown to induce "inside-out" changes in cells to influence migration, stiffness and differentiation via adjusting the physical characteristics of the microenvironment [18,21]. Moreover, our synthetic material and the two-dimensional set-up of the experiments do not mimic the complex organic three-dimensional environments in which cells are imbedded in vivo. In addition, the contribution of the integrin-FAX axis in the graphene-induced osteogenic differentiation was elucidated in vitro, rather than in the animal. In addition, the osteogenic potential was evaluated in an ectopic model. Future studies shall evaluate the potential of graphene scaffold in situ and benchmark its potential to induce osteogenesis to other materials used for bone tissue engineering research. On other hand, these caveats provide us future avenues for investigation. Future studies will investigate the contribution of other integrin-relevant links (e.g., serine/threonine kinase and Rac pathways) and pathways involved in the differentiation of stem cells into osteoblasts (e.g., TGF-β/SMAD, Wnt and BMP-2). Despite of these limitations, our work provides the evidence that graphene induces the osteogenic differentiation by the upregulation of proteins sensitive to physical stimuli involved in the integrin-FAK axis. Thus, the molecular properties of graphene are capable of activating the integrin-FAK transmembrane complex that recruit the activity of both ROCK1 and F-actin that, in turn, stimulate the phosphorylation of Smad p1/5, upstream of RUNX2, OPN and OCN expression to bring osteogenesis closer to fruition (Figure 6).

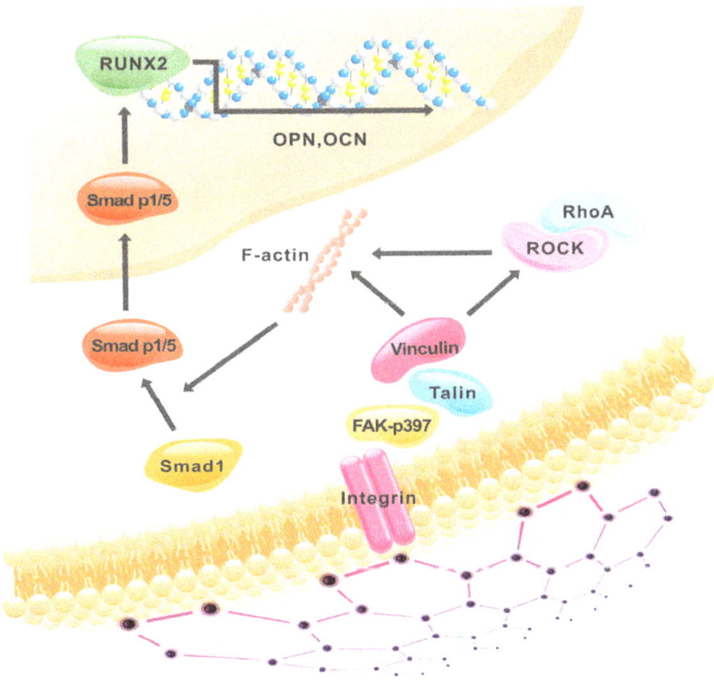

Figure 6. Mono-atomic graphene film promotes osteogenic differentiation of human MSCs via activation the integrin-FAK axis.

4. Material and Methods

4.1. Graphene Films and Scaffold Preparation

Graphene samples were produced by CVD using a custom-built furnace in a Class 1000 clean room facility at the NUS Centre for Advanced 2D Materials and Graphene Research Centre.

For single-layer graphene films, copper foils (Graphene Platform, Tokyo, Japan) were placed in a quartz tube. Thereafter, hydrogen gas (8 sccm) was introduced into the chamber and the temperature was increased to 1010 °C (25 °C/min) and maintained for 35 min. The graphene films were grown by flowing 16 sccm of CH_4 into the tube for 30 min at 500 mTorr. Finally, the tube was cooled to room temperature with H_2. The graphene-coated copper foils were spin-coated with polymethyl methacrylate (PMMA, Sigma, Saint Louis, MO, USA) and maintained at 180 °C for 10 min. The uncoated surface of the copper foil was etched with oxygen plasma (3 min, 50 W, 50 sccm, Vita-mini reactive ion etching, FEMTO Science Inc., Gyeonggi-Do, Korea). Following this, the copper was etched with 1.5% ammonium persulphate solution for 8 h and the graphene/PMMA transferred to deionized water for 2 h. Thereafter, the floating membrane was gently scooped onto the target polydimethylsiloxane (PDMS) substrates and the PMMA dissolved in acetone for 12 h. Finally, the graphene-coated samples were washed in isopropyl alcohol for 3 h.

The graphene scaffold was grown using nickel templates (density 320 ± 25 g/m^2, pore size ~500 μm, Alantum Advanced Technology Materials, Seongnam, Korea) with the same CVD protocol. Thereafter, the nickel was removed with $FeCl_3$ solution for 72 h at room temperature and washed with deionized water for 72 h.

Raman spectra of graphene films and scaffolds were obtained at room temperature, with an excitation laser source of 532 nm and power of 0.1 mW (Raman Microscope CRM 200, Witec, Ulm, Germany) and confirmed the production of single-layer films and multi-layer graphene scaffolds (Figure 7A).

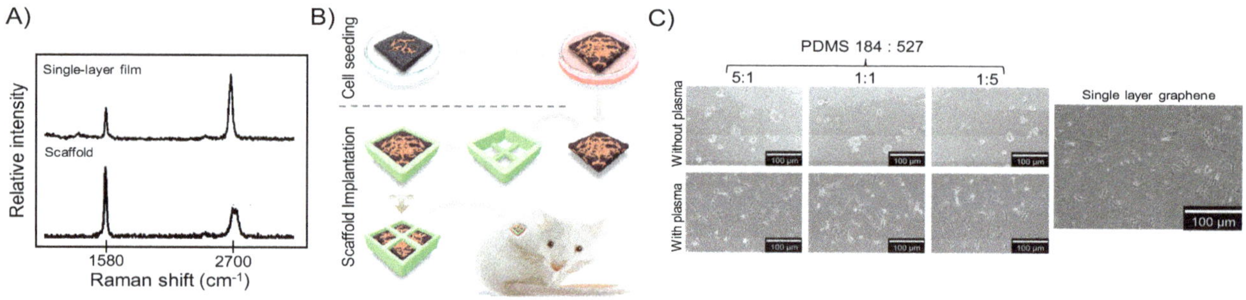

Figure 7. (**A**) Raman characterization. The Raman fingerprints confirmed the successful production of single layer graphene films and multilayer graphene scaffolds. (**B**) Graphene scaffold transplantation in vivo. MSC were seeded in the chemical vapor deposition (CVD)-grown graphene scaffolds (10 × 10 × 1 mm) and maintained in suspension plates at 37 °C for seven days to allow for attachment and proliferation. The scaffolds were placed in three-dimensionally (3D)-printed polylactide protection containers and implanted subcutaneously into immunodeficient mice for four weeks. (**C**) Cell attachment on PDMS with tunable elastic properties and graphene. Cells attached and proliferated on the surface of the oxygen plasma-etched PDMS substrates and single layer CVD-grown graphene.

4.2. Graphene Scaffold Transplantation In Vivo

The use of human cells and animals were approved by the NUS Institutional Review Board, Institutional Biosafety Committee and Institutional Animal Care and Use Committee (R17-0956, 12/12/2017).

Human dental pulp stem cells (DP003F, Alcells, Alameda, USA) were cultured in basal growth culture medium ((Dulbecco's modified Eagle's medium (DMEM, Invitrogen, Carlsbad, CA, USA), 10% fetal bovine serum (Invitrogen) and 1% penicillin/streptomycin (Invitrogen)) until 70~80% confluence and harvested (TrypLE, Invitrogen). As shown in Figure 7B, MSC (2 × 10^4, passage 3) were seeded in the graphene scaffold (0.8 × 0.8 × 0.2 cm) and maintained undisturbed for seven days. Following that, the scaffolds (n = 6) were placed inside 3D-printed polylactide protection containers (Cube, 3D Systems, Columbia, SC, USA) and transplanted into the subcutaneous space of immunodeficient mice (CB-17 SCID, Invivos, Singapore). After 28 days, specimens were retrieved, fixed with 4%

formaldehyde solution in phosphate-buffered saline at 4 °C for 24 h and stained with hematoxylin and eosin (H&E). Immunohistochemical analyses of the tissues formed were performed for OPN and RUNX2 (1:1000, Abcam, Cambridge, UK), and anti-human mitochondria antibodies (1:500, Abcam). Controls were tissue sections stained with an isotype-matched non-specific IgG antibody.

4.3. Role of Integrin-FAK Axis in the Graphene-Induced Osteogenic Differentiation

4.3.1. Substrate Preparation

To create the PDMS substrates with tunable modulus of elasticity, we blended Sylgard 184 and 527 (Dow Corning, Midland, TX, USA) in different proportions (5:1 = 1.3 MPa, 1:1 = 830 kPa, and 1:5 = 130 kPa [41]). Glass slides (22 mm × 22 mm) were covered with the freshly mixed PDMS and spin-coated (2000 rpm, 90 s). The PDMS substrates were maintained at 120 °C for 1 h followed by 60 °C overnight. To improve cell attachment, the PDMS substrates were treated with oxygen plasma (3 min, 5 W, 20 sccm, Vita-mini reactive ion etching, Figure 7C). Thereafter, half of the PDMS substrates were coated with a single layer of graphene (Gp) by the scooping method.

4.3.2. Inhibitor Concentration Optimization

Echistatin, Y27632 and DMH1 were used to selectively inhibit the expression of key proteins expressed in the integrin-FAK axis namely integrin, Rho-associated kinase 1 (ROCK1) and Smad.

To optimize the concentration of the inhibitors, MSC were seeded in 96-well flat-bottom plate (800/well) and maintained undisturbed in basal growth culture medium for 24 h. Thereafter, the culture medium was completely removed and 100 μL of DMEM with different concentrations of the inhibitors were added and changed every 48 h. Cell proliferation was evaluated for seven days by an MTS assay (CellTiter 96 AQueous One Solution Assay, Promega, Madison, WI, USA). The inhibitory ratio of cell proliferation was calculated based on the absorbance at 490 nm (Multiskan GO Microplate Spectrophotometer, Thermo Fisher Scientific, Waltham, MA, USA) obtained for the untreated cells (control). Statistical analyses were performed with Mann–Whitney test (α = 5%, SPSS Statistics 22, IBM, Armonk, NY, USA). The concentrations that inhibited cell proliferation by ~30% were selected for the subsequent tests.

4.3.3. Role of Integrin-FAK Axis on Graphene Osteogenic Differentiation

MSC (7×10^3) were seeded on the PDMS substrates alone (5:1, 1:1 and 5:1) or coated with graphene (Gp) and cultured for 10 days. Thereafter, the expression of integrin-FAK axis-related (FAK-p397, F-actin, ROCK, Smad p1/5) and bone-related proteins (RUNX2, OCN and OPN) were assessed by Western blot (all antibodies from Abcam) and gels imaged using ChemiDoc MP Imaging System (Bio-Rad, Hercules, CA, USA). Cells cultured with echistatin (10 nM), Y27632 (50 μM) or DMH1 (50 μM) were the controls. Three independent samples were evaluated per group. The intensity of the bands was quantified with ImageJ (NIH, Bethesfa, MD, USA). For the relative quantification, we firstly confirmed that the housekeeping protein (GAPDH) was constant across the groups. Secondly, we obtained the lane normalization factor (LNF) by dividing the housekeeping bands on the blot by the highest signal for the housekeeping protein identified. The NFs were approximately 1.0 for all groups indicating homogeneous housekeeping protein expression. Thirdly, the protein density (PD) of all the proteins of interest (e.g., FAK) was normalized to their respective housekeeping protein in each lane. Finally, the normalized signal of each PD was divided by the LNF and the relative expression was calculated as $[(Gp - PDMS)/PDMS] \times 100$.

5. Conclusions

CVD-grown graphene induces osteogenic differentiation of MSCs due to its molecular and physical properties (e.g., elastic properties, surface features) without the assistance of the conventional cocktail of osteogenic inducers considered necessary in other platforms. Here, we extended these findings by showing that graphene scaffolds also promote the osteogenic differentiation of MSCs in vivo. Osteogenesis was corroborated with the positive expression of RUNX2 and OPN, classical markers for osteogenic differentiation. Complementary in vitro tests demonstrated that the osteogenic differentiation was mediated by the activation of the mechanosensitive integrin-FAK axis. These developmental attributes appear to be inherent to the mono-atomic graphene sheet as changing the elastic modulus of the underlying PDMS had little effect on their ability to induce osteogenesis. Our findings deepen the understanding of the effects of graphene on biological systems and broaden the potential avenues for the use of this single-atom thin material to promote osteogenesis without the delivery limitations of exogenous chemical inducers.

Author Contributions: Conceptualization, V.R. and H.X.; Methodology, V.R. and H.X. Investigation, H.X.; Draft Preparation, Revision, H.X., T.C., A.F.O. and V.R.; Supervision, V.R.; Project Administration, V.R.; Funding Acquisition, V.R.

Acknowledgments: This research is supported by the National Research Foundation, Prime Minister' Office, Singapore, under its Medium Sized Centre Programme. V.R. was supported by the grants from the Singapore Ministry of Education, Singapore (Academic Research Fund Tier 1, R-221-000-091-112 and R-221-000-104-114) and the National University Health System, Singapore (NUHS Open Collaborative Research Grant NUHS O-CRG 2016 Oct-25).

References

1. Geim, A.K.; Novoselov, K.S. The rise of graphene. *Nat. Mater.* **2007**, *6*, 183–191. [CrossRef]
2. Xie, H.; Chua, M.; Islam, I.; Bentini, R.; Cao, T.; Viana-Gomes, J.C.; Castro Neto, A.H.; Rosa, V. CVD-grown monolayer graphene induces osteogenic but not odontoblastic differentiation of dental pulp stem cells. *Dent. Mater.* **2017**, *33*, e13–e21. [CrossRef] [PubMed]
3. Lee, W.C.; Lim, C.H.Y.X.; Shi, H.; Tang, L.A.L.; Wang, Y.; Lim, C.T.; Loh, K.P. Origin of enhanced stem cell growth and differentiation on graphene and graphene oxide. *ACS Nano* **2011**, *5*, 7334–7341. [CrossRef] [PubMed]
4. Xie, H.; Cao, T.; Gomes, J.V.; Castro Neto, A.H.; Rosa, V. Two and three-dimensional graphene substrates to magnify osteogenic differentiation of periodontal ligament stem cells. *Carbon* **2015**, *93*, 266–275. [CrossRef]
5. Xie, H.; Cao, T.; Rodríguez-Lozano, F.J.; Luong-Van, E.K.; Rosa, V. Graphene for the development of the next-generation of biocomposites for dental and medical applications. *Dent. Mater.* **2017**, *33*, 765–774. [CrossRef] [PubMed]
6. Li, J.; Wang, G.; Geng, H.; Zhu, H.; Zhang, M.; Di, Z.; Liu, X.; Chu, P.K.; Wang, X. CVD growth of graphene on NiTi alloy for enhanced biological activity. *ACS Appl. Mater. Interfaces* **2015**, *7*, 19876–19881. [CrossRef] [PubMed]
7. Dubey, N.; Ellepola, K.; Decroix, F.E.D.; Morin, J.L.P.; Castro Neto, A.H.; Seneviratne, C.J.; Rosa, V. Graphene onto medical grade titanium: An atom-thick multimodal coating that promotes osteoblast maturation and inhibits biofilm formation from distinct species. *Nanotoxicology* **2018**, *12*, 274–289. [CrossRef] [PubMed]
8. Nayak, T.R.; Andersen, H.; Makam, V.S.; Khaw, C.; Bae, S.; Xu, X.; Ee, P.L.; Ahn, J.H.; Hong, B.H.; Pastorin, G.; et al. Graphene for controlled and accelerated osteogenic differentiation of human mesenchymal stem cells. *ACS Nano* **2011**, *5*, 4670–4678. [CrossRef] [PubMed]
9. Dubey, N.; Bentini, R.; Islam, I.; Cao, T.; Castro Neto, A.H.; Rosa, V. Graphene: A versatile carbon-based material for bone tissue engineering. *Stem Cells Int.* **2015**, *2015*, 804213. [CrossRef]
10. Kusuma, G.D.; Carthew, J.; Lim, R.; Frith, J.E. Effect of the Microenvironment on Mesenchymal Stem Cell Paracrine Signaling: Opportunities to Engineer the Therapeutic Effect. *Stem Cells Dev.* **2017**, *26*, 617–631. [CrossRef]
11. Crowder, S.W.; Prasai, D.; Rath, R.; Balikov, D.A.; Bae, H.; Bolotin, K.I.; Sung, H.J. Three-dimensional graphene foams promote osteogenic differentiation of human mesenchymal stem cells. *Nanoscale* **2013**, *5*, 4171–4176. [CrossRef] [PubMed]
12. Lu, J.; He, Y.-S.; Cheng, C.; Wang, Y.; Qiu, L.; Li, D.; Zou, D. Self-supporting graphene hydrogel film as an experimental platform to evaluate the potential of graphene for bone regeneration. *Adv. Funct. Mater.* **2013**, *23*, 3494–3502. [CrossRef]

13. Nuttall, M.E.; Patton, A.J.; Olivera, D.L.; Nadeau, D.P.; Gowen, M. Human trabecular bone cells are able to express both osteoblastic and adipocytic phenotype: Implications for osteopenic disorders. *J. Bone Miner. Res.* **1998**, *13*, 371–382. [CrossRef]
14. Carragee, E.J.; Hurwitz, E.L.; Weiner, B.K. A critical review of recombinant human bone morphogenetic protein-2 trials in spinal surgery: Emerging safety concerns and lessons learned. *Spine J.* **2011**, *11*, 471–491. [CrossRef] [PubMed]
15. Reid, I.R. Glucocorticoid-induced osteoporosis. *Baillieres Best Pract. Res. Clin. Endocrinol. Metab.* **2000**, *14*, 279–298. [CrossRef] [PubMed]
16. Lin, F.; Du, F.; Huang, J.; Chau, A.; Zhou, Y.; Duan, H.; Wang, J.; Xiong, C. Substrate effect modulates adhesion and proliferation of fibroblast on graphene layer. *Colloids Surf. B Biointerfaces* **2016**, *146*, 785–793. [CrossRef]
17. Chandran, R.; Knobloch, T.J.; Anghelina, M.; Agarwal, S. Biomechanical signals upregulate myogenic gene induction in the presence or absence of inflammation. *Am. J. Physiol. Cell Physiol.* **2007**, *293*, C267–C276. [CrossRef]
18. Engler, A.J.; Sen, S.; Sweeney, H.L.; Discher, D.E. Matrix elasticity directs stem cell lineage specification. *Cell* **2006**, *126*, 677–689. [CrossRef]
19. Lu, Q.; Pandya, M.; Rufaihah, A.J.; Rosa, V.; Tong, H.J.; Seliktar, D.; Toh, W.S. Modulation of dental pulp stem cell odontogenesis in a tunable peg-fibrinogen hydrogel system. *Stem Cells Int.* **2015**, *2015*, 525367. [CrossRef]
20. Shih, Y.-R.V.; Tseng, K.-F.; Lai, H.-Y.; Lin, C.-H.; Lee, O.K. Matrix stiffness regulation of integrin-mediated mechanotransduction during osteogenic differentiation of human mesenchymal stem cells. *J. Bone Miner. Res.* **2011**, *26*, 730–738. [CrossRef]
21. Holle, A.W.; Engler, A.J. More than a feeling: Discovering, understanding, and influencing mechanosensing pathways. *Curr. Opin. Biotechnol.* **2011**, *22*, 648–654. [CrossRef] [PubMed]
22. Lee, J.U.; Yoon, D.; Cheong, H. Estimation of Young's modulus of graphene by Raman spectroscopy. *Nano Lett.* **2012**, *12*, 4444–4448. [CrossRef]
23. Kalbacova, M.; Broz, A.; Kong, J.; Kalbac, M. Graphene substrates promote adherence of human osteoblasts and mesenchymal stromal cells. *Carbon* **2010**, *48*, 4323–4329. [CrossRef]
24. Akhavan, O.; Ghaderi, E.; Shahsavar, M. Graphene nanogrids for selective and fast osteogenic differentiation of human mesenchymal stem cells. *Carbon* **2013**, *59*, 200–211. [CrossRef]
25. Kern, B.; Shen, J.; Starbuck, M.; Karsenty, G. Cbfa1 contributes to the osteoblast-specific expression of type I collagen genes. *J. Biol. Chem.* **2001**, *276*, 7101–7107. [CrossRef] [PubMed]
26. Sodek, J.; Chen, J.; Nagata, T.; Kasugai, S.; Todescan, R., Jr.; Li, I.W.; Kim, R.H. Regulation of osteopontin expression in osteoblasts. *Ann. N. Y. Acad. Sci.* **1995**, *760*, 223–241. [CrossRef] [PubMed]
27. Katsumi, A.; Orr, A.W.; Tzima, E.; Schwartz, M.A. Integrins in mechanotransduction. *J. Biol. Chem.* **2004**, *279*, 12001–12004. [CrossRef] [PubMed]
28. Michael, K.E.; Dumbauld, D.W.; Burns, K.L.; Hanks, S.K.; García, A.J. Focal Adhesion Kinase Modulates Cell Adhesion Strengthening via Integrin Activation. *Mol. Biol. Cell* **2009**, *20*, 2508–2519. [CrossRef]
29. Paszek, M.J.; Zahir, N.; Johnson, K.R.; Lakins, J.N.; Rozenberg, G.I.; Gefen, A.; Reinhart-King, C.A.; Margulies, S.S.; Dembo, M.; Boettiger, D.; et al. Tensional homeostasis and the malignant phenotype. *Cancer Cell* **2005**, *8*, 241–254. [CrossRef]
30. Salasznyk, R.M.; Klees, R.F.; Boskey, A.; Plopper, G.E. Activation of FAK is necessary for the osteogenic differentiation of human mesenchymal stem cells on laminin-5. *J. Cell. Biochem.* **2007**, *100*, 499–514. [CrossRef]
31. Wang, Y.K.; Yu, X.; Cohen, D.M.; Wozniak, M.A.; Yang, M.T.; Gao, L.; Eyckmans, J.; Chen, C.S. Bone morphogenetic protein-2-induced signaling and osteogenesis is regulated by cell shape, RhoA/ROCK, and cytoskeletal tension. *Stem Cells Dev.* **2012**, *21*, 1176–1186. [CrossRef] [PubMed]
32. Kumar, C.C.; Nie, H.; Rogers, C.P.; Malkowski, M.; Maxwell, E.; Catino, J.J.; Armstrong, L. Biochemical characterization of the binding of echistatin to integrin alphavbeta3 receptor. *J. Pharmacol. Exp. Ther.* **1997**, *283*, 843–853.
33. Shah, P.P.; Fong, M.Y.; Kakar, S.S. PTTG induces EMT through integrin $\alpha V\beta 3$-focal adhesion kinase signaling in lung cancer cells. *Oncogene* **2011**, *31*, 3124–3135. [CrossRef] [PubMed]
34. Hanna, S.; El-Sibai, M. Signaling networks of Rho GTPases in cell motility. *Cell. Signal.* **2013**, *25*, 1955–1961. [CrossRef] [PubMed]

35. Amano, M.; Nakayama, M.; Kaibuchi, K. Rho-Kinase/ROCK: A Key Regulator of the Cytoskeleton and Cell Polarity. *Cytoskeleton* **2010**, *67*, 545–554. [CrossRef] [PubMed]
36. Yamamoto, T.; Ugawa, Y.; Yamashiro, K.; Shimoe, M.; Tomikawa, K.; Hongo, S.; Kochi, S.; Ideguchi, H.; Maeda, H.; Takashiba, S. Osteogenic differentiation regulated by Rho-kinase in periodontal ligament cells. *Differentiation* **2014**, *88*, 33–41. [CrossRef]
37. Afzal, F.; Pratap, J.; Ito, K.; Ito, Y.; Stein, J.L.; van Wijnen, A.J.; Stein, G.S.; Lian, J.B.; Javed, A. Smad function and intranuclear targeting share a Runx2 motif required for osteogenic lineage induction and BMP2 responsive transcription. *J. Cell. Physiol.* **2005**, *204*, 63–72. [CrossRef]
38. Lee, K.S.; Hong, S.H.; Bae, S.C. Both the Smad and p38 MAPK pathways play a crucial role in Runx2 expression following induction by transforming growth factor-beta and bone morphogenetic protein. *Oncogene* **2002**, *21*, 7156–7163. [CrossRef]
39. Zouani, O.F.; Kalisky, J.; Ibarboure, E.; Durrieu, M.C. Effect of BMP-2 from matrices of different stiffnesses for the modulation of stem cell fate. *Biomaterials* **2013**, *34*, 2157–2166. [CrossRef]
40. Song, B.; Estrada, K.D.; Lyons, K.M. Smad signaling in skeletal development and regeneration. *Cytokine Growth Factor Rev.* **2009**, *20*, 379–388. [CrossRef]
41. Palchesko, R.N.; Zhang, L.; Sun, Y.; Feinberg, A.W. Development of polydimethylsiloxane substrates with tunable elastic modulus to study cell mechanobiology in muscle and nerve. *PLoS ONE* **2012**, *7*, e51499. [CrossRef]

6

Influence of Implant Material and Surface on Differentiation and Proliferation of Human Adipose-Derived Stromal Cells

Susanne Jung, Lauren Bohner, Marcel Hanisch, Johannes Kleinheinz and Sonja Sielker *

Department of Cranio-Maxillofacial Surgery, Research Unit Vascular Biology of Oral Structures (VABOS), University Hospital Muenster, 48149 Muenster, Germany; Susanne.Jung@ukmuenster.de (S.J.); Lauren.Oliveiralimabohner@ukmuenster.de (L.B.); Marcel.Hanisch@ukmuenster.de (M.H.); Johannes.Kleinheinz@ukmuenster.de (J.K.)

* Correspondence: Sonja.Sielker@ukmuenster.de

Abstract: For the guided regeneration of periimplant hard and soft tissues, human adipose-derived stromal cells (hADSC) seem to be a promising source for mesenchymal stromal cells. For this, the proliferation and differentiation of hADSC were evaluated on titanium and zirconia dental implants with different surface treatments. Results were compared to edaphic cells as human osteoblasts (hOB) and human gingival fibroblasts (HGF). Primary cells were cultured on (1) titanium implants with a polished surface (Ti-PT), (2) sandblasted and acid-etched titanium (Ti-SLA), (3) sandblasted and alkaline etched zirconia (ZrO_2-ZLA) and (4) machined zirconia (ZrO_2-M). The cell proliferation and differentiation on osteogenic lineage were assessed after 1, 7 and 14 days. Statistical analysis was performed by one-way ANOVA and a modified Levene test with a statistical significance at $p = 0.05$. PostHoc tests were performed by Bonferroni-Holm. Zirconia dental implants with rough surface (ZrO_2-ZLA) showed the highest proliferation rates ($p = 0.048$). The osteogenic differentiation occurred early for zirconia and later for titanium implants, and it was enhanced for rough surfaces in comparison to polished/machined surfaces. Zirconia was more effective to promote the proliferation and differentiation of hADSCs in comparison to titanium. Rough surfaces were able to improve the biological response for both zirconia and titanium.

Keywords: hADSC; tissue regeneration; implants; titanium; zirconia

1. Introduction

The treatment of periimplant bone defects usually requires a reconstructive surgical procedure, with autogenous bone or biomaterial-based bone grafting to stimulate bone regeneration [1–3]. Despite the favorable clinical results showed by these techniques, disadvantages arise, such as high morbidity, limited availability and risk of infection [2–4].

Bone regeneration pathway involves the proliferation and differentiation of mesenchymal stem cells into the osteogenic lineage [5]; thus, bone tissue engineering makes it a suitable option to treat periimplant defects. The application of osteogenic cells in combination with physiological components involved on bone remodeling have shown improved outcomes in comparison to biomaterials alone [3].

A promising source for the stem cells is the adipose tissue, since it is easily collected using a low invasive approach. Human adipose-derived cells (hADSCs) differentiate into osteogenic and angiogenic lineage and represent for potential bone regeneration [6]. Additionally, extrinsic and intrinsic osteogenic inducers are recommended to optimize the culture environment and increase the cell regeneration potential [7,8]. Nonetheless, the imperative need of this osteogenic inducer is unclear and the efficacy of osteogenic differentiation without the use of an osteogenic medium has been assessed [9].

The cell biological response in periimplant defects is influenced by the dental implant material and surface [10–13]. Hempel et al. [10] showed a greater cell proliferation and differentiation on zirconia than titanium. A rough surface improved and accelerated the osteogenic response, by increasing the surface area to mimic the bone morphology [11–15].

Previous studies showed the osteoinduction and osteoconduction capability of hADSCs [16,17], however, the influence of the dental implant material and surface treatment has not yet been well established. The present study evaluated the proliferation and differentiation of hADSCs over titanium and zirconia with various surface treatments. The hADSCs were cultured without inducing factors and their biological response was evaluated using human primary osteoblasts (hOBs) and human gingiva fibroblasts (HGF).

2. Results

2.1. Cell Viability

Cell viability among experimental and control groups after 14 days is shown in Figure 1. Zirconia dental implants with a rough surface showed the highest vitality ($p = 0.022$) and proliferation rates ($p = 0.041$). Rough surfaces showed better results compared to polished or machined surfaces. Titanium implants showed higher cytotoxicity than zirconia dental implants ($p = 0.0016$), although minor, and did not affect the cell viability.

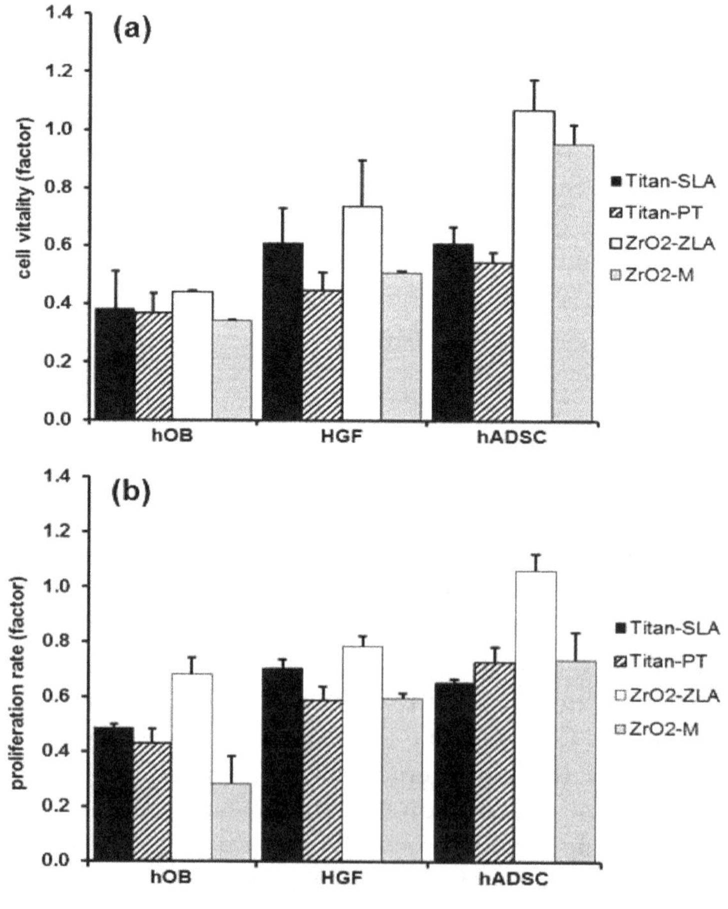

Figure 1. *Cont.*

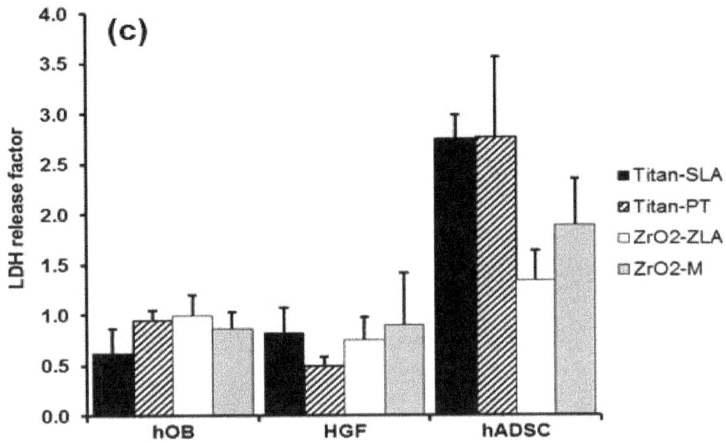

Figure 1. Cell Viability at day 14 correlated to control for human osteoblasts (hOB), human gingival fibroblasts (HGF), and human adipose-derived stromal cells (hADSC) (**a**) cell vitality $p = 0.021$; (**b**) proliferation rate, $p = 0.041$, (**c**) LDH release factor, $p = 0.0016$; standard abbreviation as error marks.

2.2. Expression of Stem Cell and Osteogenic Marker

Figure 2 shows the change in stem cells markers compared to day 1 ($p = 0.04$). Gene expression of stem cell markers differed strongly between zirconia and titanium implants (PostHoc analysis $p = 0.017$). For zirconia, gene expression was lower and decreased from day 7 to day 14. In contrast, for titanium and the control group, gene expression was higher and increased from day 7 to day 14 (Figure 2).

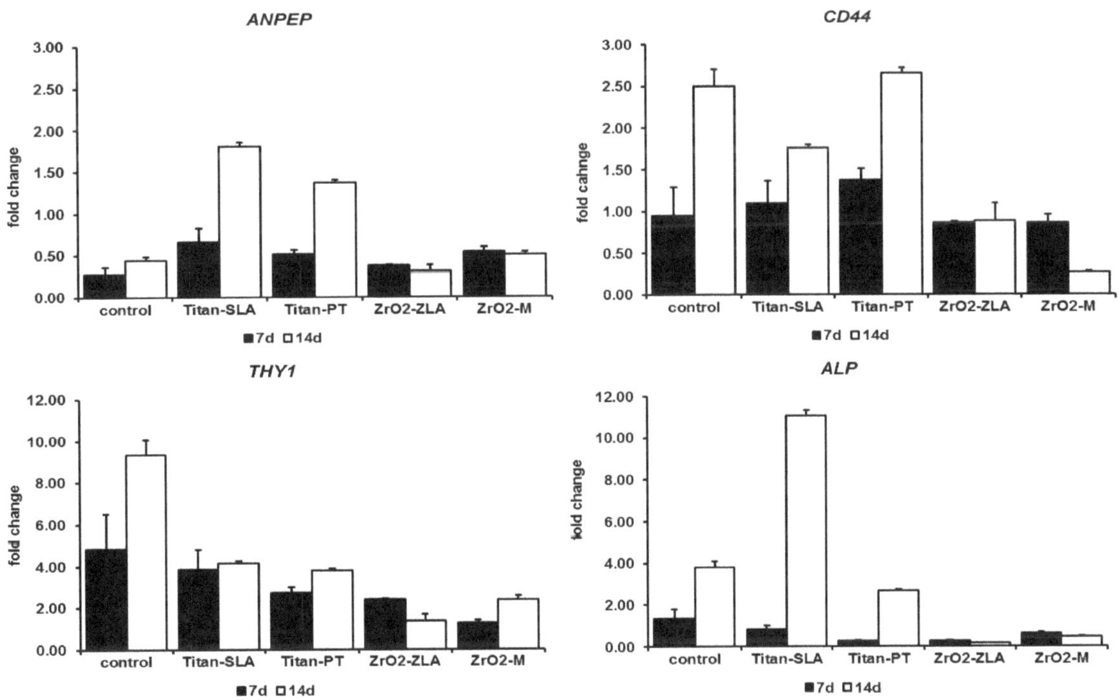

Figure 2. Fold change of stem cell marker compared to day 1 (*ANPEP* $p = 0.038$, *CD44* $p = 0.18$, *THY1* $p = 0.004$, *ALP* $p = 0.17$; standard abbreviation as error marks).

Figure 3 shows the change of osteogenic marker compared to day 1 for hADSC ($p = 0.0083$) and hOB ($p = 0.022$). Gene expression of *RANKL* was not detectable in any sample. Expression of osteogenic markers did not show a consistent picture, unlike the stem cell marker. In hOB, expression of *RUNX2* and osteoprotegerin increased from day 7 to day 14 with a low fold change, and expression of osteopontin remained constant (Figure 3). In hADSC, expression of osteogenic marker increased strongly and fold change was stronger on rough surfaces except for *RUNX2* on zirconia dental implants. Changes in expression of osteocalcin were remarkable, because no dexamethasone was added to hADSC. Expression of osteocalcin increased strongly, whereas the expression in hOB remained constant (Figure 3).

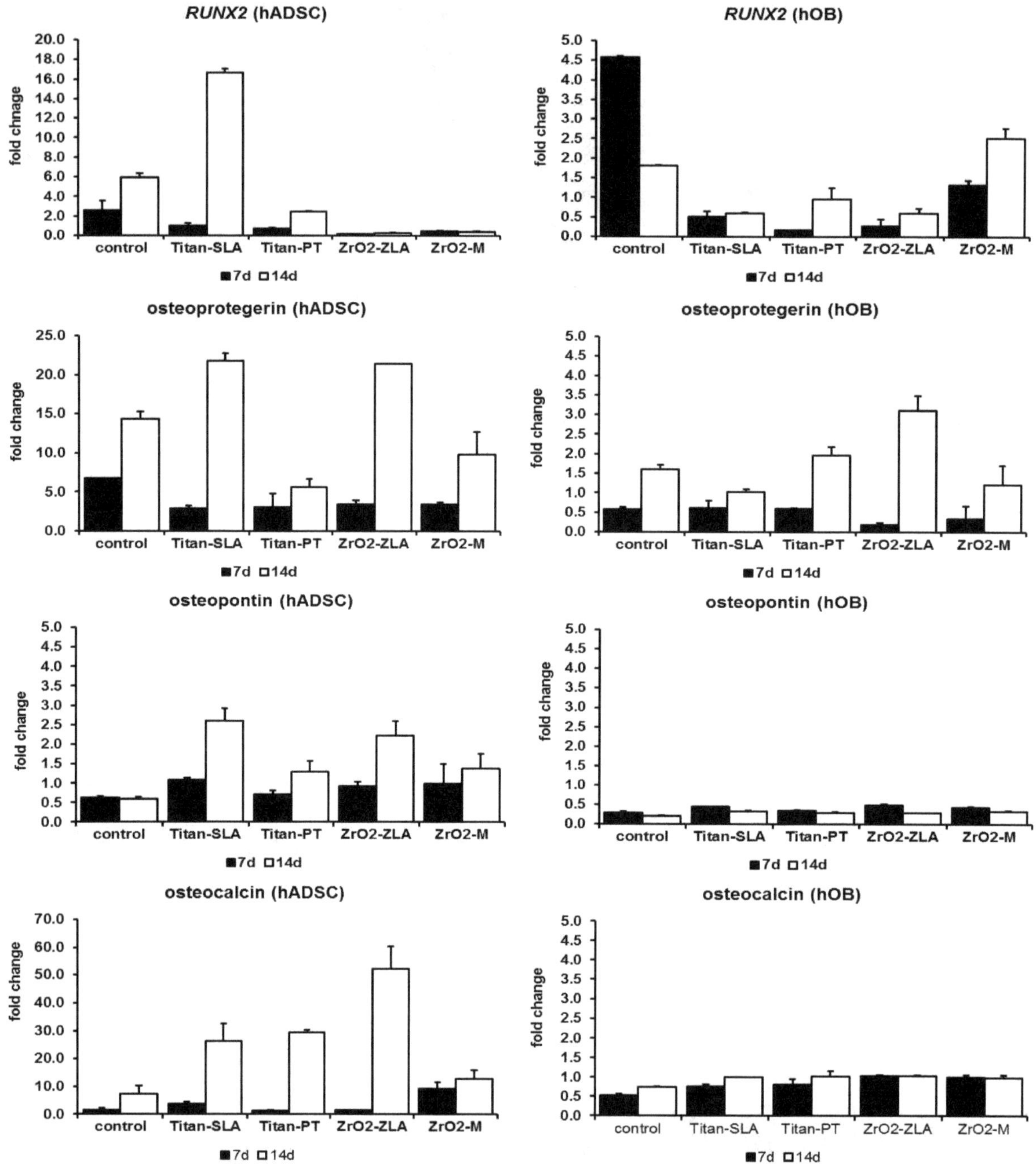

Figure 3. Fold change of osteogenic markers compared to day 1 (*RUNX2* $p = 021$ for hADSC, $p = 0.135$ for hOB; osteoprotegerin $p = 0.011$ for hADSC, $p = 0.008$ for hOB; osteopontin $p = 0.07$ for hADSC, $p = 0.024$ for hOB, osteocalcin $p = 0.024$ for hADSC, $p = 0.25$ for hOB; standard abbreviation as error marks).

3. Discussion

Zirconia implants showed higher cell viability than titanium implants. From all groups, zirconia dental implants with a machined surface showed the greatest metabolic activity and differentiation. The potential of zirconia to stimulate the osteogenic differentiation was confirmed by the decrease of stem cell markers over time, on rough and machined surfaces, which indicated the trans-differentiation into osteogenic lineage. This effect was not observed for the titanium implants. Similar findings have been reported by Hempel et al. [10], who showed that the metabolic activity was significantly greater for zirconia than for titanium implants 24 and 48 h after plating. Zirconia dental implants seem to be capable of inducing cell proliferation and accelerating the differentiation toward osteogenesis.

The findings of the present study showed that *RUNX2* (the master regulator of osteoblast differentiation) was early expressed in hADSCs over zirconia surfaces. Expression of *RUNX2* takes place at an early stage of osteogenic differentiation, followed by the inhibition of the process at later stages [18]. As the expression of *RUNX2* was not significant for zirconia dental implants after 14 days, it was assumed that the differentiation occurred predominantly during the first 24 h, and remained constant on the following days.

According to Carinci et al. [19], zirconia materials are correlated with an early gene expression, which occurs within the first 24 h of stimulation. Similar findings were shown by Altmann et al. [20], whose osteogenic marker *RUNX2* had higher levels on zirconia after 1 and 7 days. The authors claimed that this response was not only time-dependent, but a function of biomaterial. This hypothesis was confirmed in the present study, since the differentiation of hADSCs was different between titanium and zirconia implants. The titanium implants showed a late response for cell differentiation, resulting in a higher change on the expression of osteogenic markers after 14 days. The late response of titanium to cell viability and differentiation in comparison to zirconia implants had already been shown in previous studies [10,21].

The same hypothesis may be applied to the surface treatment [22]. In this study, rough surfaces showed an early expression of osteogenic markers compared to smooth surfaces. The expression of osteoprotegerin, a receptor related with the osteoclastogenesis [23], was higher on rough surfaces and lower on machined and polished surfaces. Osteogenic markers showed similar results.

Regarding to the use of inducing factors, the expression of osteocalcin did not significantly change over time for osteoblasts with inducing media, whereas for hADSCs, it decreased after 14 days without the use of inducing factors. Thus, albeit the expression of osteogenic markers may be accelerated when an inducing media is used, it seems not to be essential for the osteogenic differentiation.

Previous studies have been controversial regarding the role of inducing factors on osteogenesis. Cecchinato et al. [14] showed the osteogenic differentiation of hADSCs cells on titanium surfaces after 2 weeks; however, Abagnale et al. [21] showed no differentiation of hADSCs without osteogenic medium. For Faia-Torres et al. [9], the osteogenic differentiation only occurred with rough surfaces [9]. Thus, although the findings of this study suggested that material and surface treatment alone may induce the osteogenic differentiation, additional researche is required to confirm this hypothesis.

4. Materials and Methods

4.1. Study Design and Ethical Approval

The study evaluated the cell viability of hADSCs, primary human osteoblasts (hOB) and human gingiva fibroblasts (HGF) on titanium and zirconia with polished/machined and rough surfaces. The differentiation into osteogenic lineage was assessed for hADSCs and hOBs. The cell viability was assessed based on cell vitality, proliferation and cytotoxicity, whereas the differentiation in osteogenic lineage was measured using on the protein expression analysis. The experiment was designed according to the "Declaration of Helsinki" and approved by the Ethics Committee of the Faculty of Medicine, University of Muenster (#2016-624-f-S, 07 December 2016). Previous to the cell isolation, a written informed consent was obtained from all donors.

4.2. Isolation of Primary Human Cell Cultures

All cell colleting procedures were performed anonymously and under sterile conditions. Human fat tissue was collected from leftover tissue of patients who had undergone elective abdominal surgery at the General and Visceral Surgery, University Hospital, Muenster. Oncological surgeries were not included. Human spongiosa and gingiva samples were obtained from the leftover tissue of patients treated at the Department of Craniofacial Surgery, University Hospital Muenster.

Isolation and culture techniques of human fat tissue, primary human osteoblast and human gingiva fibroblasts cells were performed as described previously [6]. Details about the culture medium are described in Table 1. The cells were cultivated in a 5% CO_2 humidified atmosphere at 37 °C, being fed every 2–3 days and passaged with 10,000 cells/cm^2 after reaching 90% of confluence.

Table 1. Culture medium.

Cells	Medium	Culture Formula
Human adipose-derived stromal cells (hADSC)	minimum essential medium–Alpha Eagle (α-MEM) (Lonza, Walkersville, MD, USA)	10% fetal bovine serum, 1% amphotericin B (250 μg/mL), 1% glutamine (200 Mm), 1% penicillin (10,000 U/mL)/streptomycin (10,000 μg/mL) (Biochrom Merck, Berlin, Germany)
Primary human osteoblast (hOBs)	Primary human osteoblast (hOBs)	12% fetal bovine serum, 1% amphotericin B (250 μg/mL), 1% glutamine (200 mM), 1% penicillin (10000 U/mL)/streptomycin (10,000 μg/mL) (Biochrom Merck, Germany). For osteogenic differentiation, 16 ng/mL dexamethasone (Merck Pharma, Darmstadt, Germany) was added to the medium.
Primary human gingiva fibroblasts (HGF)	DMEM medium (high glucose and L-glutamine; Gibco, USA) with 1/4 Ham's F12 nutrient mixtures (Sigma, Hamburg, Germany)	10% fetal bovine serum, 1% amphotericin B (250 μg/mL), 1% penicillin (10,000 U/mL)/streptomycin (10,000 μg/mL) (all Biochrom Merck, Berlin, Germany)

4.3. Main Cell Culture

Cells were cultured on various titanium and zirconia discs (Straumann, Basel, Switzerland) measuring 5 mm diameter, the groups were: (1) titanium implants with polished surface (Ti-PT); (2) sandblasted and acid-etched titanium (Ti-SLA); (3) sandblasted and alkaline etched zirconia (ZrO_2-ZLA) and (4) machined zirconia (ZrO_2-M). For hADSCs, no inducing factor was used, whereas the hOB culture was supplemented by an osteogenic medium. The samples were placed in 48-well cell culture plates (Greiner Bio One; Bad Nenndorf, Germany) with a 5% CO_2 humidified atmosphere at 37 °C. Culturing medium was replaced every 2–3 days during cell culture study. In addition, cells for control group were cultivated as a monolayer in 48-well cell culture plates. Samples were analyzed 1, 7 and 14 days after the beginning of the experiment. Cell culture part was repeated three times.

4.4. Cell Viability

The living cell count was performed with the LUNA II system (Logos Biosystems Inc., Villeneuve d'Ascq, France). Proliferation rate was estimated with an in-house MTT assay, which determines the metabolic activity of vital cells. The conversion of the yellow thiazolyl blue tetrazolium bromide (0.5 mg/mL; Sigma-Aldrich, Hamburg, Germany) to the purple formazan was measured at a wavelength of 570 nm. Cytotoxic effects were determined with the Pierce™ LDH Cytotoxicity Assay (ThermoFisher Scientific; Wesel, Germany). All assays were performed according to manufacture protocols and done in triplicates.

4.5. Protein Expression Analysis

For protein expression analysis, cells were lysed with the Pierce™ IP Lysis Buffer (ThermoFisher Scientific, Waltham, MA, USA) according to the manufacture's protocol. The supernatant was frozen at −80 °C for subsequent assays. To determinate secreted proteins, part of the culturing medium was taken before lysis and frozen at −80 °C. Quantification protein determination was performed with the Pierce™ BCA Protein Assay (ThermoFisher Scientific, Wesel, Germany) according to the manufacture's protocol. The μQuant reader (BioTek, Bad Friedrichshall, Germany) was used for protein determination and ALP assay. Protein expression analysis was evaluated with enzyme-linked immunosorbent assay (ELISA). The ELISAs are listed in Table 2 (abcam, Cambridge, England). ELISAs were performed according to the manufacture's protocol. Absorbance was measured at a wavelength of 450 nm with the μQuant reader (BioTek, Bad Friedrichshall, Germany). Protein expression was normalized in two steps. The first step was a correlation to whole protein, and the second step was a correlation to day 1. Changes in expression related to day 1 are shown.

Table 2. Used and primer (Qiagen, Hilden, Germany) and enzyme-linked immunosorbent assay (ELISA)-Kits (abcam, Cambridge, England).

Gene/Protein	Primer	Protein Assay/ELISA
	Stem Cell Marker	
ANPEP/CD13	PPH05672A	
CD44	PPH00114A	
THY1/CD90	PPH02406G	
alkaline phosphatase	PPH01311F	
	Osteogenic Marker	
RUNX2	PPH01897C	
TNFSF11/RANKL	PPH01048F	
osteoprotegerin		ab189580
osteopontin		ab192143
osteocalcin		ab195214
	Housekeeping Genes	
RPLP0	PPH21138F	
B2M	PPH01094E	
GAPDH	PPH00150F	
HPRT1	PPH01018C	
ACTB	PPH00073G	

4.6. RNA Extraction and Real-Time qPCR

For RNA isolation and purification, an RNeasy Micro Kit (Qiagen, Hilden, Germany) was used and performed according to the manufacture's protocol. Purity and concentration of the isolated RNA was determined by a spectrophotometric reading (NanoDrop™ 2000; ThermoFisher Scientific, Wesel, Germany). For RT-qPCR, a custom-designed RT2 PCR Array (Qiagen, Hilden, Germany) was used (Table 2). For each sample 50 ng RNA was transcripted in complementary DNA (cDNA) with the RT2 First Strand Kit (Qiagen, Hilden, Germany). A DNase treatment to eliminate existent genomic DNA was part of this step. RT-qPCR was performed with the RT2 SYBR Green ROX pPCR Mastermix (Qiagen, Hilden, Germany) according to the manufacture's protocol in Eppendorf mastercycler ep realplex 4S (Eppendorf, Hamburg, Germany). One μL cDNA was used as template for each reaction. The PCR protocol was: activation of hot start Taq-polymerase for 10 min at 95 °C, followed by 40 cycles with a denaturation step for 15 sec at 95 °C and an annealing/elongation step for 60 s at 60 °C. A melting curve between 65 and 95 °C with a time ramp of 2 min for 1 °C was connected. The ΔΔCT method was used for data analysis with the RT2 Profiler PCR array data analysis web portal (https://www.qiagen.com/de/shop/genes-and-path-ways/data-analysis-center-overview-page/custom-rt2-pcr-arrays-data-analysis-center, accessed on 28 March 2018). Fold changes related to day 1 are shown.

4.7. Statistical Analysis

Statistical analysis of expression factors and protein expression factors was carried out by one-way ANOVA and a modified Levene test with a statistical significance at $p = 0.05$. PostHoc tests were performed by Bonferroni-Holm test (Daniel's XL Toolbox version 6.53; https://www.xltoolbox.net/).

5. Conclusions

Zirconia promoted the proliferation and differentiation of hADSCs more than titanium. Rough surfaces improve the biological response for both zirconia and titanium.

Author Contributions: Conceptualization, S.J., J.K. and S.S.; methodology, S.S.; validation, S.S.; formal analysis, S.S.; investigation, S.S.; writing—original draft preparation, L.B. and S.S.; writing—review and editing, S.J., M.H., L.B. and S.S.; visualization, S.S..; supervision, J.K.; project administration, S.J. and J.K.; funding acquisition, S.J. and J.K. All authors gave final approval and agree to be accountable for all aspects of the work.

Acknowledgments: This study was supported by Professor Senninger, the head of the department of Visceral Surgery of the University Hospital Muenster. Special thanks go to L.B. for her work in manuscript drafting (ITI Scholar 2017–2018).

Abbreviations

hADSC	Human adipose-derived stromal cells
hOB	Human osteoblasts
HGF	Human gingival fibroblasts

References

1. Mercado, F.; Hamlet, S.; Ivanovski, S. Regenerative surgical therapy for peri-implantitis using deproteinized bovine bone mineral with 10% collagen, enamel matrix derivative and Doxycycline-A prospective 3-year cohort study. *Clin. Oral Implants Res.* **2018**, *29*, 583–591. [CrossRef] [PubMed]
2. Renvert, S.; Roos-Jansaker, A.M.; Persson, G.R. Surgical treatment of peri-implantitis lesions with or without the use of a bone substitute—A randomized clinical trial. *J. Clin. Periodontol.* **2018**, *45*, 1266–1274. [CrossRef] [PubMed]
3. Shanbhag, S.; Pandis, N.; Mustafa, K.; Nyengaard, J.R.; Stavropoulos, A. Bone tissue engineering in oral peri-implant defects in preclinical in vivo research: A systematic review and meta-analysis. *J. Tissue Eng. Regen. Med.* **2018**, *12*, e336–e349. [CrossRef] [PubMed]
4. Maglione, M.; Salvador, E.; Ruaro, M.E.; Melato, M.; Tromba, G.; Angerame, D.; & Bevilacqua, L. Bone regeneration with adipose derived stem cells in a rabbit model. *J. Biomed. Res.* **2018**. [CrossRef]
5. Valenti, M.T.; Dalle Carbonare, L.; Mottes, M. Osteogenic Differentiation in Healthy and Pathological Conditions. *Int. J. Mol. Sci.* **2016**, *18*, 41. [CrossRef]
6. Jung, S.; Kleineidam, B.; Kleinheinz, J. Regenerative potential of human adipose-derived stromal cells of various origins. *J. Craniomaxillofac. Surg.* **2015**, *43*, 2144–2151. [CrossRef] [PubMed]
7. Chen, Q.; Yang, Z.; Sun, S.; Huang, H.; Sun, X.; Wang, Z.; Zhang, Y.; Zhang, B. Adipose-derived stem cells modified genetically in vivo promote reconstruction of bone defects. *Cytotherapy* **2010**, *12*, 831–840. [CrossRef]
8. Shiraishi, T.; Sumita, Y.; Wakamastu, Y.; Nagai, K.; Asahina, I. Formation of engineered bone with adipose stromal cells from buccal fat pad. *J. Dent. Res.* **2012**, *91*, 592–597. [CrossRef]
9. Faia-Torres, A.B.; Charnley, M.; Goren, T.; Guimond-Lischer, S.; Rottmar, M.; Maniura-Weber, K.; Spencer, D.D.; Reis, R.; Textor, M. Osteogenic differentiation of human mesenchymal stem cells in the absence of osteogenic supplements: A surface-roughness gradient study. *Acta Biomater.* **2015**, *28*, 64–75. [CrossRef]
10. Hempel, U.; Hefti, T.; Kalbacova, M.; Wolf-Brandstetter, C.; Dieter, P.; Schlottig, F. Response of osteoblast-like SAOS-2 cells to zirconia ceramics with different surface topographies. *Clin. Oral Implants Res.* **2010**, *21*, 174–181. [CrossRef]
11. Hirano, T.; Sasaki, H.; Honma, S.; Furuya, Y.; Miura, T.; Yajima, Y.; Yoshinari, M. Proliferation and osteogenic differentiation of human mesenchymal stem cells on zirconia and titanium with different surface topography. *Dent. Mater. J.* **2015**, *34*, 872–880. [CrossRef] [PubMed]
12. Ito, H.; Sasaki, H.; Saito, K.; Honma, S.; Yajima, Y.; Yoshinari, M. Response of osteoblast-like cells to zirconia with different surface topography. *Dent. Mater. J.* **2013**, *32*, 122–129. [CrossRef] [PubMed]
13. Pandey, A.K.; Pati, F.; Mandal, D.; Dhara, S.; Biswas, K. In vitro evaluation of osteoconductivity and cellular response of zirconia and alumina based ceramics. *Mater. Sci. Eng. C Mater. Biol. Appl.* **2013**, *33*, 3923–3930. [CrossRef] [PubMed]
14. Abagnale, G.; Steger, M.; Nguyen, V.H.; Hersch, N.; Sechi, A.; Joussen, S.; Denecke, B.; Merkel, R.; Hoffmann, B.; Dreser, A.; et al. Surface topography enhances differentiation of mesenchymal stem cells towards osteogenic and adipogenic lineages. *Biomaterials* **2015** *61*, 316–326. [CrossRef] [PubMed]

15. Faia-Torres, A.B.; Guimond-Lischer, S.; Rottmar, M.; Charnley, M.; Goren, T.; Maniura-Weber, K.; Spencer, N.D.; Reis, R.L.; Textor, M.; Neves, N.M. Differential regulation of osteogenic differentiation of stem cells on surface roughness gradients. *Biomaterials* **2014**, *35*, 9023–9032. [CrossRef] [PubMed]
16. Lee, H.R.; Kim, H.J.; Ko, J.S.; Choi, Y.S.; Ahn, M.W.; Kim, S.; Do, S.H. Comparative characteristics of porous bioceramics for an osteogenic response in vitro and in vivo. *PLoS ONE* **2013**, *8*, e84272. [CrossRef] [PubMed]
17. Lu, W.; Ji, K.; Kirkham, J.; Yan, Y.; Boccaccini, A.R.; Kellett, M.; Jin, Y.; Yang, X.B. Bone tissue engineering by using a combination of polymer/Bioglass composites with human adipose-derived stem cells. *Cell Tissue Res.* **2014**, *356*, 97–107. [CrossRef] [PubMed]
18. Bruderer, M.; Richards, R.G.; Alini, M.; Stoddart, M.J. Role and regulation of RUNX2 in osteogenesis. *Eur. Cell Mater.* **2014**, *28*, 269–286. [CrossRef] [PubMed]
19. Carinci, F.; Pezzetti, F.; Volinia, S.; Francioso, F.; Arcelli, D.; Farina, E.; Piattelli, A. Zirconium oxide: Analysis of MG63 osteoblast-like cell response by means of a microarray technology. *Biomaterials* **2004**, *25*, 215–228. [CrossRef]
20. Altmann, B.; Rabel, K.; Kohal, R.J.; Proksch, S.; Tomakidi, P.; Adolfsson, E.; Bernsmann, F.; Palermo, P.; Fürderer, T.; Steinberg, T. Cellular transcriptional response to zirconia-based implant materials. *Dent. Mater.* **2017**, *33*, 241–255. [CrossRef]
21. Cecchinato, F.; Karlsson, J.; Ferroni, L.; Gardin, C.; Galli, S.; Wennerberg, A.; Zavan, B.; Andeersson, M.; Jimbo, R. Osteogenic potential of human adipose-derived stromal cells on 3-dimensional mesoporous TiO_2 coating with magnesium impregnation. *Mater. Sci. Eng. C Mater. Biol. Appl.* **2015**, *52*, 225–234. [CrossRef] [PubMed]
22. Miranda, R.B.P.; Grenho, L.; Carvalho, A.; Fernandes, M.H.; Monteiro, F.J.; Cesar, P.F. Micropatterned Silica Films with Nanohydroxyapatite for Y-TZP Implants. *J. Dent. Res.* **2018**, *97*, 1003–1009. [CrossRef] [PubMed]
23. Liu, W.; Zhang, X. Receptor activator of nuclear factor-kappaB ligand (RANKL)/RANK/osteoprotegerin system in bone and other tissues (review). *Mol. Med. Rep.* **2015**, *11*, 3212–3218. [CrossRef] [PubMed]

7

Physicochemical and Microbiological Assessment of an Experimental Composite Doped with Triclosan-Loaded Halloysite Nanotubes

Diana A. Cunha [1], Nara S. Rodrigues [1], Lidiane C. Souza [1], Diego Lomonaco [1,2], Flávia P. Rodrigues [1,3], Felipe W. Degrazia [4], Fabrício M. Collares [4], Salvatore Sauro [5,6,*] and Vicente P. A. Saboia [1,7]

1 Post-Graduate Programme in Dentistry, Federal University of Ceará, Rua Monsenhor Furtado S/N, Rodolfo Teófilo, Fortaleza 60430-355, Ceará, Brazil; araujo.diana@gmail.com (D.A.C.); nara.sousa.rodrigues@gmail.com (N.S.R.); lidiane_costa26@hotmail.com (L.C.S.); lomonaco@ufc.br (D.L.); flapiro@gmail.com (F.P.R); vpsaboia@yahoo.com (V.P.A.S.)

2 Department of Organic and Inorganic Chemistry, Federal University of Ceará, Fortaleza 60440-900, Ceará, Brazil

3 School of Dentistry, Paulista University—UNIP, R. Dr. Bacelar 1212, Vila Clementino, São Paulo 04026-002, SP, Brazil

4 Laboratório de Materiais Dentários, Faculdade de Odontologia, Universidade Federal do Rio Grande do Sul, Rua Ramiro Barcelos, 2492, Rio Branco, Porto Alegre 90035-003, Rio Grande do Sul, Brazil; fdegrazia@hotmail.com (F.W.D.); fabricio.collares@ufrgs.br (F.M.C.)

5 Departamento de Odontología, Facultad de Ciencias de la Salud, Universidad CEU-Cardenal Herrera, C/Del Pozos/n, Alfara del Patriarca, 46115 Valencia, Spain

6 Tissue Engineering and Biophotonics Research Division King's College London Dental Institute (KCLDI), London SE1 9RT, UK

7 Department of Restorative Dentistry, School of Dentistry, of Ceará, Fortaleza 60430-355, Ceará, Brazil

* Correspondence: salvatore.sauro@uchceu.es

Abstract: This study is aimed at evaluating the effects of triclosan-encapsulated halloysite nanotubes (HNT/TCN) on the physicochemical and microbiological properties of an experimental dental composite. A resin composite doped with HNT/TCN (8% *w/w*), a control resin composite without nanotubes (HNT/TCN-0%) and a commercial nanofilled resin (CN) were assessed for degree of conversion (DC), flexural strength (FS), flexural modulus (FM), polymerization stress (PS), dynamic thermomechanical (DMA) and thermogravimetric analysis (TGA). The antibacterial properties (M) were also evaluated using a 5-day biofilm assay (CFU/mL). Data was submitted to one-way ANOVA and Tukey tests. There was no significant statistical difference in DC, FM and RU between the tested composites ($p > 0.05$). The FS and CN values attained with the HNT/TCN composite were higher ($p < 0.05$) than those obtained with the HNT/TCN-0%. The DMA analysis showed significant differences in the TAN δ ($p = 0.006$) and Tg ($p = 0$) between the groups. TGA curves showed significant differences between the groups in terms of degradation ($p = 0.046$) and weight loss ($p = 0.317$). The addition of HNT/TCN induced higher PS, although no significant antimicrobial effect was observed ($p = 0.977$) between the groups for CFUs and ($p = 0.557$) dry weight. The incorporation of HNT/TCN showed improvements in physicochemical and mechanical properties of resin composites. Such material may represent an alternative choice for therapeutic restorative treatments, although no significance was found in terms of antibacterial properties. However, it is possible that current antibacterial tests, as the one used in this laboratory study, may not be totally appropriate for the evaluation of resin composites, unless accompanied with aging protocols (e.g., thermocycling and load cycling) that allow the release of therapeutic agents incorporated in such materials.

Keywords: mechanical properties; nanotubes; resin composite; *Streptococcus mutans*; triclosan

1. Introduction

Resin dental composites (RDCs) have been widely modified in the last few decades. Indeed, in order to increase their clinical performance, especially in terms of wear resistance and lower polymerization shrinkage, modern RDCs are formulated with a high amount of glass/ceramic fillers (60–80 wt.%) [1]. Moreover, inorganic nanoparticles and nanofibers have also been incorporated within the composition of RDCs to advance their mechanical and esthetic properties [2], as well as their biological and bioactive properties [3].

Nowadays, the formation of secondary caries remains one of the main reasons for the replacement of resin composite restorations [4–6]. Carious lesions along the margins of our restorations present an important causal relationship with the accumulation of a cariogenic biofilm; this is probably facilitated by gaps formed at the tooth-restoration interface, as well as by excessive roughness of resin composite [7]. *Streptococcus mutans* is one of the main species of a cariogenic biofilm responsible for secondary caries [8], hence, restorative materials with bioactive and antimicrobial properties are needed in order to improve the clinical outcome in daily practice [9].

Triclosan (TCN) is a well-known antibacterial agent used in a wide range of products such as toothpastes and mouthwashes. Several studies demonstrated the efficiency of such therapeutic substances against gram-positive microorganisms, (e.g., *Streptococcus mutans* [10,11], *Staphylococcus aureus* [12], *Lactobacillus* spp. [13], and *Actinomyces* spp. [14]). Indeed, due to such antimicrobial potential, along with its low molecular weight, uses and applications of TCN have radically increased in the last 30 years [12]. However, neat TCN incorporation in resin-based materials could lead to a high leachability that can cause a rapid decrease of the antimicrobial properties of such materials. To overcome this issue, TCN was previously incorporated in specific "vehicles" known as nanotubes, in order to achieve a slower and more controlled release of such an antibacterial agent [3,11].

Halloysite nanotubes (HNT) are natural aluminosilicates with a hollow tubular structure [3], which are typically used as a reinforcing nano-filler to improve some mechanical properties of resin-composites [15] such as tensile strength, flexural strength, storage modulus [16], as well as microhardness and bond strength [17]. HNT is a "green" biocompatible nanomaterial characterized by very low cytotoxicity [18]. Furthermore, it acts as "biologically-safe" reservoirs for the encapsulation and controlled release of a variety of therapeutic drugs [15,19], bioactive molecules [20] and matrix metalloproteinase inhibitors [21,22]. Active principles released by halloysite may last 30 to 100 times more than when these were incorporated alone or using some different nanocarriers in polymer nanocomposite [23,24].

Thus, the aim of the present study was to evaluate in vitro the effects of triclosan-encapsulated halloysite nanotubes (HNT/TCN) on the physical-chemical and microbiological properties of an experimental micro-hybrid resin dental composite.

The null hypothesis tested in this study was that the inclusion of HNT-TCN would not influence the physicochemical and microbiological properties of such an experimental resin composite.

2. Material and Methods

2.1. Material

Halloysite nanotubes ($Al_2Si_2O_5(OH)_4{\cdot}2H_2O$) with a diameter of 30–70 nm and length of 1–3 μm (Sigma-Aldrich, St. Louis, MO, USA) were treated with a silane solution (5 wt.% of 3-metacryloxypropyltrimetoxysilane and 95 wt.% acetone) at 110 °C for 24 h. Subsequently, these were mixed [1:1 ratio] with 2,4,4-Trichloro-2-hydroxydiphenyl ether (TCN: Triclosan, Fagron, Rotterdam, SH, The Netherlands) under constant shaking for 1 h [3]. The mixture was then dispersed in 95 wt.% pure ethanol (0.03 mg/mL^{-1}) and ultasonicated for 1 h. The nanoparticles were finally desiccated for 10 days at 30 °C to ensure complete evaporation of the residual solvents. The HNT/TCN nanoparticles obtained after such processing method were finally prepared and characterized using a Transmission Electron Microscope (TEM) JEM 120 Exll (JEOL, Tokyo, Japan) at 80 kV at a magnification X 300,000.

An experimental resin composite was created by mixing 75 wt.% Bis-GMA (2,2-bis-[4-(hydroxyl-3-methacryloxy-propyloxy)phenyl]propane) and 25 wt.% triethylene glycol dimethacrylate (TEGDMA) (Sigma-Aldrich, St. Louis, MO, USA) under continuous agitation and sonication for 30 min. Camphorquinone (CQ), ethyl4-dimethylaminobenzoate (EDAB), and diphenyliodoniumhexafluorophosphate (DPIHFP; Milwaukee, MI, USA) were also added at 1 mol % to obtain a light-curable resin-based material. Incorporation of 8 wt.% of HNT/TCN and 72 wt.% silica micro-hybrid filler was performed by stirring for 12 h under continuous sonication of the experimental resin composite.

The control experimental resin composite was formulated with the same organic matrix and silica micro-hybrid filler (80 wt.%), but without the use of the HNT/TCN nanotubes (HNT/TCN-0%) (Table 1).

Table 1. Composition of the resin composite used in this study.

Name of the Composite	Type of Composite	Manufacturer/Lot No.	Composition
HNT/TCN-0%	Experimental resin-composite	—	**Organic matrix:** Bis-GMA, TEGDMA.
			Filler type: Silica micro-hybrid filler 80 wt.%
			Filler content: 80 wt.%
HNT/TCN	Experimental resin-composite	—	**Organic matrix:** Bis-GMA, TEGDMA.
			Filler type: Silica micro-hydrid filler 72 wt.% and halloysite nanotubes 8 wt.%.
			Filler content: 80 wt.%
Filtek Z-350XT (Shade A1D)	Commercial nano-filled composite	3M ESPE (St Paul, MN, USA)/N702257	**Organic matrix:** Bis-GMA, Bis-EMA, UDMA, TEGDMA
			Filler type: Silica and zirconia nanofillers, agglomerated zirconia-silica nanoclusters
			Filler content: 82 wt.%

A commercial nano-filled resin composite was used in this study as a control group. According to the manufacturer (3M ESPE), this material has nanoclusters of zirconia (4–11 nm) and silica (20 nm) nanoparticles, along with micro-filled silica/zirconia particles (0.6 mm) (Table 1).

2.2. Degree of Conversion (DC)

Three discs were created for each composite used in this study using teflon molds (6 mm in diameter × 2 mm thick) and light-cured in the absence of oxygen for 40 s under an acetate transparent strip using a light-curing system (1200 mW/cm^2, Bluephase, Ivoclar Vivadent, Schaan, Liechtenstein), at a standardized 2-mm distance. The degree of conversion (DC) of each material tested in this study was evaluated through micro-Raman spectroscopy (Xplora Horiba, Paris, France) in the range between 1590 and 1670 cm^{-1} using the 638 nm laser emission wavelength, 5 s acquisition time and 10 accumulations [11,25]. Three specimens for each group were analyzed at a standardized room temperature of 23 ± 1 °C. DC was calculated as described in a previous study by Rodrigues et al. [25] on the intensity of the C=C stretching vibrations (peakheight) at 1635 cm^{-1} and using the symmetric ring stretching at 1608 cm^{-1} from the polymerized and non-polymerized specimens.

$$DC\% = \left(1 - \left(\frac{R\ cured}{R\ uncured}\right)\right) \times 100 \quad (1)$$

2.3. Flexural Strength and Flexural Modulus

The flexural strength (FS) and flexural modulus (FM) ($n = 5$) evaluation was performed according to ISO 4049/2000 [26] using a universal mechanical testing machine (Instron 3345, Canton, MA, EUA). Specimens with standard dimensions of 25 × 2 × 2 mm were prepared using a Teflon split mold. A polyester strip and a glass slide covered the resin-composite, and the light tip guide was placed over the center of the mold, to light-cure the specimens for 40 s as described in Section 2.2. After irradiation, the specimens were removed from the molds and carefully polishedusing a 320 grit SiC abrasive paper. All of the specimens were stored in water at 37 °C for 24 h. The specimens were positioned in a 3-point bending apparatus with 2 parallel supports with a distance of 20 mm. The specimens were loaded until fracture with a 500 Kgf load cell at a cross-head speed of 0.05 mm/min. The flexural strength (MPa) was calculated using the following formula:

$$\sigma = \frac{3L \times F_{max}}{2w \times h^2} \tag{2}$$

L is the distance between the parallel supports (mm); F_{max} is the load at fracture (N); w is the width (mm), and h is the height (mm).

The flexural modulus (GPa) was calculated using the following formula:

$$E_f = \frac{F \times L^3}{4wh^3d} \tag{3}$$

F and d stands for the load and deflection increment, respectively, between 2 specific points in the elastic portion of the curves (N and mm); L is the distance between the parallel supports (mm); w is the width (mm), h is the height (mm).

2.4. Dynamic Thermomechanical Analysis (DMA)

Three specimens (8 mm × 2 mm × 2 mm) were prepared for each group (Table 1) and light-cured as previously described. A DMA system (Mettler Toledo, Columbus, OH, USA), equipped with a single bending cantilever was used to determine the mechanical properties in clamped mode. The viscoelastic properties were characterized by applying a sinusoidal deformation force to the material under dynamic conditions: Temperature, time, frequency, stress, or a combination of these parameters. The storage modulus (E′), glass transition temperature (Tg) and tangent delta (TAN-δ) of the tested materials were evaluated at different temperatures under cyclic stress (frequency of 2.0 Hz and amplitude of 10 μm) and from 50 to 800 °C at the heating rate of 2 °C min^{-1}. The TAN-δ value represents the damping properties of the material, serving as an indicator of all types of molecular motions and phase transitions.

2.5. Thermogravimetric Analysis (TGA)

A further three specimens were prepared for each group (Table 1) (mass of 10 mg). A thermogravimetric analysis was performed to determine the thermal degradation and the weight percentage of fillers resin-composites. A thermal program from 30 to 193 °C at the heating rate of 2 °C min^{-1} in nitrogen atmosphere determined the weight changes as a function of time and temperature. Thermogravimetric analysis was performed using the Pyris 1 TGA (SDTA851—Mettler Toledo) thermal analyzer.

2.6. Polymerization Stress Measurements (PS)

Poly(methyl methacrylate) rods, 5 mm in diameter and 13 or 28 mm in length, had one of their flat surfaces sandblasted with 250 μm alumina. On the shorter rod, to allow for the highest possible light transmission during photoactivation, the opposite surface was polished with silicone SiC papers (600, 1200, and 2000 grit) followed by felt disks with 1μm alumina paste (Alumina 3, ATM, Altenkirchen, Germany). The sandblasted surfaces received a layer of methylmethacrylate

(JET Acrilico Auto Polimerizante, Sao Paulo, Brazil), followed by two thin layers of unfilled resin (Scotchbond Multi-Purpose Plus, bottle 3, 3M ESPE).

The resin composite was light-cured as previously described for 40 s. The rods were attached to the opposing clamps of a universal testing machine (Instron 5565, Canton, MA, USA) with the treated surfaces, facing each other with a 1-mm gap. The resin composite was inserted into the gap and shaped into a cylinder following the perimeter of the rods. An extensometer (0.1 μm resolution), attached to the rods (Instron 2630-101, Bucks, UK) in order to assess the height of the specimen, provided the feedback to the testing machine to keep the height constant. Therefore, the force registered by the load cell was necessary to counteract the polymerization shrinkage to maintain the specimen's initial height. A hollow stainless steel fixture with a lateral slot attached the short rod to the testing machine, allowing the tip of the light guide to be positioned in contact with the polished surface of the rod. Force development was monitored for 10 min from the beginning of the photoactivation; the nominal stress was calculated by dividing the maximum force value by the cross-section area of the rod. Five specimens were tested for each tested material [27].

2.7. Microbiology Assay

Streptococcus mutans (*S. mutans*) UA159 (ATTCC) was obtained from single colonies isolated on blood agar plates, inoculated in Tryptone yeast-extract broth containing 1% glucose (*w*/*v*) and incubated for 18 h at 37 °C under micro-aerophilic conditions in partial atmosphere of 5% CO_2.

To analyze antimicrobial effects, blocks (4 × 4 × 2 mm) of each group were produced (Table 1). Materials were dispensed in a silicone mold, covered with a polyester tape and then submitted to digital pressure for 2 s to better accommodate the material, with curing light being activated for 40 s. Specimens were sterilized by exposure to Plasma Hydrogen Peroxide before starting biofilm formation. Mono-species *S. mutans* biofilms were formed on blocks placed in bath cultures at 37 °C in 5 % CO_2 up to 5 days in 24-well polystyrene plates. The biofilms grew in tryptone yeast-extract broth containing 1% sucrose (*w*/*w*) and were kept undisturbed for 24 h to allow an initial biofilm formation. During the biofilm formation period, once daily the discs were dip-washed three times in a plate containing NaCl 0.89% solution to remove the loosely bound biofilm and they were transferred to new 24-well plates with sterile medium. The blocks of each experimental group were removed after 5 days of initial biofilm formation and transferred to pre-weighed microtubes containing 1 mL of NaCl 0.89 % solution. Biofilms were then dispersed with 3 pulses of 15 s with 15 s of interval at a 7-W output (Branson Sonifier 150; Branson Ultrasonics, Danbury, CT, USA). An aliquot (0.05 mL) of the homogenized biofilm was serially diluted (10^{-1}–10^{-7}) and plated onto blood agar plates. Plates were then incubated at 37 °C, 5% CO_2 for 48 h, before enumerating viable microorganisms. Results were expressed as colony forming units (CFU)/mL and transformed in log_{10} CFU to reduce variance heterogeneity [28].

To determine the biofilm dry weight, 200 μL aliquots of the initial biofilm suspension were transferred to pre-weighed tubes and dehydrated with ethanol solutions (99 %). The tubes were centrifuged, and the supernatants were discarded before the pellet was dried into a desiccator (P_2O_5) for 24 h and weighted (±0.00001 mg). The dry weight of the biofilm was determined by calculating the weight in the tube (initial weight − final weight) and in the original suspension (dry weight in 1 mL = dry weight in 200 μL × 5) [29].

2.8. Statistical Analysis

Physicochemical properties data was submitted to analysis of variance with one factor (One way-ANOVA), followed by Tukey test. For analyzing antimicrobial effects was performed analysis of variance with one factor (One way-ANOVA). Significance level was set at 5%. The program used to perform the analyses was IBM SPSS Statistics Version 20.0 (Armonk, NY, USA).

3. Results

TEM analysis showed that TCN was successfully deposited inside the lumen of the HNTs (Figure 1A,B). Means and standard deviations of physicochemical properties of the tested materials are presented in Tables 2 and 3. To summarize, the degree of conversion (DC) test showed that there was no significant difference between the tested materials ($p = 0.879$). The flexural strength of HNT/TCN and that of Z350XT was greater than attained with the control HNT/TCN-0% ($p = 0.005$) composite. However, no significant difference was encountered between the storage modulus (E_f) of the three tested groups (Figure 2). The maximum polymerization stress obtained in the specimens created with HNT/TCN composite was significantly ($p < 0.05$) greater than that observed in the control HNT/TCN-free resin composite. The DMA assessment showed no significant differences between the three tested composites for the TAN δ at Tg ($p = 0.006$) and Tg ($p = 0$) (Table 3). The TGA curves (Figure 3) obtained in nitrogen atmosphere showed that there was no significant difference between the three tested composites on the first degradation step ($p > 0.05$): HNT/TCN (296 °C), HNT/TCN-0% (301 °C) and the commercial resin composite (286 °C). Moreover, on the second degradation step, no significant difference was observed: HNT/TCN (419 °C), HNT/TCN-0% (426 °C) and the commercial resin composite (415 °C). There was no difference ($p = 0.317$) between the weight loss of the composites HNT/TCN (25.7%), HNT/TCN (24.5%) and the commercial resin composite (30%) (Table 3).

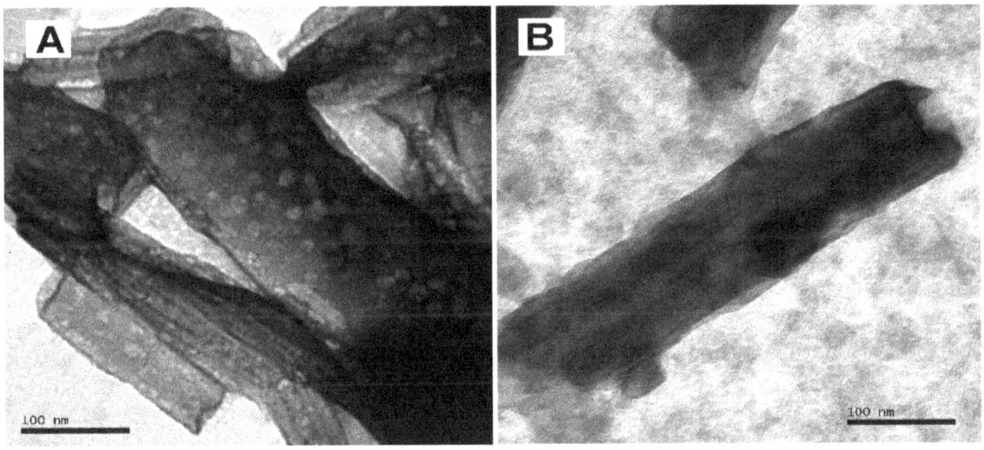

Figure 1. (**A**) TEM image that shows the presence of TCN nanoparticles with diameter of 5–10 nm. (**B**) TEM image of a nanotube with its inner-surface of 40–50 nm diameter range and outer-surface of 90 nm diameter.

Table 2. Results Degree of Conversion (DC), Flexural Modulus (E) and Flexural Strength (FS), Maximum polymerization stress (PS).

Composite	DC (%)	E (GPa)	FS (MPa)	PS (MPa)
HNT/TCN-0%	75.9 (5.4) ^{A}	6.8 (0.9) ^{A}	75.9 (10.1) ^{B}	3.6 (0.3) ^{B}
HNT/TCN	78.5 (2.2) ^{A}	7.5 (0.2) ^{A}	107.2 (6.6) ^{A}	5.4 (0.9) ^{A}
Z350XT	72.5 (10.6) ^{A}	6.8 (0.4) ^{A}	101.4 (18.4) ^{A}	3.6 (0.3) ^{B}

* Different capital letters in column indicate statistical difference ($p < 0.05$).

Table 3. Results Glass Transition Temperature (Tg), TAN-δ and Thermogravimetric analysis (TGA).

Composite	Tg (°C)	Tanδ (×10³) at Tg	TGA Weight Loss (%)	TGA Temperature of the First Degradation Step (°C)	TGA Temperature of the Second Degradation Step (°C)
HNT/TCN-0%	102 (6.56) B	156.7 (0.15) A	27.3 (0.58) A	301 (1.73) A	426 (3.6) A
HNT/TCN	154 (4.36) A	106.7 (0.11) B	26.3 (0.58) A	296 (1.0) B	419 (1.15) A,B
Z350XT	105.3 (3.51) B	103.3 (0.15) B	27 (1.0) A	286 (2.64) C	415 (5.72) B

* Different capital letters in column indicate statistical difference ($p < 0.05$).

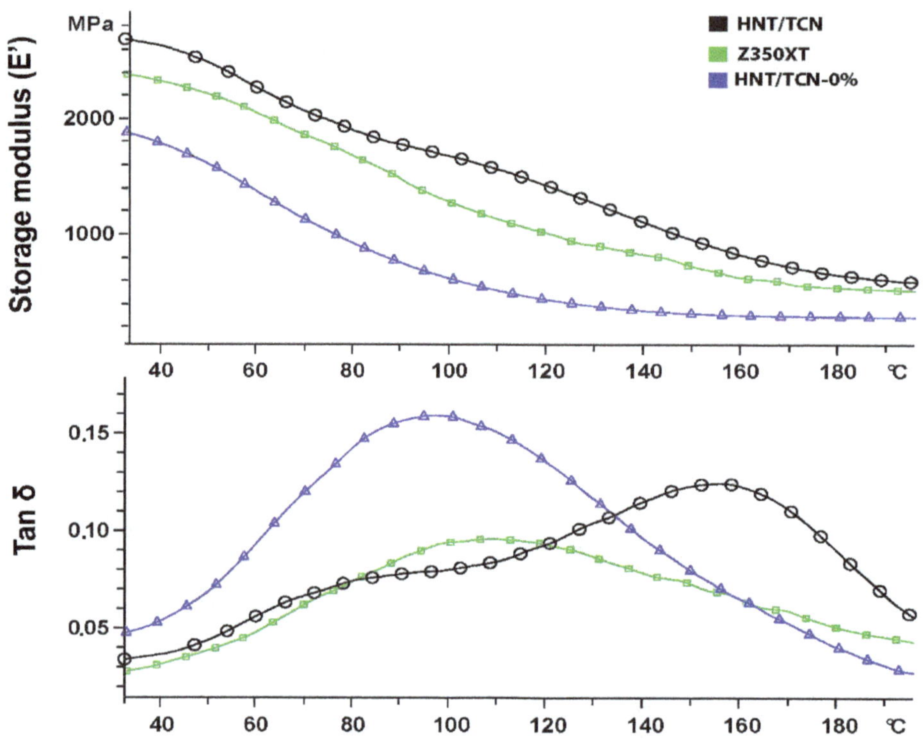

Figure 2. DMA curves of the specimens showed that the MPa, TAN δ at Tg for HNT/TCN resin composite presented a lower TAN δ at Tg when compared to the control composite containing no HNT/TCN-0%. The glass transition temperature (Tg) of HNT/TCN is higher than the other resin composite.

The results of the microbiological test are presented in Table 4. There were no statistically significant differences ($p = 0.977$) between the experimental groups for CFUs and ($p = 0.557$) for dry weight.

Table 4. Results microbiological tests, as colony forming units after 5 days (CFU)/mL/mm^2 and biofilm dry weight. This test showed no statistical difference between experimental groups and commercial resin composite ($p = 0.977$).

Composite	(CFU)/mL/mm^2	Dry Weight (g)
HNT/TCN-0%	6.9267 (0.35) A	0.0004 (0.00025) A
HNT/TCN	6.8733 (0.28) A	0.0008 (0.00082) A
Z350XT	6.8867 (0.28) A	0.0003 (0.00006) A

* The same capital letters indicate absence of statistical difference ($p < 0.05$).

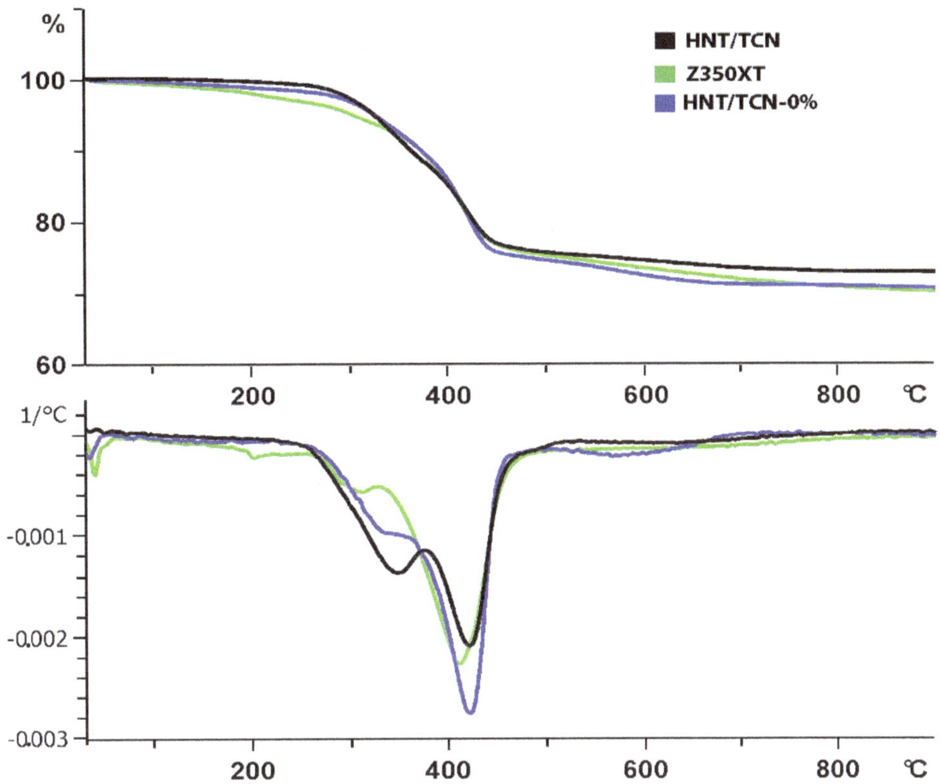

Figure 3. TGA curves of the specimens. Curve of the weight loss (%) showing that HNT/TCN resin composite presented a lower weight loss than other groups. The second curve below shows that there were two steps of degradation for each group.

4. Discussion

Recent studies have demonstrated that the incorporation of HNTs (5 wt.%) in resin-based materials (i.e., dental adhesive systems and enamel infiltrants) could improve their micro-hardness, flexural strength [15] and maximum polymerization rate [11]. However, if the concentration of HNTs is higher than 10 wt.% it is likely to attain a decrease of both flexural strength [15] and maximum polymerization rate [11]. The reason of such outcomes has been attributed to the behavior of such nanotubes to agglomerate in micro-cluster; this causes interference in the mechanism of interaction between nanotubes and the polymer matrix [30]. The null hypothesis that the inclusion of HNT-TCN at concentration of 8% into an experimental resin composite would have increased the physicochemical and microbiological properties must be partially accepted since some physicochemical properties were improved, although no significant differences were attained in terms of antibacterial activity (CFUs) and dry weight after 5 days of initial biofilm formation.

The physicochemical results obtained in this study are in agreement with those recently presented by Degrazia et al. [11]. Indeed, the organic matrix structure and the characteristic of fillers employed in the formulation of composite materials exert a direct influence on the surface roughness, degree of conversion, finishing, and polishing procedures; this may influence the surface quality of resin composite when applied in clinical scenarios [31]. Moreover, it is believed that if a higher degree of conversion is achieved, it is possible to extend the long-term stability and longevity of resin composites, especially in those cases when relatively "short" light-curing periods are performed [32]. However, despite the absence of statistical significance, the HNT/TCN composite presented greater numerical degree of conversion compared to the two control composites tested in this study. It is important to consider that for monomers with the same functionality, the higher the conversion of double bond monomers, the greater the mechanical strength of the cured resin [33]. Indeed, it has been already demonstrated that during the light-curing process HNT/TCN nanotubes may increase the intermolecular interactions between monomers during polymerization [30], due to the C=O and Al-O-H groups present on the inner and outer surface of the HNTs [34]. In general, in case of greater cross-link conversion degree, the conversion of monomers may advance and increase the density of the polymer network [35].

The dynamic mechanical analysis is usually employed for the evaluation of the glass transition temperature (Tg) of resin-based materials, since this allows a more "in-depth" knowledge of the network homogeneity and cross-linking density [36]. As previously stated, the addition of nanotubes in resin-based materials may cause the formation of intermolecular interactions (hydrogen bond formation between hydroxyl groups) between the outer surface of HNTs and Bis-GMA molecule by hydroxyl groups [30].

It has been reported that, low values of TAN δ at specific Tg values indicate a better interfacial adhesion between the organic matrix and the filler [35]. In the present study, the glass transition temperature of the tested materials showed that the HNT/TCN composite presented a lower TAN δ at Tg when compared to the control composite containing no HNT. This outcome indicates that the nanotubes may enhance the chemical interaction during polymerization reaction between the organic matrix and the inorganic fillers (Figures 2 and 3).

Furthermore, the strength, modulus and impact resistance of resin-based materials can be increased when these are doped with HNTs, even at relative low concentration (5 wt.%) [23]. According to the ISO 4049/2000 standard [26], the flexural strengths of universal resin-based restorative materials should be higher than 80 MPa. The Flexural strength test (Table 2) showed that FS of the commercial nanofilled composite and that of the experimental composite HNT/TCN were statistically higher than FS obtained with the control composite HNT/TCN-0%; the latter did not meet the minimal required values of ISO 4049/2000. High flexural strength is necessary to prevent cohesive fractures within the bulk material, especially when considering posterior restorations [37,38]. However, HNT/TCN presented FS values similar to that of the modern commercial composite used in this study. However, although the similarity in flexural strength, the elastic modulus of the Filtek Z350 XT attained in our study was lower than that reported by Rosa et al., 2012 [39]. The main reason for such a difference can be attributed to the different light-curing protocol used in our study.

A further important characteristic that may influence the stress development is the flexural modulus (FM); this is often associated with the composition of the tested material. In this study, the FM tests showed no significant difference between the tested groups (Table 2). Correlation between the FM and the polymerization stress values is a valid simplified approach [38]. However, the limitations of this in vitro test are related to the fact that the light needed to pass through the acrylic rod, as well as the 1 mm thick material before reaching the upper rod in order to create the bonding between the materials and the rods [40]. Indeed, in this study the high standard deviation of polymerization stress test obtained in the HNT/TCN resin composite may be related to the compliance of the test. Tensilometer test configurations can also present some limitations when considering a clinical scenario and the configuration of the cavities [41]. Nonetheless, it was previously reported that it is a valid method to simulate the conditions present in small cavities, where the volume of the resin composite is restricted; this may represent the clinical situation in minimally invasive restorative procedures [42].

Resin composites with lower values of the polymerization stress are those having the lowest elastic modulus; this is probably due to the greater deformation capacity of these latter materials [43]. The addition of HNT/TCN in the experimental resin composite resulted in a significant increase in PS (Table 2). It is known that resin-composites with high modulus of elasticity may generate stiffer restorations; such conditions may increase the effect of the polymerization stress on the tooth-composite interfaces [44]. Conversely, resin composites with a lower elastic modulus create less stress on the interface, although these may lack full dimensional recovery to withstand the masticatory load [44]. Indeed, it can be observed that despite the higher polymerization stress value of HNT/TCN, FM values had the tendency to be higher than the other two materials tested in this study. Another reason HNT/TCN composite showed higher polymerization stress may be associated with the lower micro-hybrid silica filler content (72%) compared to the HNT-free control composite, which had 80 wt.% of micro-hybrid filler.

To test the antibacterial effect, a test was carried out with 5 days of biofilm growth. Degrazia and collaborators [11], showed that their resin-based material doped with HNT/TCN had antibacterial effect up to 72h; antibacterial properties can be also evaluated after 24 h of biofilm growth. It is suggested that the antibacterial effect can be obtained by direct contact of *S. mutans* with the inhibitory agent present in the resin composite (TCN in case of the present work). In agreement with this idea, Feitosa and collaborators [22] demonstrated strong antibacterial activity when *S. mutans* was in direct contact with doxycycline-encapsulated nanotube-modified dentin adhesive after 24 h. In the present study, no statistically significant difference was found between the CFUs values of the 3 tested composites biofilm formed over a 5-day period ($p = 0.977$) (Table 4). It seems that the decrease in the inhibitory antibacterial effect overtime might be related to the inability of such agent from the resin composite to reach the whole thickness of the plaque, in particular the outer layers of bacteria. Probably, the absence in degradation and wearing of the material seems to be considered as an advantage. Due to the interestingly low CFU of the HNT/TCN, in the present work, we believe that the daily removal of the biofilm can reduce its thickness and allow the direct contact of the agent with the bacteria and promoting a more effective antibacterial action. Furthermore, it is possible that current antibacterial tests performed in a laboratory may not be totally appropriate for the evaluation of resin composites, unless accompanied with aging protocols that allow the release of therapeutic agents such as the TCN.

Future studies are suggested to improve the development of antimicrobial materials and the understanding of the relationship between their formulations, morphology and properties, to promote the longevity (shelf-life and ageing) of resin-based materials restorations. Moreover, studies including its rheological properties with alternative methods for synthesis and nanotubes can extend the range of application of such materials as well the satisfaction of as patients and clinicians.

5. Conclusions

It can be concluded that:

- Incorporation of 8 wt.% seems to be a satisfactory formulation of halloysite nanotube for achieving appropriate mechanical properties for an experimental resin micro-hybrid composite without affecting the viscosity and the material and increase the risk for phase separation;
- The experimental resin composite containing 8 wt.% halloysite nanotube doped with triclosan, from a physicochemical point of view, seems to be a suitable restorative material such as the current commercial nano-filled resin-composite;
- Incorporation of triclosan seems to be test-dependent, since it showed no response in mature biofilms as used in this study.

Author Contributions: D.A.C. performed the experiments and wrote the manuscript; N.S.R. and L.C.S. performed the experiments; D.L. analyzed the data and contributed materials/analysis tools; F.P.R. wrote part of the manuscript and revised the manuscript; F.W.D. revised the manuscript; F.M.C. analyzed the data and revised the manuscript; S.S. conceived of and designed the experiments. Revised the manuscript at all the steps; V.P.A.S. conceived of and designed the experiments.

Acknowledgments: We would like to acknowledge the "Departamento de Biomateriais e Biologia Oral" from Universidade de São Paulo for all the technical support offered on polymerization stress measurements test. In addition to Coordenação de Aperfeiçoamento de Pessoal de Nível Superior—CAPES, by granting the scholarship.This work was also supported by the research grant INDI—"Programa de Consolidación de Indicadores: Fomento Plan Estatal CEU-UCH" 2017–2018 to Salvatore Sauro. We would also like to thank all those members of the group "Dental Biomaterials Science & Research (https://www.facebook.com/groups/985792791507045/?ref=bookmarks) who helped us in enriching the background and the references of our study.

References

1. Padovani, G.C.; Feitosa, V.P.; Sauro, S.; Tay, F.R.; Durán, G.; Paula, A.J.; Durán, N. Advances in dental materials through nanotechnology: Facts, perspectives and toxicological aspects. *Trends Biotechnol.* **2015**, *33*, 621–636. [CrossRef] [PubMed]
2. Wang, X.; Cai, Q.; Zhang, X.; Wei, Y.; Xu, M.; Yang, X.; Ma, Q.; Cheng, Y.; Deng, X. Improved performance of Bis-GMA/TEGDMA dental composites by net-like structures formed from SiO_2 nanofiber fillers. *Mater. Sci. Eng. C* **2016**, *59*, 464–470. [CrossRef] [PubMed]
3. Degrazia, F.W.; Leitune, V.C.B.; Takimi, A.S.; Collares, F.M.; Sauro, S. Physicochemical and bioactive properties of innovative resin-based materials containing functional halloysite-nanotubes fillers. *Dent. Mater.* **2016**, *32*, 1133–1143. [CrossRef] [PubMed]
4. Murdoch-Kinch, C.A.; McLean, M.E. Minimally invasive dentistry. *J. Am. Dent. Assoc.* **2003**, *134*, 87–95. [CrossRef] [PubMed]
5. Bernardo, M.; Luis, H.; Martin, M.D.; Leroux, B.G.; Rue, T.; Leitão, J.; DeRouen, T.A. Survival and reasons for failure of amalgam versus composite posterior restorations placed in a randomized clinical trial. *J. Am. Dent. Assoc.* **2007**, *138*, 775–783. [CrossRef] [PubMed]
6. Demarco, F.F.; Corrêa, M.B.; Cenci, M.S.; Moraes, R.R.; Opdam, N.J.M. Longevity of posterior composite restorations: Not only a matter of materials. *Dent. Mater.* **2012**, *28*, 87–101. [CrossRef] [PubMed]
7. Khvostenko, D.; Hilton, T.J.; Ferracane, J.L.; Mitchell, J.C.; Kruzic, J.J. Bioactive glass fillers reduce bacterial penetration into marginal gaps for composite restorations. *Dent. Mater.* **2016**, *32*, 73–81. [CrossRef] [PubMed]
8. Loesche, W.J. Role of streptococcus mutans in human dental decay. *Microbiol. Rev.* **1986**, *50*, 353–380. [PubMed]
9. Fugolin, A.P.P.; Pfeifer, C.S. New resins for dental composites. *J. Dent. Res.* **2017**, *96*, 1085–1091. [CrossRef] [PubMed]
10. Wu, H.-X.; Tan, L.; Tang, Z.-W.; Yang, M.-Y.; Xiao, J.-Y.; Liu, C.-J.; Zhuo, R.-X. Highly efficient antibacterial surface grafted with a triclosan-decorated poly(n-hydroxyethylacrylamide) brush. *ACS Appl. Mater. Interfaces* **2015**, *7*, 7008–7015. [CrossRef] [PubMed]
11. Degrazia, F.W.; Genari, B.; Leitune, V.C.B.; Arthur, R.A.; Luxan, S.A.; Samuel, S.M.W.; Collares, F.M.; Sauro, S. Polymerisation, antibacterial and bioactivity properties of experimental orthodontic adhesives containing triclosan-loaded halloysite nanotubes. *J. Dent.* **2017**. [CrossRef] [PubMed]
12. Kaffashi, B.; Davoodi, S.; Oliaei, E. Poly(ϵ-caprolactone)/triclosan loaded polylactic acid nanoparticles composite: A long-term antibacterial bionanocomposite with sustained release. *Int. J. Pharm.* **2016**, *508*, 10–21. [CrossRef] [PubMed]
13. Rathke, A.; Staude, R.; Muche, R.; Haller, B. Antibacterial activity of a triclosan-containing resin composite matrix against three common oral bacteria. *J. Mater. Sci. Mater. Med.* **2010**, *21*, 2971–2977. [CrossRef] [PubMed]
14. Wicht, M.; Haak, R.; Kneist, S.; Noack, M. A triclosan-containing compomer reduces spp. predominant in advanced carious lesions. *Dent. Mater.* **2005**, *21*, 831–836. [CrossRef] [PubMed]
15. Feitosa, S.A.; Münchow, E.A.; Al-Zain, A.O.; Kamocki, K.; Platt, J.A.; Bottino, M.C. Synthesis and characterization of novel halloysite-incorporated adhesive resins. *J. Dent.* **2015**, *43*, 1316–1322. [CrossRef] [PubMed]
16. Guimarães, L.; Enyashin, A.N.; Seifert, G.; Duarte, H.A. Structural, electronic, and mechanical properties of single-walled halloysite nanotube models. *J. Phys. Chem. C* **2010**, *114*, 11358–11363. [CrossRef]
17. Bottino, M.C.; Batarseh, G.; Palasuk, J.; Alkatheeri, M.S.; Windsor, L.J.; Platt, J.A. Nanotube-modified dentin adhesive—Physicochemical and dentin bonding characterizations. *Dent. Mater.* **2013**, *29*, 1–8. [CrossRef] [PubMed]
18. Cavallaro, G.; Lazzara, G.; Milioto, S.; Parisi, F. Halloysite nanotubes for cleaning, consolidation and protection. *Chem. Rec.* **2018**. [CrossRef] [PubMed]
19. Alkatheeri, M.S.; Palasuk, J.; Eckert, G.J.; Platt, J.A.; Bottino, M.C. Halloysite nanotube incorporation into adhesive systems—Effect on bond strength to human dentin. *Clin. Oral Investig.* **2015**, *19*, 1905–1912. [CrossRef] [PubMed]

20. Ghaderi-Ghahfarrokhi, M.; Haddadi-Asl, V.; Zargarian, S.S. Fabrication and characterization of polymer-ceramic nanocomposites containing drug loaded modified halloysite nanotubes. *J. Biomed. Mater. Res. Part A* **2018**. [CrossRef] [PubMed]
21. Palasuk, J.; Windsor, L.J.; Platt, J.A.; Lvov, Y.; Geraldeli, S.; Bottino, M.C. Doxycycline-loaded nanotube-modified adhesives inhibit MMP in a dose-dependent fashion. *Clin. Oral Investig.* 2017. [CrossRef] [PubMed]
22. Feitosa, S.A.; Palasuk, J.; Kamocki, K.; Geraldeli, S.; Gregory, R.L.; Platt, J.A.; Windsor, L.J.; Bottino, M.C. Doxycycline-encapsulated nanotube-modified dentin adhesives. *J. Dent. Res.* **2014**, *93*, 1270–1276. [CrossRef] [PubMed]
23. Liu, M.; Jia, Z.; Jia, D.; Zhou, C. Recent advance in research on halloysite nanotubes-polymer nanocomposite. *Prog. Polym. Sci.* **2014**, *39*, 1498–1525. [CrossRef]
24. Svizero Nda, R.; Silva, M.S.; Alonso, R.C.; Rodrigues, F.P.; Hipólito, V.D.; Carvalho, R.M.; D'Alpino, P.H. Effects of curing protocols on fluid kinetics and hardness of resin cements. *Dent. Mater. J.* **2013**, *32*, 32–41. [CrossRef] [PubMed]
25. Rodrigues, N.S.; de Souza, L.C.; Feitosa, V.P.; Loguercio, A.D.; D'Arcangelo, C.; Sauro, S.; Saboia, V.d.P.A. Effect of different conditioning/deproteinization protocols on the bond strength and degree of conversion of self-adhesive resin cements applied to dentin. *Int. J. Adhes. Adhes.* **2017**. [CrossRef]
26. ISO 4049. *Dentistry—Polymer-Based Filling, Restorative and Luting Materials; 7.10 Depth of cure, Class 2 materials;* International Organization for Standardization: Geneva,Switzerland, 2000.
27. Gonçalves, F.; Boaro, L.C.; Ferracane, J.L.; Braga, R.R. A comparative evaluation of polymerization stress data obtained with four different mechanical testing systems. *Dent. Mater.* **2012**, *28*, 680–686. [CrossRef] [PubMed]
28. Duarte, S.; Gregoire, S.; Singh, A.P.; Vorsa, N.; Schaich, K.; Bowen, W.H.; Koo, H. Inhibitory effects of cranberry polyphenols on formation and acidogenicity of streptococcus mutans biofilms. *FEMS Microbiol. Lett.* **2006**, *257*, 50–56. [CrossRef] [PubMed]
29. Peralta, S.L.; Carvalho, P.H.A.; van de Sande, F.H.; Pereira, C.M.P.; Piva, E.; Lund, R.G. Self-etching dental adhesive containing a natural essential oil: Anti-biofouling performance and mechanical properties. *Biofouling* **2013**, *29*, 345–355. [CrossRef] [PubMed]
30. Chen, Q.; Zhao, Y.; Wu, W.; Xu, T.; Fong, H. Fabrication and evaluation of Bis-GMA/TEGDMA dental resins/composites containing halloysite nanotubes. *Dent. Mater.* **2012**, *28*, 1071–1079. [CrossRef] [PubMed]
31. Abzal, M.; Rathakrishnan, M.; Prakash, V.; Vivekanandhan, P.; Subbiya, A.; Sukumaran, V. Evaluation of surface roughness of three different composite resins with three different polishing systems. *J. Conserv. Dent.* **2016**, *19*. [CrossRef]
32. Sauro, S.; Osorio, R.; Watson, T.F.; Toledano, M. Therapeutic effects of novel resin bonding systems containing bioactive glasses on mineral-depleted areas within the bonded-dentine interface. *J. Mater. Sci. Mater. Med.* **2012**, *23*, 1521–1532. [CrossRef] [PubMed]
33. Braga, R.R.; Ballester, R.Y.; Ferracane, J.L. Factors involved in the development of polymerization shrinkage stress in resin-composites: A systematic review. *Dent. Mater.* **2005**, *21*, 962–970. [CrossRef] [PubMed]
34. Luo, R.; Sen, A. Rate enhancement in controlled radical polymerization of acrylates using recyclable heterogeneous lewis acid. *Macromolecules* **2007**, *40*, 154–156. [CrossRef]
35. Karabela, M.M.; Sideridou, I.D. Synthesis and study of properties of dental resin composites with different nanosilica particles size. *Dent. Mater.* **2011**, *27*, 825–835. [CrossRef] [PubMed]
36. Bacchi, A.; Yih, J.A.; Platta, J.; Knight, J.; Pfeifer, C.S. Shrinkage/stress reduction and mechanical properties improvement in restorative composites formulated with thio-urethane oligomers. *J. Mech. Behav. Biomed. Mater.* **2018**, *78*, 235–240. [CrossRef] [PubMed]
37. Aydınoğlu, A.; Yoruç, A.B.H. Effects of silane-modified fillers on properties of dental composite resin. *Mater. Sci. Eng. C* **2017**, *79*, 382–389. [CrossRef] [PubMed]
38. Boaro, L.C.C.; Gonalves, F.; Guimarães, T.C.; Ferracane, J.L.; Versluis, A.; Braga, R.R. Polymerization stress, shrinkage and elastic modulus of current low-shrinkage restorative composites. *Dent. Mater.* **2010**, *26*, 1144–1150. [CrossRef] [PubMed]
39. Rosa, R.S.; Balbinot, C.E.; Blando, E.; Mota, E.G.; Oshima, H.M.; Hirakata, L.; Pires, L.A.; Hübler, R. Evaluation of mechanical properties on three nanofilled composites. *Stomatologija* **2012**, *14*, 126–130. [PubMed]

40. Gonçalves, F.; Boaro, L.C.C.; Miyazaki, C.L.; Kawano, Y.; Braga, R.R. Influence of polymeric matrix on the physical and chemical properties of experimental composites. *Braz. Oral Res.* **2015**, *29*, 1–7. [CrossRef] [PubMed]
41. Boaro, L.C.C.; Fróes-Salgado, N.R.; Gajewski, V.E.S.; Bicalho, A.A.; Valdivia, A.D.C.M.; Soares, C.J.; Miranda Júnior, W.G.; Braga, R.R. Correlation between polymerization stress and interfacial integrity of composites restorations assessed by different in vitro tests. *Dent. Mater.* **2014**, *30*, 984–992. [CrossRef] [PubMed]
42. Rodrigues, F.P.; Lima, R.G.; Muench, A.; Watts, D.C.; Ballester, R.Y. A method for calculating the compliance of bonded-interfaces under shrinkage: Validation for Class i cavities. *Dent. Mater.* **2014**, *30*, 936–944. [CrossRef] [PubMed]
43. Labella, R.; Lambrechts, P.; Van Meerbeek, B.V.G. Polymerization shrinkage and elasticity of flowable adhesives and filled composites. *Dent. Mater.* **1999**, *15*, 128–137. [CrossRef]
44. Rosatto, C.M.P.; Bicalho, A.A.; VerÃssimo, C.; BraganÃ§a, G.F.; Rodrigues, M.P.; Tantbirojn, D.; Versluis, A.; Soares, C.J. Mechanical properties, shrinkage stress, cuspal strain and fracture resistance of molars restored with bulk-fill composites and incremental filling technique. *J. Dent.* **2015**, *43*, 1519–1528. [CrossRef] [PubMed]

8

Influence of Fractionation Methods on Physical and Biological Properties of Injectable Platelet-Rich Fibrin: An Exploratory Study

Prakan Thanasrisuebwong [1,2], Rudee Surarit [3], Sompop Bencharit [4,5] and Nisarat Ruangsawasdi [6,*]

1 Department of Oral and Maxillofacial Surgery, Faculty of Dentistry, Mahidol University, Bangkok 10400, Thailand; ae13ea@gmail.com
2 Ph.D. program in Oral Biology, Faculty of Dentistry, Mahidol University, Bangkok 10400, Thailand
3 Department of Oral Biology, Faculty of Dentistry, Mahidol University, Bangkok 10400, Thailand; rudee.sur@mahidol.ac.th
4 Department of General Dentistry, School of Dentistry, Virginia Commonwealth University, Richmond, VA 23298, USA; sbencharit@vcu.edu
5 Department of Biomedical Engineering, College of Engineering, Virginia Commonwealth University, Richmond, VA 23298, USA
6 Department of Pharmacology, Faculty of Dentistry, Mahidol University, Bangkok 10400, Thailand
* Correspondence: nisarat.rua@mahidol.ac.th

Abstract: Injectable platelet-rich fibrin (i-PRF) has been used as an autografting material to enhance bone regeneration through intrinsic growth factors. However, fractionation protocols used to prepare i-PRF can be varied and the effects of different fractionation protocols are not known. In this study, we investigated the influence of different fractions of i-PRF on the physical and biological properties derived from variations in i-PRF fractionation preparation. The i-PRF samples, obtained from the blood samples of 10 donors, were used to harvest i-PRF and were fractioned into two types. The yellow i-PRF fractionation was harvested from the upper yellow zone, while the red i-PRF fractionation was collected from both the yellow and red zone of the buffy coat. The viscoelastic property measurements, including the clot formation time, α-angle, and maximum clot firmness, were performed by rotational thromboelastometry. The fibrin network was examined using a scanning electron microscope. Furthermore, the concentration of growth factors released, including VEGF, TGF-β1, and PDGF, were quantified using ELISA. A paired *t*-test with a 95% confidence interval was used. All three viscoelastic properties were statistically significantly higher in the yellow i-PRF compared to the red i-PRF. The scanning electron microscope reviewed more cellular components in the red i-PRF compared to the yellow i-PRF. In addition, the fibrin network of the yellow i-PRF showed a higher density than that in the red i-PRF. There was no statistically significant difference between the concentration of VEGF and TGF-β1. However, at Day 7 and Day 14 PDGF concentrations were statistically significantly higher in the red i-PRF compared to the yellow group. In conclusion, these results showed that the red i-PRF provided better biological properties through the release of growth factors. On the other hand, the yellow i-PRF had greater viscoelastic physical properties. Further investigations into the appropriate i-PRF fractionation for certain surgical procedures are therefore necessary to clarify the suitability for each fraction for different types of regenerative therapy.

Keywords: bone regeneration; fractionation; growth factors; i-PRF; PRF; ROTEM®

1. Introduction

Platelet-rich fibrin (PRF) derived from the centrifugation of whole blood has long been used successfully in regenerative dentistry and medicine [1–5]. A centrifugation speed of 2700 rpm for 12 min in PRF with a glass or glass-coated tubes permits the use of PRF material without any additional anticoagulants. The fibrin matrix scaffold network in PRF appears to be beneficial in tissue regeneration [6]. PRF has shown to enhance regeneration of bone [1,7], cartilage [8], soft tissue [5,9–11], and nerve fiber [12]. However, the application of solid PRF, resulting from a blood sample preparation at 400 g relative centrifugal force (RCF) or 2700 round per minute (rpm) for 12 min, has its limitations. For instance, it cannot be mixed with a particulate bone substitute. To mix with particulate bone, the biomaterials in a liquid form are more suitable. Both injectable platelet-rich fibrin (i-PRF) and PRF-predecessor platelet-rich plasma (PRP) are the liquid formula within the platelet concentrated group that can be used efficiently for mixing with the particulate bone graft. PRP is traditionally prepared from whole blood using a higher speed centrifugation compared to PRF [1–5]. Unfortunately, PRP has some drawbacks because it requires either synthetic anticoagulants, such as citrate dextrose-A (ACD-A) and citrate phosphate dextrose (CPD), or other activating agents, such as thrombin. Although those additive agents allow for appropriate clinical working time and manipulation, they can inhibit healing and regeneration due to the lack of biocompatibility [9–11,13–15].

The concept of low speed centrifugation is central to the preparation of the liquid form of i-PRF as well as to create a material rich in leukocytes, platelets, and growth factors, including the vascular endothelial growth factor (VEGF), transforming growth factor-beta 1 (TGF-β1), and platelet-derived growth factor (PDGF), compared to the first generation platelet-derived PRP [9–11,16]. According to the low speed centrifugation concept, i-PRF can be obtained by using a centrifugation speed at 60 g RCF or 700 rpm for 3 min [10,16,17]. Blood harvesting is similar to the PRF membrane method, however, the non-coating plastic tube was recommended in order to prevent the formation of early clotting in the tube. After centrifugation, whole blood is separated into three main parts based on the buffy coat layer: A yellow upper part, a buffy coat middle part, and a red blood cell containing lower part. A small syringe with an 18G hypodermic needle is used for collecting the i-PRF to be used. The harvesting method of i-PRF after centrifugation has been described as harvesting only the whole upper layer above the buffy coat [16,17], however, the amount of the upper layer harvested can vary among individuals and the position of needle tips during harvesting can also be varied based on different clinical practice. To the best of our knowledge, there is no study examining the different properties of yellow and red i-PRF.

The aim of this study was to investigate the influence of different separation techniques of i-PRF on its mechanical and biological properties. We further hypothesize that fractionation of the centrifuged plasma for i-PRF is central to the i-PRF's physical properties and biological components. We proposed to examine two fractionation protocols producing yellow i-PRF and red i-PRF based on the fraction of centrifuged plasma above and within the buffy coat, respectively. We expected that the yellow i-PRF would have less cellular components, a denser fibrin network, and therefore have better physical properties than the red i-PRF. On the contrary, we expected that the red i-PRF would have more cellular components and therefore have better biological properties reflecting the greater release of known PRF-related growth factors, including VEGF, TGF-β1, and PDGF.

2. Results

Rotational thromboelastometry (ROTEM®, Tem International GmbH, Munich, Germany) [18] was applied to examine the viscoelastic properties of red and yellow i-PRF. The means and standard deviations for the clot formation time (CFT), α-angle, and maximum clot firmness (MCF) were 52.8 ± 13.14 s, 81.2 ± 1.81 degree, and 85.3 ± 3.56 mm, respectively, for the yellow i-PRF and 68.2 ± 12.31 s, 77.8 ± 2.82 degree, and 81.6 ± 4.50 mm, respectively, for the red i-PRF as shown in Figure 1. The results showed statistically significant differences (paired t-test) between the two types of i-PRF in all three properties: CFT, α-angle, and MCF, with p-value = 0.008, 0.004, and 0.001, respectively, as shown in

Figure 1. The CFT for the yellow i-PRF was shorter than the red i-PRF. The α-angle was higher in the yellow i-PRF compared to the red i-PRF. The MCF was also higher in the yellow i-PRF compared to the red i-PRF.

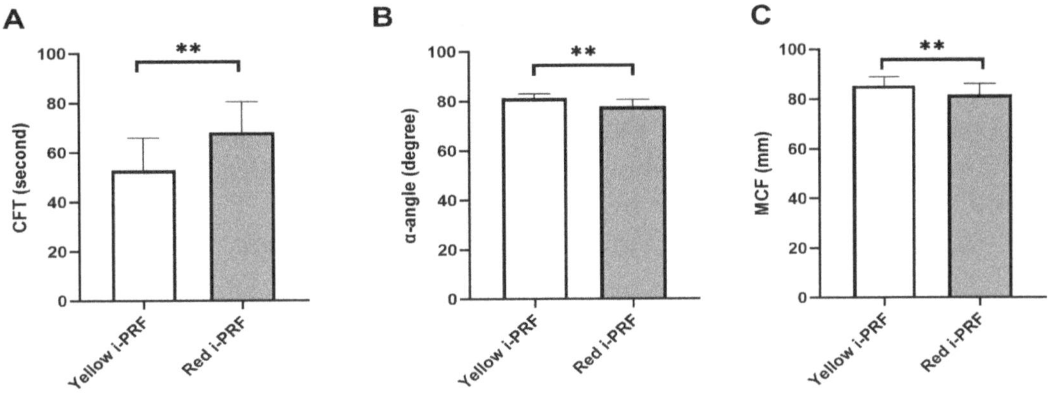

Figure 1. Rotational thromboelastometry (ROTEM®) analysis demonstrating (**A**) clot formation time (CFT), (**B**) α-angle, and (**C**) maximum clot firmness (MCF) of the yellow injectable platelet-rich fibrin (i-PRF) and the red i-PRF. ** $p < 0.01$.

The examination of the i-PRF by SEM showed the fibrin network architecture and cellular components. In the yellow i-PRF, a dense fibrin network with less cellular components than the red i-PRF was observed (Figure 2). On the contrary, SEM showed that more cellular components, such as leukocyte, platelets, and erythrocytes, were in the red i-PRF compared to the yellow i-PRF. In addition, the numerous erythrocytes were enmeshed in the fibrin network. The shapes of these erythrocytes were normal, but the fibrin network appeared at a lower density and was less organized compared to the yellow i-PRF (Figure 2).

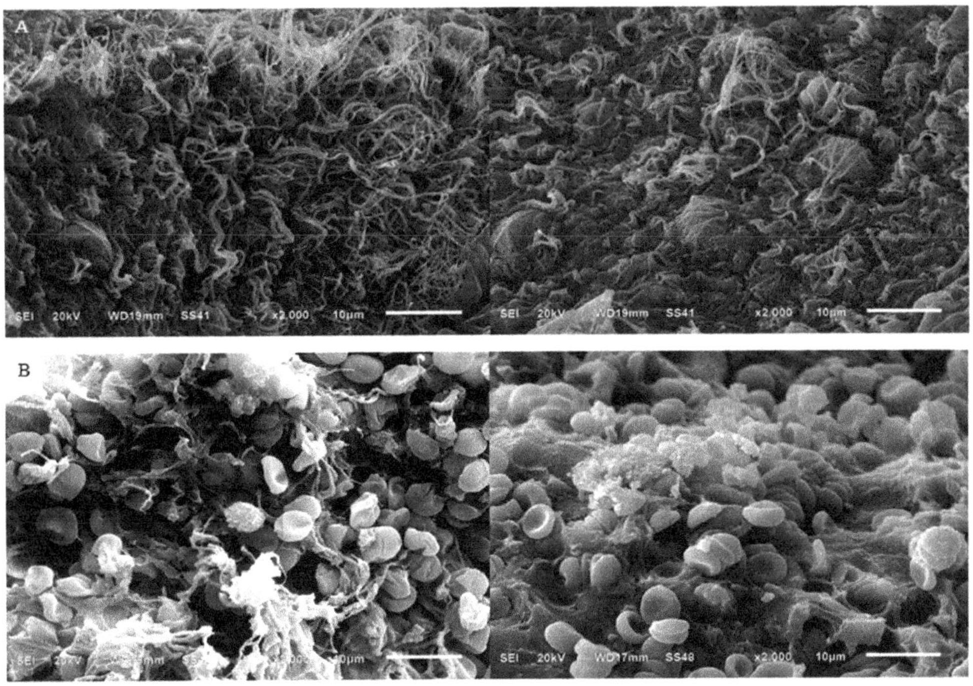

Figure 2. Scanning electron microscope images of i-PRF using different fraction methods. A different position of the harvesting needle led to two types of i-PRF: The yellow and red i-PRF. (**A**) The yellow i-PRF showed a dense and highly organized fibrin network. (**B**) On the other hand, the red i-PRF demonstrated more cellular components of leukocyte, platelets, and erythrocytes than the yellow i-PRF.

The growth factor concentrations were quantified at 3 h, 24 h, 72 h (3 days), 168 h (7 days), and 336 h (14 days) after preparation. There was a distinct difference between the releasing patterns for VEGF, TGF-β1, and PDGF (Figure 3). At 3 h, 24 h, and 3 days, the VEGF concentrations were increased. Three hours after preparation, the VEGF concentration of both i-PRFs was at a similar level. This level presented in the yellow i-PRF was similar at 24 h again while the red i-PRF dramatically increased. The concentrations of VEGF peaked at Day 3 for both the yellow and red i-PRF. There was a slightly higher concentration of VEGF in the red i-PRF compared to the yellow i-PRF but the difference was not statistically significant (Figure 3A). Different results were detected at Day 7 and 14 after clotting. At this time point, both i-PRFs showed a decreasing VEGF concentration. In conclusion, the released accumulation of VEGF showed a higher concentration in the red i-PRF than the yellow i-PRF (Figure 3B).

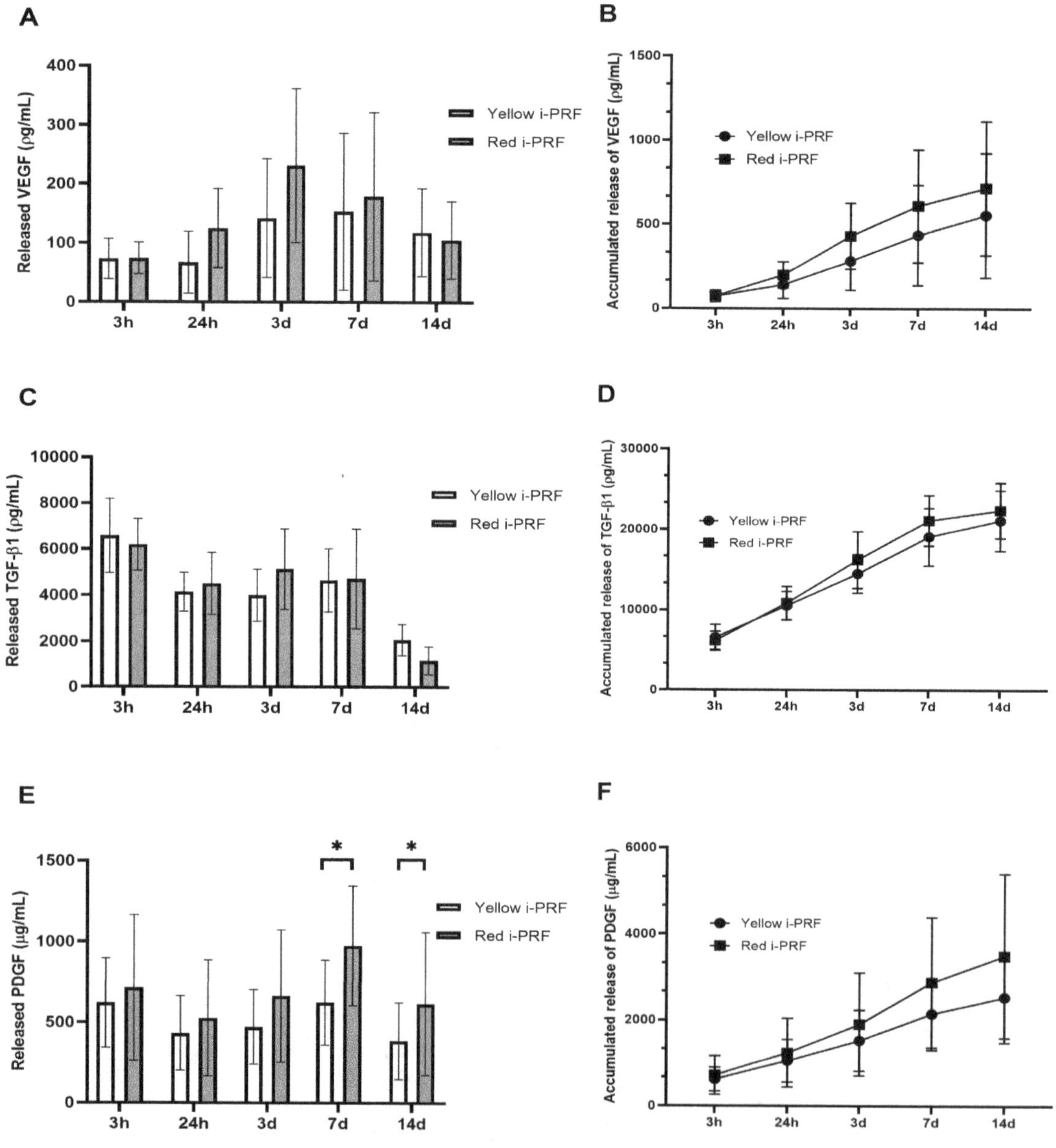

Figure 3. Time point releases and accumulated releases of three growth factors: (**A,B**) vascular endothelial growth factor (VEGF), (**C,D**) transforming growth factor-β1 (TGF-β1), and (**E,F**) platelet-derived growth factor (PDGF). * $p < 0.05$.

The growth factor concentration for the human TGF-β1 showed a general trend at all time points. The highest concentration was recorded at 3 h for the yellow and red i-PRF then decreased and was stable at 24 h, 3 days, and 7 days. There was a dramatic decrease of the TGF-β1 concentration for both i-PRFs at Day 14 (Figure 3C). Note that the released accumulation of TGF-β1 presented a similar trend and value for the yellow and red i-PRFs (Figure 3D). Using a paired *t*-test, there was however no statistically significant difference between the concentration of VEGF and TGF-β1 (Figure 3).

The release of PDGF was more constant throughout the experimental timeline. Analysis of the PDGF release (Figure 3E) revealed that more PDGF was released from the red i-PRF at 7 and 14 days (975.47 ± 371.24 μg/mL and 615.98 ± 443.59 μg/mL) compared with the yellow i-PRF (623.46 ± 263.30 μg/mL and 385.59 ± 237.53 μg/mL). These data were statistically significant for Day 7 ($p = 0.02$) and Day 14 ($p = 0.03$). Cumulatively, PDGF continued to release at all time points and a stronger releasing trend was observed for the red i-PRF over the yellow i-PRF (Figure 3F).

Analysis of the kinetics of the growth factors released showed that VEGF, TGF-β1, and PDGF reached peak release at Day 3, 3 h, and Day 7, respectively. On top of that, TGF-β1 was almost completely released within the first 7 days while VEGF and PDGF showed a longer releasing over 14 days.

3. Discussion

The main difference of i-PRF from solid PRF is the lower speed and time in centrifugation for i-PRF [10,19]. The idea of a slower centrifugation is to allow some cellular and growth factor components to stay in the final product [6,9–11,17,20–24]. The i-PRF can be used in combination with particulate bone allograft or autograft materials [25]. This advantage of a liquid formula of i-PRF allows a more efficient incorporation of the bone graft material and increases the signaling molecules throughout the whole graft.

Little information is known about the physical properties of i-PRF, which are important either when being used alone or in combination with grafting materials. This study is one of the first to apply ROTEM® technology, which is commonly used in hematology research [18,26–31], to examine i-PRF. We hypothesized that compared to the lower layer—red i-PRF, the upper layer—yellow i-PRF would have superior physical properties because of its lack of cellular components. All physical properties confirmed our hypothesis. Although the yellow i-PRF was statistically superior compared to the red i-PRF in viscoelastic properties, the value of the CFT, α-angle, and MCF of both i-PRFs were similar to the reference value or slightly better compared to the standard whole blood that was measured using ROTEM® [32]. In addition, the value of the CFT, α-angle, and MCF showed only a minor difference between both i-PRFs. The SEM analysis demonstrated a dense, organized, acellular fibrin network as a reason for the superior physical properties in the yellow i-PRF compared to the red i-PRF. This clinically suggests that if i-PRF is to be used mainly as filler material or enhancement stability and handling of grafting material, the yellow and red i-PRF may achieve a similar outcome.

A previous SEM analysis of leukocyte-PRF showed multi-different plasma layers that constituted of a fibrin-rich layer at the uppermost layer, followed by an enriched platelet layer, and the buffy coat layer with numerous leukocytes before the base layer of erythrocytes [33]. The SEM in our analysis demonstrated a dense, organized, acellular fibrin network as in the fibrin-rich layer at the plasma top layer of leukocyte-PRF. This characteristic might be a reason for the superior physical properties in the yellow i-PRF compared to the red i-PRF. Meanwhile, the red i-PRF showed a greater number of cells and platelets attached to the fibrin network similar to a combination of all the middle layers and the erythrocyte base layer of leukocyte-PRF together. This additional cell and platelet content in the red i-PRF might lead to better biological properties as we could observe a greater release of the growth factors.

Contrary to the physical properties, we hypothesized that the red i-PRF, which has more cellular components, would have higher release of growth factors. While there was no statistically significant difference in the releases of VEGF and TGF-β1, PDGF at later time points were significantly higher in the red i-PRF compared to the yellow i-PRF. This may be a result of the remaining platelet and cellular components shown in the SEM in the red i-PRF. Note also that the releasing level of all three growth factors was similar to previously reported levels [10]. In addition, we found that the growth factors continue to release even at Day 14. This result is similar to other PRF studies [9–11,17,20–24]. Self-cooperation of the fibrin network slowly forms the high fibrillar aggregation in PRF, which also entraps proteins and growth factors to the binding domains of fibrin molecules. In contrast, PRP is rapidly activated to gelation from a load of thrombin. Therefore, an unstable fibrin network of PRP is formed, which results in lower growth factor retention and incompatible cell homing. PRP therefore only releases growth factors in the early stage. Unlike the PRP, the kinetic release of growth factors from i-PRF is longer, up to 14 days, because of its preserved valuable components, including platelets and leukocytes. The growth factor release from this component can be sustained over a longer period of time from the cellular and acellular component trapped in a naturally progressive polymerization of the fibrin matrix [34]. On top of this, i-PRF potentially allows more growth factor attachment to the heparin-binding domain, which is the high-affinity growth factor-binding site of the fibrinogen that causes prolonged retention of the growth factor within fibrin [35]. This result suggests that when i-PRF is used in combination with particulate bone grafts, the signaling molecules for bone tissue engineering can be achieved. The red i-PRF may therefore have more benefits than the yellow i-PRF because of the greater release of the growth factor shown. In such cases, clinicians should harvest the red i-PRF just with the buffy coat.

This study demonstrated for the first time that minimal changes in the fractionation protocol for i-PRF could alter the physical and biological properties of the final product. This in turn may change the clinical outcomes/applications. These techniques need to be examined further through cell culture analysis and human clinical studies. In any case clinicians should pay particular attention to centrifugation and fractionation protocols. Deviations from the published protocols can result in variations of physical properties and biological components as seen in this study and in others [17]. In addition, further research to develop a novel biomaterial product from i-PRF is an interesting topic, where the freeze-dried or lyophilized technique may be used for sterilization [36,37].

4. Materials and Methods

4.1. Sample Collection and Preparation

The study protocol was approved by the Institutional Review Board of Human Ethic Committee of the Faculty of Dentistry, Mahidol University (COA. No. MU-DT/PY-IRB 2017/061.221). Blood samples were harvested from 10 healthy volunteers (age range 30–35, gender M/F = 2/8). The donors had no history of using antiplatelet or anticoagulant medications. All donors gave written consent for blood collection and for sample preparation and experiments (Figure 4).

Sample preparation was adopted from a previous published protocol, Miron et al. 2017 [10]. Immediately after the blood sample was collected, the sample was centrifuged at 60 g RCF for 3 min using a Duo Centrifuge (Process for PRF, Nice, France) at room temperature; 60 g RCF is equivalent to 700 rpm for this device, which has a 110 mm radius. After centrifugation, two types of i-PRF samples were harvested, yellow and red i-PRF. According to Wang et al. 2017 [24], about 1 mL of sample, either the yellow or red i-PRF, was collected. The yellow i-PRF referred to the sample harvested only in the upper liquid yellow zone above the buffy coat. The red i-PRF referred to the sample harvested from the zone, red and yellow, with the buffy coat. The bevel edge of the harvesting needle was used as a reference point (Figure 4). Subsequently, both types of i-PRF were used to observe the physical properties, including viscoelasticity and morphology, and the biological properties, which is the release of growth factors.

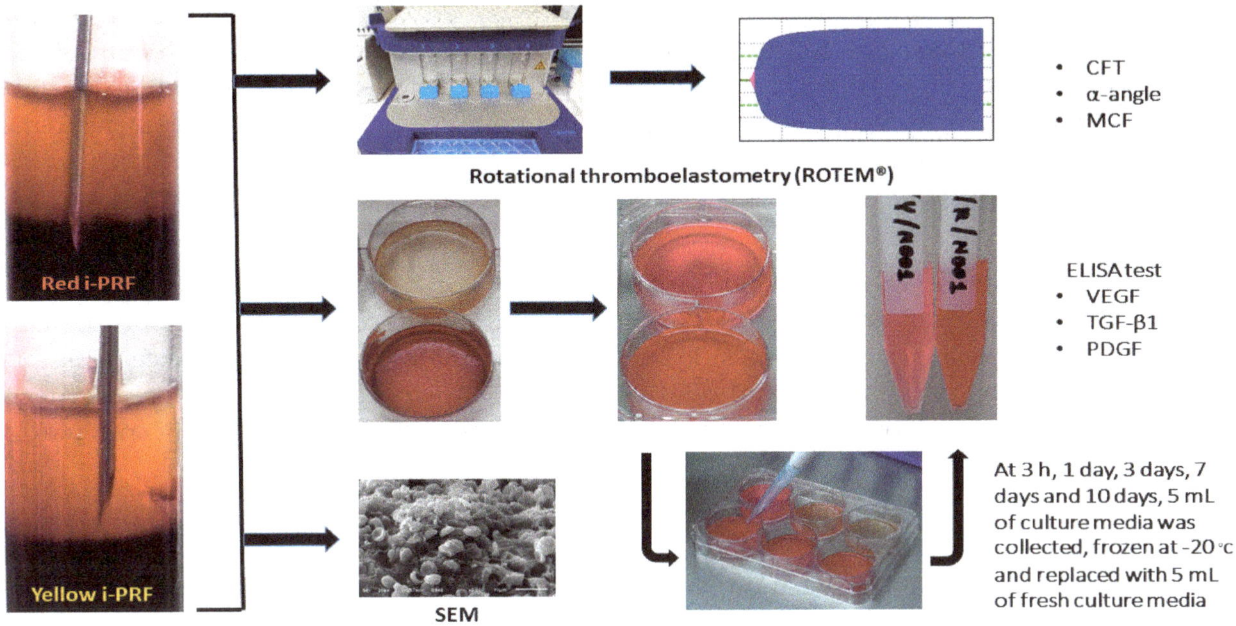

Figure 4. Study workflow of three experiments comparing the red and yellow i-PRF and their fractionation protocol used in this study.

4.2. Viscoelastic Property Analysis

The viscoelastic properties of the i-PRF samples were analyzed using rotational thromboelastometry (ROTEM®, Tem International GmbH, Munich, Germany) [18]. ROTEM® generates output from transducing changes reflecting from the viscoelastic strength of the blood sample while a constant rotational force is applied. Three parameters were analyzed and digitally recorded: Clot formation time (CFT), α-angle, and maximum clot firmness (MCF). The CFT represents the speed at which a solid clot forms, which is primarily influenced by the platelet function, fibrinogen, and coagulation factors. The CFT measures a duration from the clot initiation until it reaches the 20 mm amplitude. The α-angle is a measure to observe the dynamics of clot formation, which represents the acceleration of the fibrin network formation and the amount of cross-linking build up. The MCF is a measure for stability of the clot following the polymerization process.

4.3. Scanning Electron Microscopy (SEM)

The qualitative analysis of the morphological changes of the yellow and red i-PRF was performed using SEM (JEOL, Peabody, MA, USA). The SEM examination was used to observe blood elements present in the fibrin extracellular matrix. Cellular components such as leukocytes, platelets, and erythrocytes were examined and recorded. The density of the fibrin network was also analyzed. The i-PRF samples immediately after completing their clot formation were fixed in 2% glutaraldehyde in Dulbecco's phosphate buffered saline (DPBS) buffer with a pH of 7.4 overnight. Next, samples were dried in the desiccator, then sputtered with 20 nm gold. SEM photography was then performed at 5 to 10 kV using 100× to 2000× magnifications.

4.4. Enzyme-Linked Immunosorbent Assay (ELISA)

ELISA kits were used to quantify the released growth factors: VEGF, TGF-β1, and PDGF (R&D systems Minnesota, United States). Approximately 9 mL of collected i-PRF from each protocol was transferred into a 6-well plate. The plate was then placed in a 5% CO_2 incubator at 37 °C for 30 min to allow for complete clotting formation. Afterwards, 5 mL of Minimum Essential Medium Eagle-Alpha Modification (α-MEM) with nucleosides (Gibco, USA) was added to each sample. The samples were further incubated at 37 °C to allow for the release of growth factors during a 3 h to 14 days period of study. At 3 h, 24 h, 72 h (3 days), 168 h (7 days), and 336 h (14 days), 5 mL of culture media was collected, frozen at −20 °C, and replaced with 5 mL of additional fresh culture media. The concentrations of VEGF, TGF-β1, and PDGF were measured according to the manufacturer's instructions. Optical density was assessed using a microplate reader at 450 nm. The measurements were performed in triplicates.

4.5. Statistical Analysis

Statistical assessment was performed using SPSS version 17.0. All data were presented as the mean value ± standard deviation (SD). The data were tested for the distribution by using a Kolmogorov-Smirnov test and Levene's test to confirm the normality and equal variance assumptions of the data. The data, assuming normal distribution, were then analyzed using paired *t*-tests to compare the differences between two groups in each experiment. The level of significance used was $p < 0.05$.

5. Conclusions

This study suggests that fractionation protocols in i-PRF preparation can alter the final product's physical and biological properties. Clinicians should pay attention to the applications of i-PRF in combinational use with other grafting materials. For the handling and stability of grafting material application, the yellow and red may provide the final i-PRF product with a similar outcome. For the use of i-PRF in enhancing biological properties, the red i-PRF collected from the sample with the buffy coat, which released a higher level of growth factors, in particular, PDGF, should be used.

Author Contributions: Author P.T. designed the study, performed experiments, as well as collected and analyzed the data. Author R.S. designed the study and interpreted the data. Author S.B. helped with study designs, data interpretation, and manuscript writing. Author N.R. oversaw the entire project and supervised Author P.T. in all experiments. All authors contributed to the manuscript writing and approved the final draft.

Acknowledgments: We thank Chareerut Phruksaniyom for technical assistance and Center of Research, Faculty of Dentistry, Mahidol University for providing devices.

References

1. Choukroun, J.; Diss, A.; Simonpieri, A.; Girard, M.O.; Schoeffler, C.; Dohan, S.L.; Dohan, A.J.; Mouhyi, J.; Dohan, D.M. Platelet-rich fibrin (prf): A second-generation platelet concentrate. Part V: Histologic evaluations of prf effects on bone allograft maturation in sinus lift. *Oral Surg. Oral Med. Oral Pathol. Oral Radiol. Endod.* **2006** *101*, 299–303. [CrossRef]
2. Choukroun, J.; Diss, A.; Simonpieri, A.; Girard, M.O.; Schoeffler, C.; Dohan, S.L.; Dohan, A.J.; Mouhyi, J.; Dohan, D.M. Platelet-rich fibrin (prf): A second-generation platelet concentrate. Part IV: Clinical effects on tissue healing. *Oral Surg. Oral Med. Oral Pathol. Oral Radiol. Endod.* **2006**, *101*, e56–e60. [CrossRef]
3. Dohan, D.M.; Choukroun, J.; Diss, A.; Dohan, S.L.; Dohan, A.J.; Mouhyi, J.; Gogly, B. Platelet-rich fibrin (prf): A second-generation platelet concentrate. Part III: Leucocyte activation: A new feature for platelet concentrates? *Oral Surg. Oral Med. Oral Pathol. Oral Radiol. Endod.* **2006**, *101*, e51–e55. [CrossRef]
4. Dohan, D.M.; Choukroun, J.; Diss, A.; Dohan, S.L.; Dohan, A.J.; Mouhyi, J.; Gogly, B. Platelet-rich fibrin (prf): A second-generation platelet concentrate. Part II: Platelet-related biologic features. *Oral Surg. Oral Med. Oral Pathol. Oral Radiol. Endod.* **2006**, *101*, e45–e50. [CrossRef]
5. Dohan, D.M.; Choukroun, J.; Diss, A.; Dohan, S.L.; Dohan, A.J.; Mouhyi, J.; Gogly, B. Platelet-rich fibrin (prf): A second-generation platelet concentrate. Part I: Technological concepts and evolution. *Oral Surg. Oral Med. Oral Pathol. Oral Radiol. Endod.* **2006**, *101*, e37–e44. [CrossRef]

6. Ghanaati, S.; Booms, P.; Orlowska, A.; Kubesch, A.; Lorenz, J.; Rutkowski, J.; Landes, C.; Sader, R.; Kirkpatrick, C.; Choukroun, J. Advanced platelet-rich fibrin: A new concept for cell-based tissue engineering by means of inflammatory cells. *J. Oral Implantol.* **2014**, *40*, 679–689. [CrossRef]
7. Del Corso, M.; Vervelle, A.; Simonpieri, A.; Jimbo, R.; Inchingolo, F.; Sammartino, G.; Dohan Ehrenfest, D.M. Current knowledge and perspectives for the use of platelet-rich plasma (prp) and platelet-rich fibrin (prf) in oral and maxillofacial surgery Part 1: Periodontal and dentoalveolar surgery. *Curr. Pharm. Biotechnol.* **2012**, *13*, 1207–1230. [CrossRef]
8. Kuo, T.F.; Lin, M.F.; Lin, Y.H.; Lin, Y.C.; Su, R.J.; Lin, H.W.; Chan, W.P. Implantation of platelet-rich fibrin and cartilage granules facilitates cartilage repair in the injured rabbit knee: Preliminary report. *Clinics* **2011**, *66*, 1835–1838. [CrossRef]
9. Miron, R.J.; Fujioka-Kobayashi, M.; Bishara, M.; Zhang, Y.; Hernandez, M.; Choukroun, J. Platelet-rich fibrin and soft tissue wound healing: A systematic review. *Tissue Eng. Part B Rev.* **2017**, *23*, 83–99. [CrossRef]
10. Miron, R.J.; Fujioka-Kobayashi, M.; Hernandez, M.; Kandalam, U.; Zhang, Y.; Ghanaati, S.; Choukroun, J. Injectable platelet rich fibrin (i-prf): Opportunities in regenerative dentistry? *Clin. Oral Investig.* **2017**, *21*, 2619–2627. [CrossRef]
11. Miron, R.J.; Zucchelli, G.; Pikos, M.A.; Salama, M.; Lee, S.; Guillemette, V.; Fujioka-Kobayashi, M.; Bishara, M.; Zhang, Y.; Wang, H.L.; et al. Use of platelet-rich fibrin in regenerative dentistry: A systematic review. *Clin. Oral Investig.* **2017**, *21*, 1913–1927. [CrossRef]
12. Torul, D.; Bereket, M.C.; Onger, M.E.; Altun, G. Comparison of the regenerative effects of platelet-rich fibrin and plasma rich in growth factors on injured peripheral nerve: An experimental study. *J. Oral Maxillofac. Surg.* **2018**, *76*, 1823.e1–1823.e12. [CrossRef]
13. He, L.; Lin, Y.; Hu, X.; Zhang, Y.; Wu, H. A comparative study of platelet-rich fibrin (prf) and platelet-rich plasma (prp) on the effect of proliferation and differentiation of rat osteoblasts in vitro. *Oral Surg. Oral Med. Oral Pathol. Oral Radiol. Endod.* **2009**, *108*, 707–713. [CrossRef]
14. Borie, E.; Olivi, D.G.; Orsi, I.A.; Garlet, K.; Weber, B.; Beltran, V.; Fuentes, R. Platelet-rich fibrin application in dentistry: A literature review. *Int. J. Clin. Exp. Med.* **2015**, *8*, 7922–7929.
15. Kumar, Y.R.; Mohanty, S.; Verma, M.; Kaur, R.R.; Bhatia, P.; Kumar, V.R.; Chaudhary, Z. Platelet-rich fibrin: The benefits. *Br. J. Oral Maxillofac. Surg.* **2016**, *54*, 57–61. [CrossRef]
16. Choukroun, J.; Ghanaati, S. Reduction of relative centrifugation force within injectable platelet-rich-fibrin (prf) concentrates advances patients' own inflammatory cells, platelets and growth factors: The first introduction to the low speed centrifugation concept. *Eur. J. Trauma Emerg. Surg.* **2018**, *44*, 87–95. [CrossRef]
17. Wend, S.; Kubesch, A.; Orlowska, A.; Al-Maawi, S.; Zender, N.; Dias, A.; Miron, R.J.; Sader, R.; Booms, P.; Kirkpatrick, C.J.; et al. Reduction of the relative centrifugal force influences cell number and growth factor release within injectable prf-based matrices. *J. Mater. Sci. Mater. Med.* **2017**, *28*, 188. [CrossRef]
18. Whiting, D.; DiNardo, J.A. Teg and rotem: Technology and clinical applications. *Am. J. Hematol.* **2014**, *89*, 228–232. [CrossRef]
19. De Almeida Barros Mourao, C.F.; Calasans-Maia, M.D.; de Mello Machado, R.C.; de Brito Resende, R.F.; Alves, G.G. The use of platelet-rich fibrin as a hemostatic material in oral soft tissues. *Oral Maxillofac. Surg.* **2018**, *22*, 329–333. [CrossRef]
20. Ghanaati, S.; Herrera-Vizcaino, C.; Al-Maawi, S.; Lorenz, J.; Miron, R.J.; Nelson, K.; Schwarz, F.; Choukroun, J.; Sader, R. Fifteen years of platelet rich fibrin (prf) in dentistry and oromaxillofacial surgery: How high is the level of scientific evidence? *J. Oral Implantol.* **2018**, *44*, 471–492. [CrossRef]
21. Fujioka-Kobayashi, M.; Miron, R.J.; Hernandez, M.; Kandalam, U.; Zhang, Y.; Choukroun, J. Optimized platelet-rich fibrin with the low-speed concept: Growth factor release, biocompatibility, and cellular response. *J. Periodontol.* **2017**, *88*, 112–121. [CrossRef]
22. Abd El Raouf, M.; Wang, X.; Miusi, S.; Chai, J.; Mohamed AbdEl-Aal, A.B.; Nefissa Helmy, M.M.; Ghanaati, S.; Choukroun, J.; Choukroun, E.; Zhang, Y.; et al. Injectable-platelet rich fibrin using the low speed centrifugation concept improves cartilage regeneration when compared to platelet-rich plasma. *Platelets* **2017**, *30*, 213–221. [CrossRef]
23. Wang, X.; Zhang, Y.; Choukroun, J.; Ghanaati, S.; Miron, R.J. Effects of an injectable platelet-rich fibrin on osteoblast behavior and bone tissue formation in comparison to platelet-rich plasma. *Platelets* **2018**, *29*, 48–55. [CrossRef]

24. Wang, X.; Zhang, Y.; Choukroun, J.; Ghanaati, S.; Miron, R.J. Behavior of gingival fibroblasts on titanium implant surfaces in combination with either injectable-prf or prp. *Int. J. Mol. Sci.* **2017**, *18*, 331. [CrossRef]
25. Sohn, D.S.; Huang, B.; Kim, J.; Park, W.E.; Park, C.C. Utilization of Autologous Concentrated Growth Factors (CGF) Enriched Bone Graft Matrix (Sticky Bone) and CGF-Enriched Fibrin Membrane in Implant Dentistry. *J. Implant Adv. Clin. Dent.* **2015**, *7*, 11–29.
26. Kelly, J.M.; Rizoli, S.; Veigas, P.; Hollands, S.; Min, A. Using rotational thromboelastometry clot firmness at 5 minutes (rotem((r)) extem a5) to predict massive transfusion and in-hospital mortality in trauma: A retrospective analysis of 1146 patients. *Anaesthesia* **2018**, *73*, 1103–1109. [CrossRef]
27. Franchini, M.; Mengoli, C.; Cruciani, M.; Marietta, M.; Marano, G.; Vaglio, S.; Pupella, S.; Veropalumbo, E.; Masiello, F.; Liumbruno, G.M. The use of viscoelastic haemostatic assays in non-cardiac surgical settings: A systematic review and meta-analysis. *Blood Transfusion Trasfusione del Sangue* **2018**, *16*, 235–243.
28. Longstaff, C. Measuring fibrinolysis: From research to routine diagnostic assays. *J. Thromb. Haemost.* **2018**, *16*, 652–662. [CrossRef]
29. Meledeo, M.A.; Peltier, G.C.; McIntosh, C.S.; Voelker, C.R.; Bynum, J.A.; Cap, A.P. Functional stability of the teg 6s hemostasis analyzer under stress. *J. Trauma Acute Care Surg.* **2018**, *84*, S83–S88. [CrossRef]
30. Remy, K.E.; Yazer, M.H.; Saini, A.; Mehanovic-Varmaz, A.; Rogers, S.R.; Cap, A.P.; Spinella, P.C. Effects of platelet-sparing leukocyte reduction and agitation methods on in vitro measures of hemostatic function in cold-stored whole blood. *J. Trauma Acute Care Surg.* **2018**, *84*, S104–S114. [CrossRef]
31. Baksaas-Aasen, K.; Van Dieren, S.; Balvers, K.; Juffermans, N.P.; Naess, P.A.; Rourke, C.; Eaglestone, S.; Ostrowski, S.R.; Stensballe, J.; Stanworth, S.; et al. Data-driven development of rotem and teg algorithms for the management of trauma hemorrhage: A prospective observational multicenter study. *Ann. Surg.* **2018**. [CrossRef] [PubMed]
32. Lang, T.; Bauters, A.; Braun, S.L.; Potzsch, B.; von Pape, K.W.; Kolde, H.J.; Lakner, M. Multi-centre investigation on reference ranges for rotem thromboelastometry. *Blood Coagul. Fibrinolysis* **2005**, *16*, 301–310. [CrossRef]
33. Madurantakam, P.; Yoganarasimha, S.; Hasan, F.K. Characterization of leukocyte-platelet rich fibrin, a novel biomaterial. *J. Vis. Exp.* **2015**. [CrossRef]
34. Schar, M.O.; Diaz-Romero, J.; Kohl, S.; Zumstein, M.A.; Nesic, D. Platelet-rich concentrates differentially release growth factors and induce cell migration in vitro. *Clin. Orthop. Relat. Res.* **2015**, *473*, 1635–1643. [CrossRef]
35. Martino, M.M.; Briquez, P.S.; Ranga, A.; Lutolf, M.P.; Hubbell, J.A. Heparin-binding domain of fibrin(ogen) binds growth factors and promotes tissue repair when incorporated within a synthetic matrix. *Proc. Natl. Acad. Sci. USA* **2013**, *110*, 4563–4568. [CrossRef]
36. Ansarizadeh, M.; Mashayekhan, S.; Saadatmand, M. Fabrication, modeling and optimization of lyophilized advanced platelet rich fibrin in combination with collagen-chitosan as a guided bone regeneration membrane. *Int. J. Biol. Macromol.* **2019**, *125*, 383–391. [CrossRef] [PubMed]
37. Kardos, D.; Hornyak, I.; Simon, M.; Hinsenkamp, A.; Marschall, B.; Vardai, R.; Kallay-Menyhard, A.; Pinke, B.; Meszaros, L.; Kuten, O.; et al. Biological and mechanical properties of platelet-rich fibrin membranes after thermal manipulation and preparation in a single-syringe closed system. *Int. J. Mol. Sci.* **2018**, *19*, 3433. [CrossRef]

9

Biomimetic Mineralizing Agents Recover the Micro Tensile Bond Strength of Demineralized Dentin

Luiz Filipe Barbosa-Martins [1], Jossaria Pereira de Sousa [1], Lívia Araújo Alves [2], Robert Philip Wynn Davies [3] and Regina Maria Puppin-Rontanti [4,*]

1. Department of Pediatric Dentistry, Piracicaba Dental School, State University of Campinas, Piracicaba 13414-903; Brazil; flpmarttins@gmail.com (L.F.B.-M.); jossariasousa@gmail.com (J.P.d.S.)
2. Department of Oral Diagnosis, Piracicaba Dental School, State University of Campinas, Piracicaba 13414-903, Brazil; liviaaalves@hotmail.com
3. Division of Oral Biology, School of Dentistry, Faculty of Medicine & Health, University of Leeds, Leeds LS9 7TF, UK; R.P.W.Davies@leeds.ac.uk
4. Departments of Pediatric Dentistry and Restorative Dentistry, Piracicaba Dental School, University of Campinas, Piracicaba 13414-903, Brazil

* Correspondence: rmpuppin@unicamp.br

Abstract: Biomimetic remineralization is an approach that mimics natural biomineralization, and improves adhesive procedures. The aim of this paper was to investigate the influence of Dentin Caries-like Lesions (DCLL)-Producing Model on microtensile bond strength (μTBS) of etch and rinse adhesive systems and investigate the effect of remineralizing agents such as Sodium Fluoride (NaF), MI Paste™ (MP) and Curodont™ Repair (CR) on caries-affected dentin (n = 6). Nine groups were established: (1) Sound dentin; (2) Demineralized dentin/Chemical DCLL: (3) Demineralized dentin/Biological DCLL; (4) Chemical/DCLL + NaF; (5) Chemical/DCLL + MP; (6) Chemical/DCLL + CR; (7) Biological/DCLL + NaF; (8) Biological/DCLL + MP; (9) Biological/DCLL + CR. Then all dentin blocks were subjected to a bonding procedure with Adper™ Single Bond 2 adhesive system/Filtek Z350XT 4 mm high block, following this they were immersed in deionized water/24 h and then sectioned with ≅1 mm^2 beams. The μTBS test was conducted at 1 mm/min/500 N loading. Failure sites were evaluated by SEM (scanning electron microscopy (150×). μTBS data were submitted to factorial ANOVA and Tukey's test ($p < 0.05$). The highest values were found when demineralized dentin was treated with MP and CR, regardless caries lesion depth ($p < 0.05$). There was a predominance of adhesive/mixed in the present study. It was concluded that the use of the artificial dentin caries production models produces differences in the μTBS. Additionally MP and CR remineralizing agents could enhance adhesive procedures even at different models of caries lesion.

Keywords: dentin; desmineralization; microtensile bond strength

1. Introduction

During the execution of routine dental restorations, the hybrid structure formed by the dental bonding procedure occurs through the interaction and subsequent polymerization of monomers around the demineralized collagen matrix [1]. The oral cavity is a severe environment for the resin-dental bond to survive for a reasonable length of time, with thermomechanical changes, chemical attacks by acids and enzymes and other factors posing routine daily challenges. Therefore, to achieve effective and stable bonding, the preservation of dentin collagen is critical, since collagen represents the major organic component of the dentin matrix [2].

Caries is among the most common diseases worldwide [3], and the immediate bond strengths to caries-affected dentin are commonly 20–50% lower than to sound dentin [4–6]. The restoration of the normal conditions of the mineral content of the caries-affected dentin, prevents the action of enzymes in addition to providing an increased bond durability [7].

Biomimetic remineralization mimics the process of natural biomineralization by replacing demineralized collagen matrix water with apatite crystallites [7]. Caries-affected dentin is comprised of about 14–53% of water compared with sound dentin, which exhibits a much lower value [8]. Therefore, by replacing water with minerals at the dentin–resin interface, this would increase the mechanical properties and inhibit water-related hydrolysis [9].

It has recently been demonstrated that the use of remineralizing agents in dentin could recover the mechanical properties of the substrate [10]. In addition to sodium fluoride (NaF) and sodium phosphate (Na_3PO_4), casein phosphopeptide amorphous calcium phosphate (CPP-ACP), which is derived from milk protein, can release calcium phosphate assisting in enamel and dentin remineralization [11]. It acts mainly by inhibiting demineralization and enzymatic degradation [12]. Furthermore, recent studies have shown that the use CPP-ACP has no negative effect on bond strength [13,14]. The peptidic biomimetic matrix 'P_{11}-4', which has been incorporated into a clinical product (Curodont™ Repair) has shown encouraging results in early clinical trials. It has been shown to improve the visual appearance of carious lesions and increases the opacity on X-rays after treatment of proximal caries [15,16]. Additionally, following the application of P_{11}-4 and subsequent bonding procedures an increased resin-dentin bond strength has been observed [17].

The restructured demineralized collagen matrix found in caries-affected dentin process by interventions such as Sodium Fluoride (NaF), CPP-ACP contained in MI Paste™ (GC International) and P_{11}-4 peptide contained in Curodont™ Repair (Credentis AG), prior to adhesive procedures by an etch-and-rinse adhesive system (Adper™ Single Bond 2 (3M ESPE) in the demineralized dentin could be a promising proposal for adhesive clinical procedures.

Clinical binding procedures simulated by mechanical methods (i.e., TMBS, μTBS) often use artificial demineralized dentin. However, the lack of standardization of caries lesions creates technical difficulties for evaluation [18]. In vitro models have been used to produce demineralized dentin under controlled conditions [19–22]. Chemical methods provide superficial dentin demineralization, resulting in a substrate with similar hardness compared to natural caries-affected dentin [19]. Conversely, the microbiological method promotes an excessive softening of dentin, but with a more comparable morphological pattern of collagen degradation to natural caries lesions [19–22]. Pacheco et al., 2013 [23], evaluating molecular and structural lesions related to dental caries, produced by the chemical (GC), biological (GB), in situ (GIS) and natural (CNG) approaches, showed similar and lower surface hardness between CNG and GB of which GC and GIS, lower mineral content (Ca^{2+} and PO_4^{3-}) for GB and GNC than GC and GIS. Therefore, the structure and mechanical properties are different with respect to the caries model production and the remineralizing agents may act differently in the adhesion procedures depending on the model of caries lesions used.

To ascertain the potential efficacy of the bonding procedure carried out on remineralized dentin we aimed to evaluate different remineralization treatments and the method used in producing the simulated dentin-like caries lesions on the micro tensile bond strength of remineralized dentin. The hypothesis was that the Dentin Caries-like Lesions Producing Model and the remineralizing agents (Sodium Fluoride-(NaF), MI Paste™-(MP) and Curodont™ Repair-(CR)) affect microtensile bond strength-μTBS of etch-and-rinse adhesive system on caries-affected dentin.

2. Materials and Methods

Sixty-three sound human third molars were collected with patients' informed consent, as approved by the Ethics Committee of Piracicaba Dental School, University of Campinas (Protocol number 37634814.5.0000.5418). The teeth were stored in 0.1% thymol solution at 4 °C for no longer than 2 months after extraction. A 4.0 mm coronal dentin slice from each tooth was obtained by sectioning 2.0 mm below cement-enamel junction (CEJ), and 2.0 mm above CEJ, using a slow-speed water-cooled diamond saw (Isomet 1000, Buehler Ltd., Lake Bluff, IL, USA). Six dentin slices were used for sound dentin (control group-CG), and the others were randomly assigned into 2 groups (n = 24), according to the caries method production. The dentin surface of each specimen was wet polished with a 600-grit SiC paper (Arotec, São Paulo, Brazil) for 30 s to create a standardized smear layer. The dentin surfaces were carefully examined under a stereomicroscope at ×50 magnification to confirm the absence of enamel islets. The specimens were immediately subjected to production of caries in vitro. The group distribution is illustrated in Figure 1. To check the caries dentin depth, three teeth were chosen from each group and probed using a polarized light microscope (Figure 2).

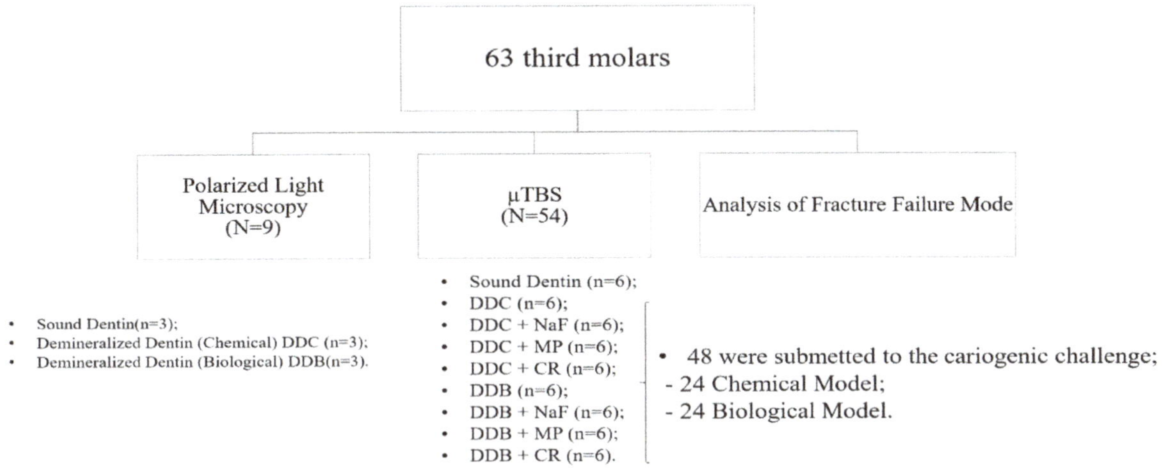

Figure 1. Experimental design. DDC—demineralized dentin provided by chemical model; DDC/NaF-DDC + 2% NaF; DDC/MP-DDC + MI Paste™; DDC/CR-DDC + Curodont™ Repair; DDB—demineralized dentin provided by biological model; DDB/NaF-DDB + 2% NaF; DDB/MP-DDB + MI Paste™; DDB/CR-DDB + Curodont™ Repair.

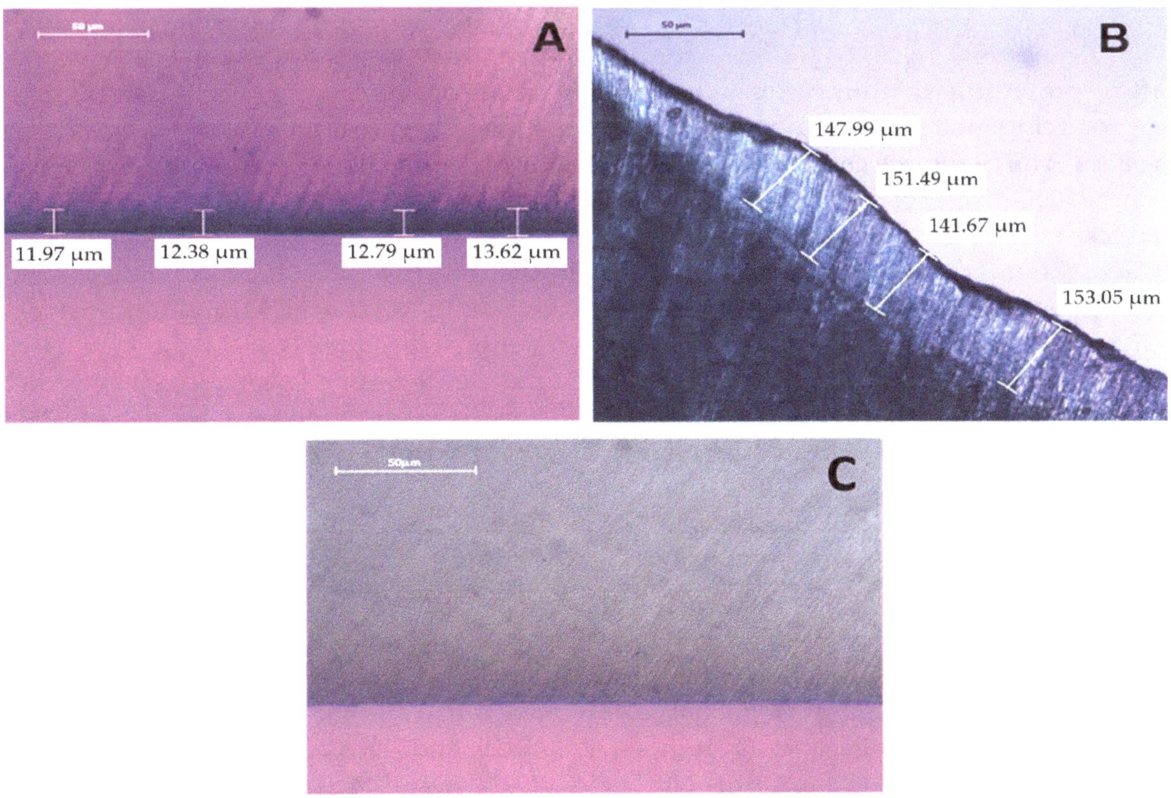

Figure 2. (**A**) Artificial caries lesions provided by Chemical Model; (**B**) Artificial caries lesions provided by Biological Model after removing the softened tissue; (**C**) Sound Dentin.

2.1. *Artificial Dentin Caries-Like Lesions (DCLL) Production Protocols*

Sixty dentin slices (54 teeth for μTBS and 6 for polarized light microscopy) were randomly assigned into 2 groups according to dentin-like caries lesions producing models: chemical (carboxymethylcellulose acid gel) and biological (Streptococcus mutans—UA159 biofilm).

2.1.1. Chemical Model

The specimens were submerged in vials containing 5 mL of 6% carboxymethylcellulose acid gel (0.1 M lactic acid titrated to pH 5.0 in a KOH solution) at pH 5.0 and 37 °C. The specimens remained in the gel for 48 h without renewal [23]. This model has been reported to supposedly provide a demineralized dentin similar to that of caries affected dentin.

2.1.2. Biological Model

The specimens were fixed with orthodontic wire on the lids of glass vials containing 250 mL of sterile deionized water and were sterilized with gamma radiation (14.5 kGy dose) for 60 h (Pacheco et al., 2013). Then, they were transferred to another glass vial containing 250 mL of sterile brain-heart infusion (BHI) broth (LabCenter, São Paulo, Brazil) supplemented with 0.5% yeast extract (LabCenter, São Paulo, Brazil), 0.5% glucose (LabCenter, São Paulo, Brazil), 1% sucrose (LabCenter, São Paulo, Brazil) and 2% *S. mutans* (UA159, ATCC, Oklahoma, OK, USA) incubated at 37 °C and supplemented with 10% CO_2, pH of around 4.0. Starter culture was transferred into 250 mL of fresh BHI and grown for 4 h at 37 °C under aerobic conditions. Optical density at 550 nm (A550) of all bacterial suspensions was adjusted to 0.05 prior to inoculation. Inoculation occurred only in the first day of the experiment, but the broth was renewed every 48 h over a 7-day period. The broth was Gram stained daily to monitor contamination. The resulting biofilm formed over the teeth was removed with gauze and the softer dentin layer was removed using #6 carbide drills; the removal ceased when dentin appearance was like that of caries-affected dentin [23].

2.2. *Polarized Light Microscopy (PLM)*

After providing dentin caries-like lesions, three specimens of each dentin caries-like lesions-producing models and control group were sectioned perpendicular to the occlusal surface to obtain slices. The two more central slices of each tooth were selected and polished with #800, #1200, #2400 and #4000-grit silicon carbide (SiC) paper (Buehler, Lake Buff, IL, USA), obtaining a 0.15 μm dentin thickness. Dentin slices were analyzed for the depth of demineralization on PLM (Leica DMLP, Leica microsystems, Wetzlar, Germany). The dentin slices were kept in 100% humidity throughout the investigation. Depth caries lesions were measured in a PLM (Leica DMLP, Leica microsystems) using 20×/0.4 (corr.) objective. Standard settings for contrast, brightness and light were used for all images. Four measurements were made in different parts of the same lesion from the lesion border to the deepest part of the lesion, for each dentin caries-like lesion model. An average depth for each specimen was calculated from the individual values based on depth difference between dentin caries-like lesions and sound dentin on the same specimen. Dentin caries-like lesions observed in the specimens subjected to Chemical Model presented x = 12.69 μm average depth and Biological Model x = 148.55 μm, measured using PLM.

2.3. *Dentin Surface Treatment*

Thirty-six teeth were assigned to 6 groups according to the remineralization treatment: demineralized dentin by chemical model (DDC) + treated with 0.2% NaF Solution (1 min)—DDC/NaF; DDC + treated with MI Paste™ (1 min)—DDC/MP; and DDC + treated with Curodont™ Repair—DDC/CR applied (5 min) plus Ca^{2+} and PO_4^{3-} Solution (1 min); demineralized dentin by biological model (DDB) + 0.2% NaF Solution—DDB/NaF; DDB + treated with MI Paste™ applied

(1 min)—DDB/MP; and DDB + treated with Curodont™ Repair—DDB/CR applied (5 min) plus Ca^{2+} and PO_4^{3-} Solution (1 min).

The specimens of groups DDC/NaF and DDB/NaF were remineralized using 0.1 mL of the 0.2% NaF. 0.2% NaF solution was applied on demineralized dentin surface and left dry for 1 min at room temperature for the groups DDC/NaF and DDB/NaF. 0.1 mL of the MI Paste™ was applied onto the surface of the specimens from DDC/MP and DDB/MP groups with microbrush for 1 min at room temperature, the excess paste was removed by washing with deionized water. For DDC/CR and DDB/CR groups, 50 μL of the Curodont™ Repair was applied and left for 5 min, then, a Ca^{2+} and PO_4^{3-} solution was applied and left onto surface for 1 min. For all treatments, the solution excess was removed with absorbent paper.

2.4. Bonding Procedures

A single operator applied the adhesive according to the manufacturer's instruction (Table 1). An LED light-curing unit (Bluephase, Ivoclar Vivadent; Schaan, Liechtenstein) was set to the low power mode with a light intensity of 650 mW/cm^2. A nanohybrid resin composite (Filtek Z350 XT, A2 (3M ESPE, St. Paul, MN, USA)) was used to create resin composite buildups in four layers of 1 mm each [17]. Each layer was light cured for 20 s, followed by a final polymerization of 60 s. The specimens were then stored at 100% humidity at 37 °C for 24 h.

Table 1. Materials, manufactures, components, batch numbers and application mode of tested materials.

Materials (Manufactures)	Main Components	Batch Number	Application Mode
0.2% NaF Solution	0.2 g of NaF in 100 mL deionized water	Made in the Lab *	1. Apply 1.0 mL of 0.2% NaF solution
Ca^{2+} and PO_4^{3-} Solution	Saturated solution of Ca^{2+} and PO_4^{3-} (1.5 mmol/L calcium, 0.9 mmol/L phosphate, and 150 mmol/L KCl in 20 mmol/L cacodylic buffer, pH 7.0) [24].	Made in the Lab	1. Apply 0.1 mL of Ca^{2+} and PO_4^{3-} solution
MI™ Paste—GC Internacional, Itabashi-ku, Tóquio, Japão	Glycerol, CPP-ACP, D-Sorbitol, Propylene glycol, Titanium dioxide and silicon	N2347319	1. Apply 0.1 mL of MI™ Paste
Curodont™ Repair—Credentis AG, Dorfstrasse, Windisch, Switzerland	P_{11}-4 peptide—amino acid sequence—(Ace-Gln-Gln-Arg-Phe-Glu-Trp-Glu-Phe-Glu-Gln-Gln-NH_2)	N342x	1. Apply 50 μL of Curodont™ Repair for 5 min 2. Apply 0.1 mL of Ca^{2+} and PO_4^{3-} solution
Scotchbond™ Universal Etchant—3M ESPE; St Paul, MN, USA	32% phosphoric acid	N345	1. Apply etchant for 15 s 2. Rinse for 10 s
Adper Single Bond 2.0—3M ESPE; St Paul, MN, USA	HEMA, water, ethanol, Bis-GMA, dimethacrylates, amines, metacrylate functional copolymer of polyacrylic and polyitaconic acids, 10% by weight of 5 nanometer-diameter spherical sílica particles	N42912	3. Blot water excess 4. Apply 2 consecutive coats of adhesive for 15 s with gentle agitation 5. Gently air dry for 5 s 6. Light-cure for 10 s
Filtek™ Z350 XT—3M ESPE; St Paul, MN, USA	BIS-GMA, Bis-EMA, UDMA, TEG-DMA, camphorquinone, non-agglomerated silica nanoparticles	N98354	1. Incremental insertion 2 mm 2. Light-cure for 20 s

* Pediatric Dentistry Laboratory.

2.5. Microtensile Bond Strength Test (μTBS)

After storage, the specimens were sectioned perpendicularly to the resin/dentin interface to produce dentin–resin beams with 1 mm^2 at cross-sectional area, using a low speed diamond saw (ISOMET 1000, Buehler Ltd., Lake Buff, IL, USA). From six to eight beams were obtained per tooth, each beam was measured with a digital caliper (Mitutoyo; Kawasaki, Japan) to determine the cross-sectional area. All beams were kept in deionized water for 24 h.

For μTBS measurements, each beam was fixed to a microtensile device with cyanocrylate glue (Super Bonder (#1883519), Loctite, Henkel Corp., Rocky Hill, CT, USA), and tested in a universal testing machine (DL 2000, EMIC, Equipment and Systems Ltda., São José dos Pinhais, Brazil). The test was carried out with a 500 N load at 1.0 mm/min cross speed until failure. The μTBS values were expressed in MPa.

2.6. Analysis of Failure Mode

All the fractured specimens from the microtensile bond strength analysis were assessed to determine the failure mode using SEM at ×50 and ×150 magnifications. The fractured surfaces of the beams were paired, air dried, mounted on aluminum stubs, gold coated, and examined by SEM (JSM-5600LV, JEOL; Tokyo, Japan), operated at 15 kV. The failure patterns were classified according to the following categories: adhesive, mixed (involving resin composite, adhesive and/ or dentin), cohesive failure in the resin composite, and cohesive failure in dentin [17,25,26].

2.7. Statistical Analysis

Bond strength values for each group were analyzed by Shapiro–Wilk test (R Software version 3.4.3, The R Foundation for Statistical Computing, Vienna, Austria) in order to assess the normality of the data distribution. Factorial ANOVA and post hoc Tukey test (R Software version 3.4.3, The R Foundation for Statistical Computing, Vienna, Austria) were used to determine statistically significant differences between factors: the dentin-like caries lesions model (two levels—chemical and biological models) and dentin remineralization treatment (four levels—SD, DD, NaF + DD, CPP-ACP + DD and P_{11}-4 + DD) on dentin/resin bond strength, and additional Dunnett test to determine statistically significant differences between the experimental groups and the control group (sound dentin). The Kruskal Wallis test was used to evaluate the failure mode. The R Software version 3.4.3 (The R Foundation for Statistical Computing, Vienna, Austria), was used to perform the tests. Statistical difference was set at $\alpha = 5\%$.

3. Results

The images of the lesions observed in Chemical Model x = 12.69 (average depth) (A) and Biological Model x = 148.55 (B) using polarized light microscopy are displayed in Figure 2.

Factorial ANOVA revealed a significant interaction between studied factors: dentin caries-like lesion model and remineralization treatment ($p < 0.001$). In addition, there was a statistically significant difference concerning artificial dentin caries-like lesion model ($p < 0.001$), and also between treatments ($p < 0.001$).

As shown in Table 2, a Tukey test (R Software version 3.4.3, The R Foundation for Statistical Computing, Vienna, Austria) revealed that μTBS values of NaF to demineralized dentin for both, chemical and biological dentin caries-like lesion models, were significantly lower than other remineralizing agents ($p < 0.001$). Biological DCLL model significantly reduced the microtensile bond strength when the dentin was treated by NaF and Curodont™ Repair ($p < 0.001$). Chemical DCLL model provided higher μTBS than the biological one, when demineralized dentin was treated by NaF and Curodont Repair ($p < 0.05$). In addition, dentin demineralized by the chemical DCLL treated with Curodont™ Repair provided the highest bond strength, and there was no significant difference from MI Paste™ for the same dentin condition, and they were significantly higher than sound dentin

($p < 0.05$). However, when DCLL was treated with MI Paste™, there was no influence regardless of the DCLL model ($p > 0.05$) and they were significantly higher than sound dentin ($p < 0.05$). However, only when NaF was used there was an observed lower µTBS than sound dentin ($p < 0.05$). For both DCLL models, demineralized dentin treated with NaF, MI Paste™ and Curodont™ Repair showed significant higher µTBS than demineralized dentin ($p < 0.01$). Demineralized dentin group showed the lowest bond strength for all groups ($p < 0.01$) (Table 2).

Table 2. Average and standard deviation of µTBS of demineralized dentin considering the Artificial Caries Development Models.

Experimental Groups	Artificial Caries Development Models	
	Chemical Model	Biological Model
Sound Dentin	43.32 ± 4.35	
Demineralized Dentin	21.96 ± 5.92 **Ca** *	22.89 ± 2.68 **Da** *
Demineralized Dentin + NaF	33.43 ± 10.42 **Ba** *	26.94 ± 6.70 **Cb** *
Demineralized Dentin + MI Paste™ (CPP-ACP)	45.25 ± 8.83 **Aa** *	47.95 ± 6.69 **Aa** *
Demineralized Dentin + Curodont™ Repair (P_{11}-4)	46.42 ± 12.03 **Aa** *	42.07 ± 7.83 **Bb**

Uppercase letters represent statistically significant difference in the column ($p < 0.001$). Lowercase letters represent no statistically significant difference in the row ($p > 0.05$). * indicates statistically significant difference with the control group (sound dentin) ($p < 0.05$) by additional Dunnett's test.

The failure modes of specimens are shown in Figure 3. The failure modes of DDC (76%) and DDB (85%) specimens were predominantly adhesive failure; Mixed failure were found for DDC-NaF (84%), DDB-NaF (61%), DDC-MI Paste™ (54%), DDB-MI Paste™ (68%), DDC-Curodont™ Repair (71%) and DDB-Curodont™ Repair (70%); cohesive failure in composite resin was observed in the DDB-NaF (4%); cohesive failure in dentin was observed in the DDC-MI Paste™ (6%) DDB-MI Paste™ (2%) and DDB-Curodont™ Repair (5%) groups. The failure patterns were often adhesive and mixed for all groups. There was no statistically significant difference between the fracture type by Kruskal-Wallis's test, concerning DCLL model ($p = 0.9967$).

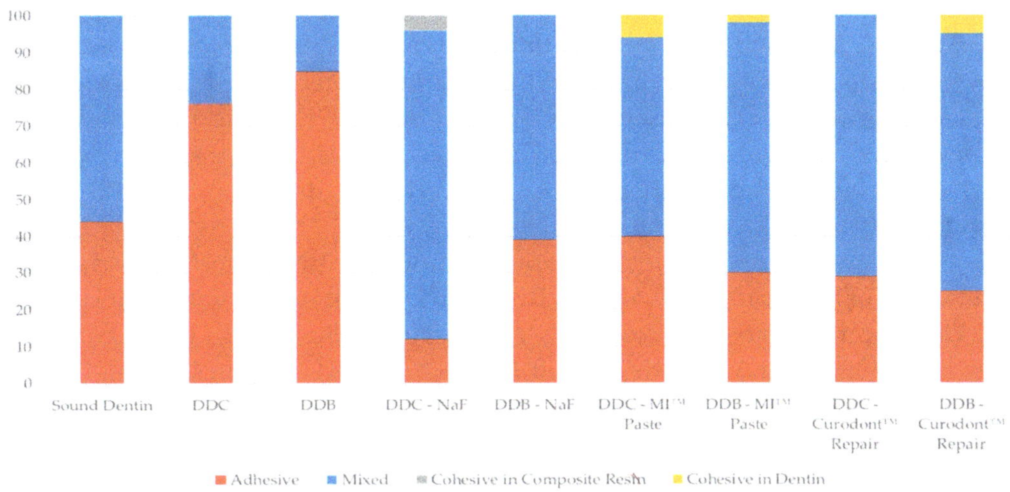

Figure 3. Distribution of failure modes. DDC—Demineralized Dentin by chemical model; DDB—Demineralized Dentin by biological model; NaF—Sodium Floride; MI Paste™-CPP-ACP—Casein phospopeptide-amorphous calcium phosphate; Curodont™ Repair—P_{11}-4—Peptide self-assembly.

Figure 4 shows representative SEMs for the fracture patterns observed for the different groups. Figure 3A—Cohesive failure on composite; 3B—Adhesive failure; 3C—Mixed failure; and 3D—cohesive failure on dentin.

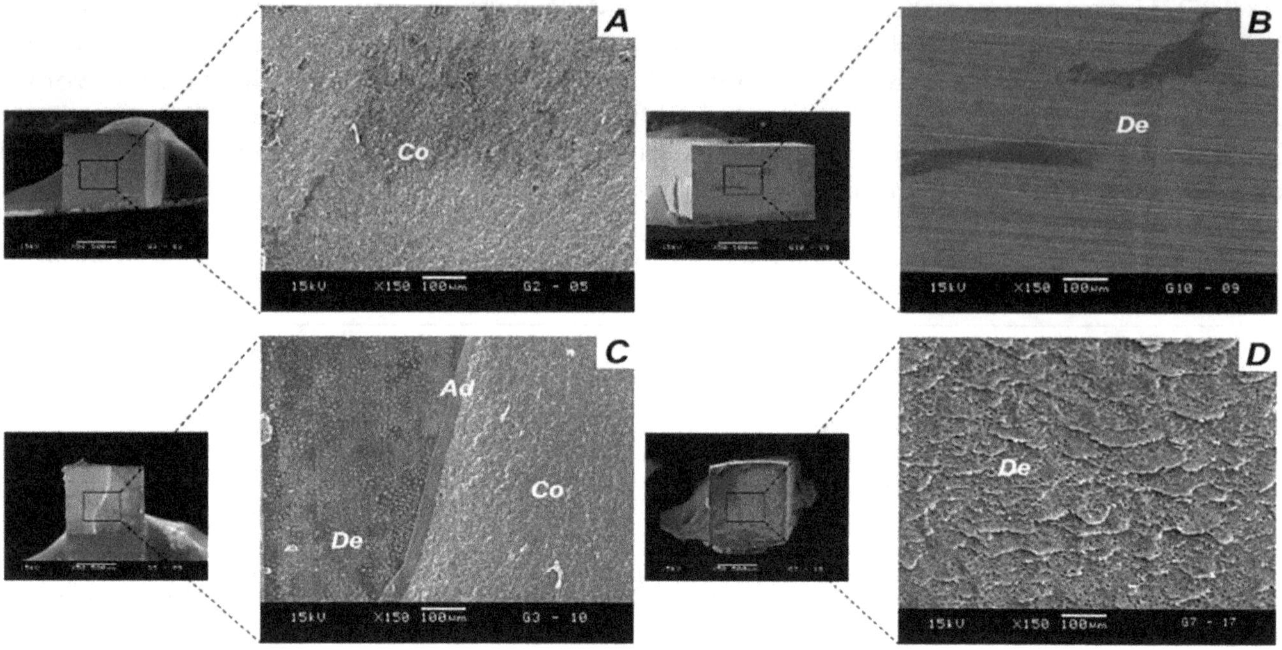

Figure 4. SEM image of failure modes. (**A**) Cohesive failure in Resin Composite; (**B**) Adhesive failure; (**C**) Mixed failure and (**D**) Cohesive failure in Dentin. Abbreviations shows areas of **Co**. Composite; **Ad**. Adhesive; **De**. Dentin.

4. Discussion

Considering the studies of bond strength on resin/dentin interfaces, the quality of the dentin substrate can play a key role in the longevity of the bonding [24,27–29]. In the present study, we have evaluated the influence of artificial caries development models (chemical and biological) and substrate conditions on resin/dentin bond strength. In this study, the first null hypothesis that there is a difference between DCLL models producing was proved, since there was no significant influence of the DCLL model on µTBS of demineralized dentin. However, the second hypothesis that there is influence of DCLL model and demineralized dentin treatment on µTBS of an etch and rinse adhesive system was rejected, since the µTBS values were dependent of DCLL model and mineralizing agent type. The highest µTBS were found when demineralized dentin was treated with for Curodont™ Repair and NaF ($p < 0.001$), although there was no significant difference on µTBS when dentin was treated with MI Paste ($p > 0.05$).

This study corroborates previous investigations demonstrating that the bonding procedures on demineralized dentin [30–32] present lower µTBS when compared to a sound one, regardless of the artificial caries development model (Table 2). Morphological changes in the substrate provided by caries production process can induce a decreased µTBS [20,33]. This reduction can be associated with changes in physical and chemical properties of the demineralized substrate when compared to sound dentin [34]. Demineralized dentin provides a high porosity in the inter-tubular dentin, exposure of collagen fibers along with decrease in mineral content [35] and partial penetration of resin monomers and a non-homogeneous hybrid layer [36]. In a porous hybrid layer, over time, mineral and organic matrix would be degraded giving rise to gaps which may be visible using a SEM which show a higher rate of degradation [36]. In addition, the demineralization of dentin surface results in a more hydrophobic surface, avoiding the wettability of the adhesive [17].

The caries lesion provided by a biological model, which uses *S. mutans* biofilm, seems to be quite similar to the natural ones, based on molecular and structural evaluations [23]. Another model used for providing dentin caries-like lesions is the chemical one, and it can be used to simulate caries-affected dentin [5].

It is desirable that bonding between mineralized tooth tissues, such as dentin, and the restorative materials must be sufficiently effective to resist varied challenges, such as biofilm attack, hydrolytic and enzymatic degradation, thermal and mechanical stress from repeated loading over many months or years [37,38]. The reinforcement of demineralized collagen matrix can be achieved using remineralizing agents [10,39]. The current biomimetic remineralization approach provides a proof-of-concept that utilizes nanotechnological principles to mimic natural biomineralization, extending the longevity of resin–dentin bonds [10]. The mineral reinforcement of collagen matrix found in demineralized dentin appears to be a strategy that restores conditions found on sound dentin, as seen in the present study. In the present study the biomimetic remineralization strategy provided a higher (CPP-ACP + Chemical and Biological DCCL models; P_{11}-4 + Biological DCCL) or similar (P_{11}-4) μTBS to demineralized dentin than sound one, while the NaF remineralization provided higher μTBS values than demineralized dentin, but lower than sound one. It can be observed that only for CCP-ACP, regardless DCLL model, the mineralizing agent provided a higher μTBS than sound dentin.

Despite it, concerning affected dentin, Bahari et al. (2014) [40] showed that 5 consecutive days of CPP-ACP application for 15 min did not have any significant effect on μTBS of SB to demineralized dentin. However, it has been considered that the methodology used in that study was quite different from that used in the present one. Firstly, according to the methodology description (Bahari et al, 2014) even sound dentin was submitted to the CPP-ACP action. Casein phosphopeptides (CPP) have been described to bind amorphous calcium phosphate, forming nano-complexes of casein phosphopeptide–amorphous calcium phosphate (CPP-ACP), thereby stabilizing in calcium phosphates [41,42]. Calcium and phosphate ions can easily diffuse into the porous lesion and deposits in the partially demineralized crystals and rebuild hydroxy-apatite crystals [43]. This further substantiates the theory that CPP-ACP is considered a biomaterial [44]. The presence of bioavailable calcium and phosphate present the MI Paste™ can maintain a supersaturated state in dental substrate [11]. Studies have demonstrated that CPP-ACP could reduce demineralization and increase remineralization of dentin [44,45]. It is possible that in that study the CPP-ACP could have been impregnated onto caries-affected dentin and sound dentin [13,46] in the same way.

It is well-established that the collagen matrix serves as a scaffold for crystal deposition but does not provide a mechanism for orderly nucleation of hydroxyapatite [39]. The results of the present study can be attributed to the ability of CPP-ACP to increase deposition of crystals on the dentin surface [47]. Furthermore, the CPP also has the capacity to stabilize nano-ACP [48]. Therefore, the deposition and stabilization may result in a restructuring of the characteristics found in sound dentin, showing the highest μTBS when demineralized dentin was treated with MI Paste. This reinforcement approach of demineralized collagen matrix structure may favor the bonding procedure. Further studies should be carried out to verify the stability of the bonding strength when CPP-ACP is used.

It is generally believed that extracellular matrix proteins, which play an important role in controlling apatite nucleation and growth in the dentin remineralization process [49], mediate a biomineralization process. Biomimetic remineralization represents a different approach to this by attempting to backfill the demineralized dentin collagen with liquid-like ACP nanoprecursor particles that are stabilized by biomimetic analogs of noncollagenous proteins [10,50]. In this way, maybe this particular nucleation would provide a regular and feasible restructuration of the demineralized dentin and also would provide a favorable substrate for bonding, due to the more hydrophyllic nature of the substrate [23].

Another interesting finding of the present study was the fact that the μTBS means of MI Paste™ group was higher than those found in sound dentin, and did not show a significant difference between either artificial caries development models. The remineralization process and the artificial caries development model, studied in this article, showed that the artificial caries development model affects only the μTBS of the demineralized dentin treated with NaF and P_{11}-4.

Similar to CCP-ACP, the P_{11}-4 approach using the DCLL chemical model provided significantly higher μTBS than sound dentin. The chemical model of DCLL provided a lower content of type I collagen and higher content of calcium and phosphate ions, than the Biological one [23]. The collagen is the precursor for mineralization, acting as a scaffold for mineral aggregation. However, when NaF is used, only a deposition of ions and CaF formation occurs on dentin surface. Possibly the high content of mineral ions decreased the surface energy of the demineralized dentin [23]. The opposite can be observed when biomimetic remineralization happens, using CPP-ACP or P_{11}-4. In this case, the mineralization occurs by organized crystal formation guided by the scaffold. This kind of surface can experience a high surface energy and a high level of wettability by resin monomers providing the highest μTBS [23].

The results of the study indicated that treatment with P_{11}-4, with a single application showed significant improvement on μTBS. Despite the fact that there was significant difference between the DCLL models, when P_{11}-4 is used, the μTBS values still show high values. For the biological model when the peptide P_{11}-4 was used no significant difference from sound dentin was observed. It is suggested that the use of the P_{11}-4 is able to nucleate hydroxyapatite and to promote repair of caries-like lesions in vitro. We have no knowledge in the literature of any report in which treatment with P_{11}-4 has been conducted in demineralized dentin, associating its effects with bonding procedures. However, research groups using other peptides, observed that this strategy mimics the functions of non-collagenous proteins (NCPs) [51,52]. This suggests that the action of the P_{11}-4 peptide reflects the reinforcing of demineralized collagen matrix.

The potential for enamel lesion repair of P_{11}-4 may mimic the functions of NPCs [15,53,54]. Several studies indicate that P_{11}-4 forms three dimensional fibrillar hierarchical structures resulting in gels in response to specific environmental triggers [53,54]. Assembled P_{11}-4 forms scaffold-like structures with negative charge domains, mirroring biological macromolecules in mineralized tissue extracellular matrices (ECM) [54].

Fluoride is well-known for its proved anti-cariogenic and antimicrobial capacity. Its ability to prevent demineralization and promote remineralization by calcium phosphate precipitation on dental surface by reducing the dissolution of hydroxyapatite [55]. Thus, the effect of demineralized dentin treated with NaF on the μTBS, improved the μTBS compared to demineralized dentin, but did not reach the sound dentin μTBS. It has to be considered that the dentin etching with 35% phosphoric acid increases the bonding efficacy of dental adhesives and removes the smear layer and the superficial part of the dentin, opening dentin tubules, demineralizing the dentin surface and increasing the microporosity of the intertubular dentin [56]. Despite the phosphoric acid used in the etching procedure removing part of the mineral deposits, possibly the reinforcement provided by NaF on demineralized dentin structure would improve the μTBS compared to demineralized dentin [57,58]. However, the differences found with μTBS of Chemical and Biological models can be explained by the deeper demineralization provided by biological model than the chemical one. Therefore, it is known that the mineral deposition of fluorides occurs on surface and generally causes hyper mineralization of the dentin and in dentin tubules [10,59–61]. The disorganized precipitation and deposit of mineral on dentin may mechanically obliterate the tubules reducing the performance of the restorative material [61], providing less efficiency of NaF treatment.

Another important aspect is that the NaF and Curodont Repair treatments showed a statistically significant difference between the DCLL. With regard to the treatment with NaF, a previous study [62] showed that this treatment is able to reduce the subsurface dentin demineralization compared with the control from 30 to 50 μm depth. At the other depths (60–220 μm) NaF showed no positive effect. Such results may be attributed to a possible reaction between NaF and demineralized dentin, producing soluble fluoride. In the present study, the demineralized dentin associated with NaF treatment exhibit mixed failure type. This result may be associated with a surface reinforcement, which was partially removed by the etching with the phosphoric acid during bonding procedures.

With the exception of the treatment with NaF, demineralized dentin treated with Curodont Repair has shown no negative influence on bond strength, as the biological DCLL did not differ from sound dentin. This behavior can be attributed to different interactions with the demineralized substrate, since the caries depth produced by the biological model DCLL was higher than chemical one. It has been reported that the P_{11}-4 scaffold can act as nucleator for hydroxyapatite, infiltrating into the porous lesions and increase the mineral diffusion within the lesion, restructuring the affected tissue [15].

Moreover, regardless of the artificial caries development model, the results presented in this study suggest that the use of remineralizing agents can reinforce the mechanical properties of demineralized dentin and would favor the durability of resin-dentin bonds, since the treated demineralized substrate provides an organized mineral surface. However, the degree of improvement in bonding strength is dependent on the artificial caries development model and dentin treatment. Further studies have to be carried out in order to observe the long-term efficacy of the remineralized dentin bonded to adhesive systems.

5. Conclusions

Based on the results of this study it can be concluded that:

MI Paste™ and Curodont™ Repair recovered higher μTBS values when compared to sound dentin. Each agent shows a different interaction with each artificial caries development model used. The remineralizing treatment of demineralized dentin is a potential approach for increasing bond strength of etch and rinse adhesive systems.

Author Contributions: Conceptualization, L.F.B.-M. and R.M.P.-R.; Data curation, L.F.B.-M.; Formal analysis, L.F.B.-M., J.P.d.S. and R.M.P.-R.; Funding acquisition, R.M.P.-R.; Investigation, L.F.B.-M. and R.M.P.-R.; Methodology, L.F.B.-M., J.P.d.S., L.A.A. and R.M.P.-R.; Project administration, L.F.B.-M., J.P.d.S. and R.M.P.-R.; Resources, R.M.P.-R.; Supervision, R.P.W.D. and R.M.P.-R.; Validation, L.F.B.-M. and J.P.d.S.; Visualization, L.F.B.-M., J.P.d.S., L.A.A. and R.M.P.-R.; Writing: original draft, L.F.B.-M., J.P.d.S., L.A.A., R.P.W.D. and Regina M.P.-R.; Writing: review and editing, L.F.B.-M., J.P.d.S., L.A.A., R.P.W.D. and R.M.P.-R.

Acknowledgments: The authors are grateful to Credentis (AG, Dorfstrasse, Windisch, Switzerland) for providing one of the materials tested.

References

1. Nakabayashi, N.; Kojima, K.; Masuhara, E. The promotion of adhesion by the infiltration of monomers into tooth substrates. *J. Biomed. Mater. Res.* **1982**, *16*, 265–273. [CrossRef] [PubMed]
2. Van, M.B.; Perdigão, J.; Lambrechts, P.; Vanherle, G. The clinical performance of adhesives. *J. Dent.* **1998**, *26*, 1–20.
3. Kassebaum, N.J.; Bernabé, E.; Dahiya, M.; Bhandari, B.; Murray, C.J.; Marcenes, W. Global burden of untreated caries: A systematic review and metaregression. *J. Dent. Res.* **2015**, *94*, 650–658. [CrossRef] [PubMed]
4. Spencer, P.; Wang, Y. Adhesive phase separation at the dentin interface under wet bonding conditions. *J. Biomed. Mater. Res.* **2002**, *62*, 447–456. [CrossRef] [PubMed]
5. de Carvalho, F.G.; de Fucio, S.B.; Sinhoreti, M.A.; Correr-Sobrinho, L.; Puppin Rontani, R.M. Confocal laser scanning microscopic analysis of the depth of dentin caries-like lesions in primary and permanent teeth. *Braz. Dent. J.* **2008**, *19*, 139–144. [CrossRef] [PubMed]
6. Perdigão, J.; Reis, A.; Loguercio, A.D. Dentin adhesion and MMPs: A comprehensive review. *J. Esthet. Restor. Dent.* **2013**, *25*, 219–241. [CrossRef] [PubMed]
7. Tjäderhane, L. Dentin bonding: Can we make it last? *Oper. Dent.* **2015**, *40*, 4–18. [CrossRef] [PubMed]
8. Nakajima, M.; Kunawarote, S.; Prasansuttiporn, T.; Tagami, J. Bonding to caries-affected dentin. *Jpn. Dent. Sci. Rev.* **2011**, *47*, 102–114. [CrossRef]
9. Niu, L.N.; Zhang, W.; Pashley, D.H.; Breschi, L.; Mao, J.; Chen, J.H.; Tay, F.R. Biomimetic remineralization of dentin. *Dent. Mater.* **2014**, *30*, 77–96. [CrossRef] [PubMed]
10. Tay, F.R.; Pashley, D.H. Biomimetic remineralization of resin-bonded acid-etched dentin. *J. Dent. Res.* **2009**, *88*, 719–724. [CrossRef] [PubMed]

11. Reynolds, E.C. Calcium phosphate-based remineralization systems: Scientific evidence? *Aust. Dent. J.* **2008**, *53*, 268–273. [CrossRef] [PubMed]
12. Brackett, M.G.; Agee, K.A.; Brackett, W.W.; Key, W.O.; Sabatini, C.; Kato, M.T.; Buzalaf, M.A.; Tjäderhane, L.; Pashley, D.H. Effect of Sodium Fluoride on the endogenous MMP Activity of Dentin Matrices. *J. Nat. Sci.* **2015**, *1*, 1–11.
13. Borges, B.C.; Souza-Junior, E.J.; da Costa Gde, F.; Pinheiro, I.V.; Sinhoreti, M.A.; Braz, R.; Montes, M.A. Effect of dentin pre-treatment with a casein phosphopeptide-amorphous calcium phosphate (CPP-ACP) paste on dentin bond strength in tridimensional cavities. *Acta Odontol. Scand.* **2013**, *71*, 271–277. [CrossRef] [PubMed]
14. Shafiei, F.; Derafshi, R.; Memarpour, M. Bond strength of self-adhering materials: Effect of dentin-desensitizing treatment with a CPP-ACP paste. *Int. J. Periodontics Restor. Dent.* **2017**, *37*, 337–343. [CrossRef] [PubMed]
15. Brunton, P.A.; Davies, R.P.; Burke, J.L.; Smith, A.; Aggeli, A.; Brookes, S.J.; Kirkham, J. Treatment of early caries lesions using biomimetic self-assembling peptides—A clinical safety trial. *Br. Dent. J.* **2013**, *215*, 1–6. [CrossRef] [PubMed]
16. Schlee, M.; Schad, T.; Koch, J.H.; Cattin, P.C.; Rathe, F. Clinical performance of self-assembling peptide P_{11}-4 in the treatment of initial proximal carious lesions: A practice-based case series. *J. Investig. Clin. Dent.* **2018**, *9*, e12286. [CrossRef] [PubMed]
17. Barbosa-Martins, L.F.; de Sousa, J.P.; de Castilho, A.R.F.; Puppin-Rontani, J.; Davies, R.P.W.; Puppin-Rontani, R.M. Enhancing bond strength on demineralized dentin by pre-treatment with selective remineralising agents. *J. Mech. Behav. Biomed. Mater.* **2018**, *81*, 214–221. [CrossRef] [PubMed]
18. Erhardt, M.C.; Rodrigues, J.A.; Valentino, T.A.; Ritter, A.V.; Pimenta, L.A. In vitro μTBS of one-bottle adhesive systems: Sound versus artificially-created caries-affected dentin. *J. Biomed. Mater. Res. B Appl. Biomater.* **2008**, *86*, 181–187. [CrossRef] [PubMed]
19. Marquezan, M.; Corrêa, F.N.; Sanabe, M.E.; Rodrigues Filho, L.E.; Hebling, J.; Guedes-Pinto, A.C.; Mendes, F.M. Artificial methods of dentine caries induction: A hardness and morphological comparative study. *Arch. Oral Biol.* **2009**, *54*, 1111–1117. [CrossRef] [PubMed]
20. Zanchi, C.H.; Lund, R.G.; Perrone, L.R.; Ribeiro, G.A.; Del Pino, F.A.; Pinto, M.B.; Demarco, F.F. Microtensile bond strength of two-step etch-and-rinse adhesive systems on sound and artificial caries-affected dentin. *Am. J. Dent.* **2010**, *23*, 152–156. [PubMed]
21. Sanabe, M.E.; de Souza Costa, C.A.; Hebling, J. Exposed collagen in aged resin–dentin bonds produced on sound and caries-affected dentin in the presence of chlorhexidine. *J. Adhes. Dent.* **2011**, *13*, 117–124. [PubMed]
22. Joves, G.J.; Inoue, G.; Nakashima, S.; Sadr, A.; Nikaido, T.; Tagami, J. Mineral density, morphology and bond strength of natural versus artificial caries-affected dentin. *Dent. Mater. J.* **2013**, *32*, 138–143. [CrossRef] [PubMed]
23. Pacheco, L.F.; Banzi, É.; Rodrigues, E.; Soares, L.E.; Pascon, F.M.; Correr-Sobrinho, L.; Puppin-Rontani, R.M. Molecular and structural evaluation of dentin caries-like lesions produced by different artificial models. *Braz. Dent. J.* **2013**, *24*, 610–618. [CrossRef] [PubMed]
24. Zancopé, B.R.; Rodrigues, L.P.; Parisotto, T.M.; Steiner-Oliveira, C.; Rodrigues, L.K.A.; Nobre-dos-Santos, M. CO_2 laser irradiation enhances CaF_2 formation and inhibits lesion progression on demineralized dental enamel—In vitro study. *Lasers Med. Sci.* **2016**, *31*, 539–547. [CrossRef] [PubMed]
25. Armstrong, S.; Breschi, L.; Özcan, M.; Pfefferkorn, F.; Ferrari, M.; Van Meerbeek, B. Academy of Dental Materials guidance on in vitro testing of dental composite bonding effectiveness to dentin/enamel using micro-tensile bond strength (μTBS) approach. *Dent. Mater.* **2017**, *33*, 133–143. [CrossRef] [PubMed]
26. Bacchi, A.; Abuna, G.; Babbar, A.; Sinhoreti, M.A.C.; Feitosa, V.P. Influence of 3-month simulated pulpal pressure on the microtensile bond strength of simplified resin luting systems. *J. Adhes. Dent.* **2015**, *17*, 265–271. [PubMed]
27. Peixoto, A.C.; Bicalho, A.A.; Isolan, C.P.; Maske, T.T.; Moraes, R.R.; Cenci, M.S.; Soares, C.J.; Faria-e-Silva, A.L. Bonding of adhesive luting agents to caries-affected dentin induced by a microcosm biofilm model. *Oper. Dent.* **2015**, *40*, 102–111. [CrossRef] [PubMed]

28. Qi, Y.P.; Li, N.; Niu, L.N.; Primus, C.M.; Ling, J.Q.; Pashley, D.H.; Tay, F.R. Remineralization of artificial dentinal caries lesions by biomimetically modified mineral trioxide aggregate. *Acta Biomater.* **2012**, *8*, 836–842. [CrossRef] [PubMed]
29. Robinson, C.; Brookes, S.J.; Kirkham, J.; Wood, S.R.; Shore, R.C. In vitro studies of the penetration of adhesive resins into artificial caries-like lesions. *Caries Res.* **2001**, *35*, 136–141. [CrossRef] [PubMed]
30. Lenzi, T.L.; Calvo, A.F.; Tedesco, T.K.; Ricci, H.A.; Hebling, J.; Raggio, D.P. Effect of method of caries induction on aged resin–dentin bond of primary teeth. *BMC Oral Health* **2015**, *15*, 79. [CrossRef] [PubMed]
31. Yoshiyama, M.; Doi, J.; Nishitani, Y.; Itota, T.; Tay, F.R.; Carvalho, R.M.; Pashley, D.H. Bonding ability of adhesive resins to caries-affected and caries-infected dentin. *J. Appl. Oral Sci.* **2004**, *12*, 171–176. [CrossRef] [PubMed]
32. Doozandeh, M.; Firouzmandi, M.; Mirmohammadi, M. The simultaneous effect of extended etching time and casein phosphopeptide-amorphous calcium phosphate containing paste application on shear bond strength of etch-and-rinse adhesive to caries-affected dentin. *J. Contemp. Dent. Pract.* **2015**, *16*, 794–799. [CrossRef] [PubMed]
33. Ceballos, L.; Camejo, D.G.; Victoria Fuentes, M.; Osorio, R.; Toledano, M.; Carvalho, R.M.; Pashley, D.H. Microtensile bond strength of total-etch and self-etching adhesives to caries-affected dentine. *J. Dent.* **2003**, *31*, 469–477. [CrossRef]
34. Fusayama, T.; Kurosaki, N. Structure and removal of carious dentin. *Int. Dent. J.* **1972**, *22*, 401–411. [PubMed]
35. Wang, S.; Huang, C.; Zheng, T.L.; Zhang, Z.X.; Wang, Y.N.; Cheng, X.R. Microtensile bond strength and morphological evaluations of total-etch and self-etch adhesives to caries-affected dentin. *Zhonghua Kou Qiang Yi Xue Za Zhi* **2006**, *41*, 323–326. [PubMed]
36. Sano, H.; Yoshiyama, M.; Ebisu, S.; Burrow, M.F.; Takatsu, T.; Ciucchi, B.; Carvalho, R.; Pashley, D.H. Comparative SEM and TEM observations of nanoleakage within the hybrid layer. *Oper. Dent.* **1995**, *20*, 160–167. [PubMed]
37. Stanislawczuk, R.; Pereira, F.; Muñoz, M.A.; Luque, I.; Farago, P.V.; Reis, A.; Loguercio, A.D. Effects of chlorhexidine-containing adhesives on the durability of resin–dentine interfaces. *J. Dent.* **2014**, *42*, 39–47. [CrossRef] [PubMed]
38. Nassar, M.; Hiraishi, N.; Shimokawa, H.; Tamura, Y.; Otsuki, M.; Kasugai, S.; Ohya, K.; Tagami, J. The inhibition effect of non-protein thiols on dentinal matrix metalloproteinase activity and HEMA cytotoxicity. *J. Dent.* **2014**, *42*, 312–318. [CrossRef] [PubMed]
39. Liu, Y.; Kim, Y.K.; Dai, L.; Li, N.; Khan, S.O.; Pashley, D.H.; Tay, F.R. Hierarchical and non-hierarchical mineralisation of collagen. *Biomaterials* **2011**, *32*, 1291–1300. [CrossRef] [PubMed]
40. Bahari, M.; Savadi Oskoee, S.; Kimyai, S.; Pouralibaba, F.; Farhadi, F.; Norouzi, M. Effect of casein phosphopeptide-amorphous calcium phosphate treatment on microtensile bond strength to carious affected dentin using two adhesive strategies. *J. Dent. Res. Dent. Clin. Dent. Prospects* **2014**, *8*, 141–147. [PubMed]
41. Reynolds, E.C. Anticariogenic complexes of amorphous calcium phosphate stabilized by casein phosphopeptides: A review. *Spec. Care Dent.* **1998**, *18*, 8–16. [CrossRef]
42. Cross, K.J.; Huq, N.L.; Reynolds, E.C. Casein phosphopeptides in oral health–chemistry and clinical applications. *Curr. Pharm. Des.* **2007**, *13*, 793–800. [CrossRef] [PubMed]
43. Kumar, V.L.; Itthagarun, A.; King, N.M. The effect of casein phosphopeptide-amorphous calcium phosphate on remineralization of artificial caries-like lesions: An in vitro study. *Aust. Dent. J.* **2008**, *53*, 34–40. [CrossRef] [PubMed]
44. Cao, Y.; Mei, M.L.; Xu, J.; Lo, E.C.; Li, Q.; Chu, C.H. Biomimetic mineralisation of phosphorylated dentine by CPP-ACP. *J. Dent.* **2013**, *41*, 818–825. [CrossRef] [PubMed]
45. Rahiotis, C.; Vougiouklakis, G. Effect of a CPP-ACP agent on the demineralization and remineralization of dentine in vitro. *J. Dent.* **2007**, *35*, 695–698. [CrossRef] [PubMed]
46. Sattabanasuk, V.; Burrow, M.F.; Shimada, Y.; Tagami, J. Resin bonding to dentine after casein phosphopeptide-amorphous calcium phosphate (CPP-ACP) treatments. *J. Adhes. Sci. Technol.* **2009**, *23*, 1149–1161. [CrossRef]
47. Adebayo, O.A.; Burrow, M.F.; Tyas, M.J. Resin-dentine interfacial morphology following CPP-ACP treatment. *J. Dent.* **2010**, *38*, 96–105. [CrossRef] [PubMed]
48. Rahiotis, C.; Vougiouklakis, G.; Eliades, G. Characterization of oral films formed in the presence of a CPP-ACP agent: An in situ study. *J. Dent.* **2008**, *36*, 272–280. [CrossRef] [PubMed]

49. Jee, S.S.; Thula, T.T.; Gower, L.B. Development of bone-like composites via the polymer-induced liquid-precursor (PILP) process. Part 1: Influence of polymer molecular weight. *Acta Biomater.* **2010**, *6*, 3676–3686. [CrossRef] [PubMed]
50. Kim, J.; Gu, L.; Breschi, L.; Tjäderhane, L.; Choi, K.K.; Pashley, D.H.; Tay, F.R. Implication of ethanol wet-bonding in hybrid layer remineralization. *J. Dent. Res.* **2010**, *89*, 575–580. [CrossRef] [PubMed]
51. Wang, D.Y.; Zhang, L.; Chen, J.H. The role of dentinal matrix metalloproteinases in collagenous degeneration of tooth tissue. *Zhonghua Kou Qiang Yi Xue Za Zhi* **2011**, *46*, 379–381. [PubMed]
52. Cao, Y.; Liu, W.; Ning, T.; Mei, M.L.; Li, Q.L.; Lo, E.C.; Chu, C.H. A novel oligopeptide simulating dentine matrix protein 1 for biomimetic mineralization of dentine. *Clin. Oral. Investig.* **2014**, *18*, 873–881. [CrossRef] [PubMed]
53. Aggeli, A.; Bell, M.; Boden, N.; Carrick, L.M.; Strong, A.E. Self-assembling peptide polyelectrolyte beta-sheet complexes form nematic hydrogels. *Angew. Chem.* **2003**, *42*, 5761–5764. [CrossRef]
54. Kirkham, J.; Firth, A.; Vernals, D.; Boden, N.; Robinson, C.; Shore, R.C.; Brookes, S.J.; Aggeli, A. Self-assembling peptide scaffolds promote enamel remineralization. *J. Dent. Res.* **2007**, *86*, 426–430. [CrossRef] [PubMed]
55. ten Cate, J.M. Remineralization of caries lesions extending into dentin. *J. Dent. Res.* **2001**, *80*, 1407–1411. [CrossRef] [PubMed]
56. Marshall, G.W., Jr.; Balooch, M.; Kinney, J.H.; Marshall, S.J. Atomic force microscopy of conditioning agents on dentin. *J. Biomed. Mater. Res.* **1995**, *29*, 1381–1387. [CrossRef] [PubMed]
57. Kato, M.T.; Bolanho, A.; Zarella, B.L.; Salo, T.; Tjäderhane, L.; Buzalaf, M.A. Sodium fluoride inhibits MMP-2 and MMP-9. *J. Dent. Res.* **2014**, *93*, 74–77. [CrossRef] [PubMed]
58. Altinci, P.; Mutluay, M.; Seseogullari-Dirihan, R.; Pashley, D.; Tjäderhane, L.; Tezvergil-Mutluay, A. NaF inhibits matrix-bound cathepsin-mediated dentin matrix degradation. *Caries Res.* **2016**, *50*, 124–132. [CrossRef] [PubMed]
59. Arends, J.; Christoffersen, J. Nature and role of loosely bound fluoride in dental caries. *J. Dent. Res.* **1990**, *69*, 601–605. [CrossRef] [PubMed]
60. Arends, J.; Christoffersen, J.; Ruben, J.; Jongebloed, W.L. Remineralization of bovine dentine in vitro. The influence of the F content in solution on mineral distribution. *Caries Res.* **1989**, *23*, 309–314. [CrossRef] [PubMed]
61. Prabhakar, A.R.; Manojkumar, A.J.; Basappa, N. In vitro remineralization of enamel subsurface lesions and assessment of dentine tubule occlusion from NaF dentifrices with and without calcium. *J. Indian Soc. Pedodontics Prev. Dent.* **2013**, *31*, 29–35. [CrossRef] [PubMed]
62. Comar, L.P.; Souza, B.M.; Gracindo, L.F.; Buzalaf, M.A.; Magalhães, A.C. Impact of experimental nano-HAP pastes on bovine enamel and dentin submitted to a pH cycling model. *Braz. Dent. J.* **2013**, *24*, 273–278. [CrossRef] [PubMed]

10

Potential for Drug Repositioning of Midazolam for Dentin Regeneration

Takeo Karakida [1], Kazuo Onuma [2], Mari M. Saito [1], Ryuji Yamamoto [1], Toshie Chiba [3], Risako Chiba [1], Yukihiko Hidaka [4], Keiko Fujii-Abe [4], Hiroshi Kawahara [4] and Yasuo Yamakoshi [1,*]

1 Department of Biochemistry and Molecular Biology, School of Dental Medicine, Tsurumi University, 2-1-3 Tsurumi, Tsurumi-ku, Yokohama 230-8501, Japan; karakida-t@tsurumi-u.ac.jp (T.K.); saito-mari@tsurumi-u.ac.jp (M.M.S.); yamamoto-rj@tsurumi-u.ac.jp (R.Y.); chiba-r@tsurumi-u.ac.jp (R.C.)
2 National Institute of Advanced Industrial Science & Technology, Central 6, 1-1-1 Higashi, Tsukuba, Ibaraki 305-8566, Japan; k.onuma@aist.go.jp
3 Research Center of Electron Microscopy, School of Dental Medicine, Tsurumi University, 2-1-3 Tsurumi, Tsurumi-ku, Yokohama 230-8501, Japan; chiba-t@tsurumi-u.ac.jp
4 Department of Dental Anesthesiology, School of Dental Medicine, Tsurumi University, 2-1-3 Tsurumi, Tsurumi-ku, Yokohama 230-8501, Japan; 2911002@stu.tsurumi-u.ac.jp (Y.H.); fujii-keiko@tsurumi-u.ac.jp (K.F.-A.); kawahara-h@tsurumi-u.ac.jp (H.K.)
* Correspondence: yamakoshi-y@tsurumi-u.ac.jp

Abstract: Drug repositioning promises the advantages of reducing costs and expediting approval schedules. An induction of the anesthetic and sedative drug; midazolam (MDZ), regulates inhibitory neurotransmitters in the vertebrate nervous system. In this study we show the potential for drug repositioning of MDZ for dentin regeneration. A porcine dental pulp-derived cell line (PPU-7) that we established was cultured in MDZ-only, the combination of MDZ with bone morphogenetic protein 2, and the combination of MDZ with transforming growth factor-beta 1. The differentiation of PPU-7 into odontoblasts was investigated at the cell biological and genetic level. Mineralized nodules formed in PPU-7 were characterized at the protein and crystal engineering levels. The MDZ-only treatment enhanced the alkaline phosphatase activity and mRNA levels of odontoblast differentiation marker genes, and precipitated nodule formation containing a dentin-specific protein (dentin phosphoprotein). The nodules consisted of randomly oriented hydroxyapatite nanorods and nanoparticles. The morphology, orientation, and chemical composition of the hydroxyapatite crystals were similar to those of hydroxyapatite that had transformed from amorphous calcium phosphate nanoparticles, as well as the hydroxyapatite in human molar dentin. Our investigation showed that a combination of MDZ and PPU-7 cells possesses high potential of drug repositioning for dentin regeneration.

Keywords: drug repositioning; cell; dentin; hydroxyapatite; nanorod; nanoparticle

1. Introduction

Tissue engineering is a multidisciplinary science. Applications of tissue engineering are founded on three components; a cell source, a scaffold, and bioactive molecules. In the field of dental tissue engineering, various soft and hard dental tissues have been regenerated in vitro using stem cells [1]. Dental pulp stem cells (DPSCs) have been isolated with various techniques and used for studies related to the cell differentiation potential and scaffolding for tissue regeneration [2,3]. DPSCs can differentiate into multiple cell types, including odontogenic and osteogenic cells, osteocytes, chondrocytes, vascular cells, neurons, and hepatocytes. In addition, DPSCs are used to generate induced pluripotent stem (iPS) cells.

In the dental research field, dental pulp-derived cells that express alkaline phosphatase (ALP) and odontoblastic marker genes, and that form precipitated nodules when cultured in a medium containing β-glycerophosphate and ascorbic acid, are generally assumed to be differentiated odontoblast-like cells. A number of odontoblastic cell lines have been established from rat [4,5], mouse [6], cattle [7], pig [8], and human [9,10] dental pulp tissues. Odontoblastic differentiation is induced by many factors, which are associated with ectoderm–mesenchyme molecular interactions. Various factors participate in the regulation of dental pulp cell differentiation, such as bone morphogenetic protein (BMP) [11,12], fibroblast growth factors (FGF) [13], and transforming growth factor beta (TGF-β) [14,15].

Drug repositioning is when new therapeutic applications are identified for existing drugs. In addition to the studies on dental pulp cells expressing cytokines, such as BMP, FGF, and TGF-β, existing drugs for treating Alzheimer's disease have been reported to promote dentin regeneration [16]. In Japan, Alzheimer's drugs such as donepezil hydrochloride (Aricept) have been widely used as acetylcholinesterase inhibitors that prevents acetylcholine, an excitatory neurotransmitter in the vertebrate nervous system. This study focuses on repositioning midazolam (MDZ), which controls gamma-aminobutyric acid (GABA), the principal inhibitory neurotransmitter in the mammalian central nervous system. Midazolam (MDZ) is a chemically synthesized imidazobenzodiazepine derivative that possesses pharmacological effects as a hypnotic, sedative, and anesthetic, has anti-anxiety and anticonvulsant properties, and acts as muscle relaxant [17]. In the dental field, MDZ has been used mainly as a sedative prior to dental anesthesia. The intravenous MDZ formulation has been recommended as a first-line drug for treating convulsive status epilepticus [18]. Intravenous MDZ has not been approved to treat status epilepticus in most countries, but it has been used off-label for patients in Japan. In tumor and cancer cells, MDZ induces cellular apoptosis by regulating the caspase pathways, endoplasmic reticulum stress, autophagy, and the cell cycle [19–22]. Few studies have focused on the effect of MDZ on dental pulp cells, although an in vitro study using human mesenchymal stem cells (hMSCs) has shown that MDZ inhibits ALP activity and calcium deposition in hMSCs, suggesting a suppressive effect on osteogenic differentiation [23]. In this study, using dental pulp cells, we examine the potential for drug repositioning of MDZ for dentin regeneration at the cell biological, genetic, protein, and crystal engineering levels.

2. Results

2.1. Combined Effect of MDZ with BMP2 or TGF-β1 on Differentiation of the PPU-7 Cell Line

MDZ is a short-acting benzodiazepine derivative with an imidazole structure and a molecular weight of 325.77 g/mol (Figure 1a). To investigate the effect of MDZ on dentin regeneration, we used a porcine animal model to establish dental pulp-derived cell lines (PPU) and ultimately selected the PPU-7 cell line for the present study (see Figures S1–S3). Because alkaline phosphatase (ALP) is considered the initial marker for the differentiation of mesenchymal cells into hard tissue-forming cells such as osteoblasts or odontoblasts [24,25], we investigated the effects of MDZ on ALP activity in the PPU-7 cell line by using a quantitative colorimetric method with a p-nitrophenylphosphate as the substrate and examined the combination of MDZ (0-10 μM) with a recombinant human BMP2 (rhBMP2) (500 ng/mL) or a recombinant human TGF-β1 (rhTGF-β1) (1 ng/mL) (Figure 1b). When the ALP activity level of the control (i.e., 0 μM MDZ, 0 ng/mL rhBMP2, 0 ng/mL rhTGF-β1) was set at 1.0, the addition of MDZ-only significantly enhanced ALP activity in PPU-7 cells in a concentration-dependent manner, especially the ALP activity at 10 μM MDZ (i.e., 10 μM MDZ, 0 ng/mL rhBMP2, 0 ng/mL rhTGF-β1), which was 1.75-fold higher than the control. BMP2-only (i.e., 0 μM MDZ, 500 ng/mL rhBMP2, 0 ng/mL rhTGF-β1) and TGF-β1-only (i.e., 0 μM MDZ, 0 ng/mL rhBMP2, 1 ng/mL rhTGF-β1) also slightly or significantly enhanced the ALP activity. The combination of rhBMP2 or rhTGF-β1 with MDZ (MDZ and BMP2 or MDZ and TGF-β1) (5 or 10 μM) slightly increased ALP activity (1.14–1.27-fold for MDZ and BMP2, and 1.28–1.29-fold for MDZ and TGF-β1) compared to the control. ALP staining for the mineral-induced PPU-7 cells displayed blue colored staining images (Figure 1c).

The cells were densely distributed on the plate of MDZ-only, whereas the combinations of MDZ and BMP2 as well as MDZ and TGF-β1 displayed a low density.

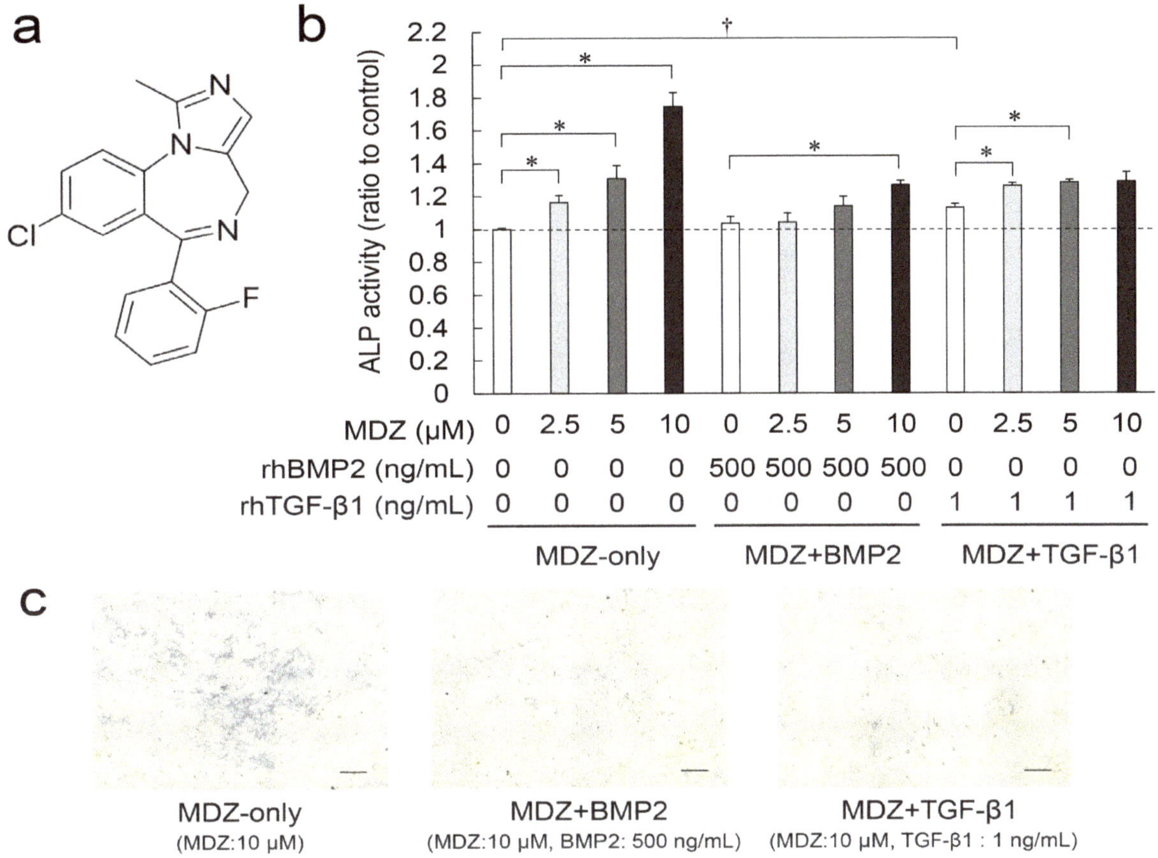

Figure 1. Combined effect of midazolam (MDZ) with bone morphogenetic protein 2 (BMP2) or transforming growth factor beta 1 (TGF-β1) on alkaline phosphatase (ALP) activity in the porcine dental pulp-derived (PPU-7) cell line. (**a**) Structure of MDZ. (**b**) ALP-inducing activity of midazolam without BMP2 or TGF-β1 (MDZ-only), midazolam with BMP2 (MDZ and BMP2) and midazolam with TGF-β1 (MDZ and TGF-β1) in PPU-7 cells. ALP activities are indicated as increasing or decreasing ratios relative to the level of the control (i.e., 0 μM MDZ, 0 ng/mL BMP2, 0 ng/mL TGF-β1), which was set at 1 (dotted line). Values are the means ± standard error of six culture wells. Significant differences are indicated by an asterisk (* $p < 0.05$, Steel's test) or a dagger († $p < 0.05$, Mann–Whitney U-test). (**c**) ALP staining for PPU-7 cells cultured with MDZ-only, MDZ and BMP2, MDZ and TGF-β1 (Scale bar: 200 μm).

2.2. *Effect of MDZ on Temporal Changes in Gene Expression of PPU-7 Cell Line*

Since the MDZ-only treatment was more effective in enhancing ALP activity and inducing mineralization in PPU-7 cells than the combination treatment of MDZ with BMP2 or TGF-β1, we investigated the effect of MDZ-only on gene expression in the PPU-7 cell line. The gene expression of a panel of odontoblastic, osteoblastic and chondrocytic markers in PPU-7 cells at one and seven days after MDZ treatment was analyzed by quantitative polymerase chain reaction (qPCR) (Figure 2). For odontoblastic markers (Figure 2a), we quantified the mRNA expression levels of matrix metalloprotease 2 (*MMP2*) and two products from the full-length *DSPP* transcript: a segment containing the dentin glycoprotein and dentin phosphoprotein (DGP and DPP) coding region (*DSPP-v1*) and a smaller segment specific for the dentin sialoprotein (DSP)-only transcript (*DSPP-v2*). At day one, the expression levels of *MMP2*, *DSPP-v1*, and *DSPP-v2* in cells cultured with MDZ were not significantly different from those in cells cultured without MDZ. In contrast, at day seven, the three mRNA expression levels in cells cultured with MDZ were significantly higher (3.8-fold for *MMP2*, 1.67-fold for *DSPP-v1*, and 2.2-fold for *DSPP-v2*) than those in cells cultured without MDZ. We also amplified osteocalcin (OC) and runt-related transcription factor 2 (*RUNX2*) as osteoblastic markers (Figure 2b) and type II collagen (Col II) and aggrecan (*ACAN*) as chondrocytic markers (Figure 2c). There were no significant differences in the four mRNA expression levels between cells cultured with and without MDZ at either day one or day seven. We interpret these findings as evidence that MDZ is required for the differentiation of PPU-7 cells into odontoblasts.

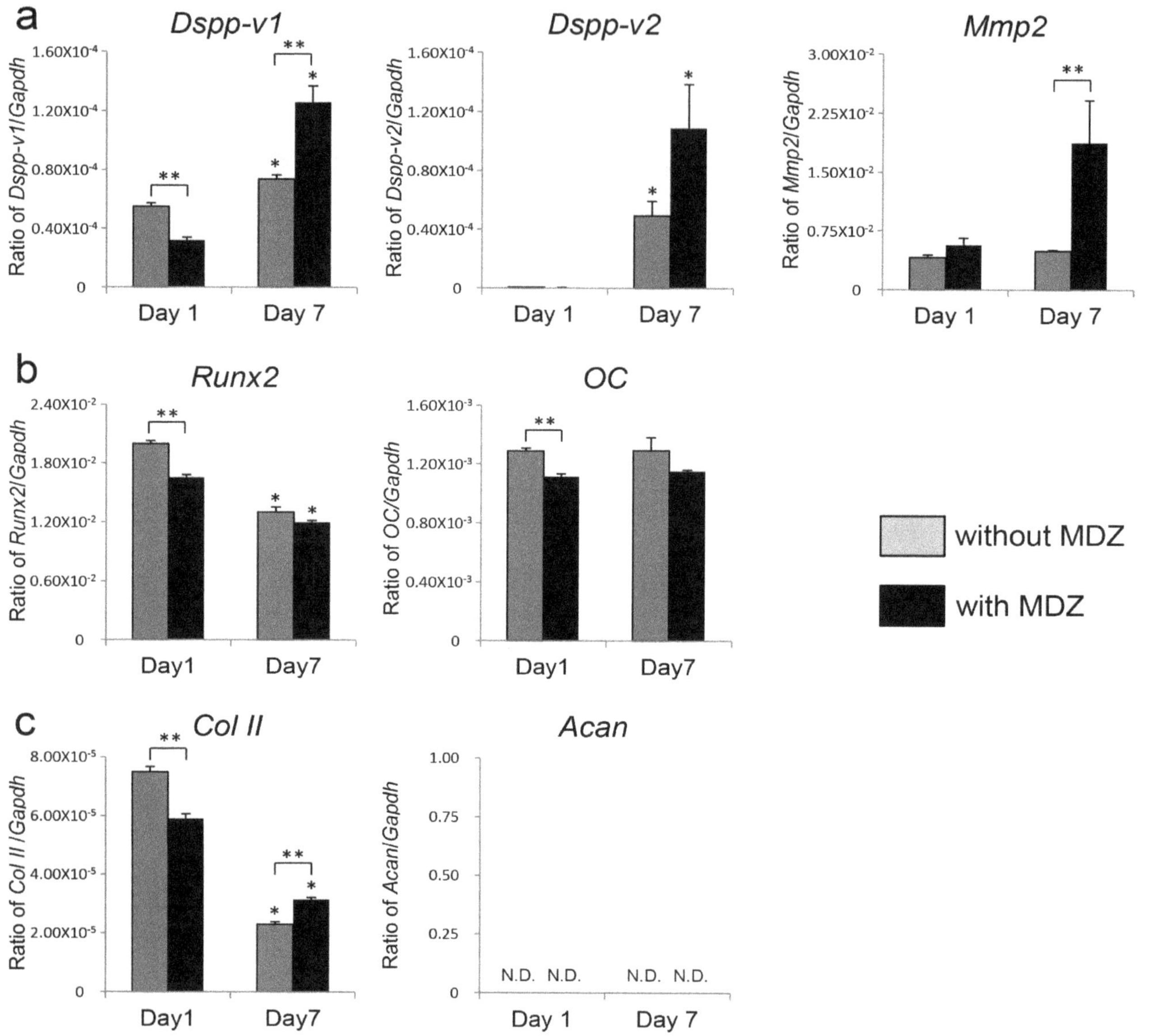

Figure 2. Effect of MDZ on temporal changes in gene expression of the PPU-7 cell line. The mRNA expression by quantitative polymerase chain reaction (qPCR) analysis of (**a**) odontoblastic differentiation markers, i.e., *DSPP*-variant 1 (*DSPP-v1*), *DSPP*-variant 2 (*DSPP-v2*) and matrix metalloprotease 2 (*MMP2*); (**b**) osteoblastic differentiation markers, i.e., osteocalcin (OC) and runt-related transcription factor 2 (*RUNX2*); and (**c**) chondrogenic differentiation markers, i.e., type II collagen (Col II) and aggrecan (*ACAN*). Each ratio was normalized to glyceraldehyde-3-phosphate dehydrogenase (*GAPDH*) as a reference gene, and the relative quantification data of *DSPP-v1*, *DSPP-v2*, *MMP2*, OC, *RUNX2*, Col II and *ACAN* in PPU-7 cell line were generated on the basis of a mathematical model for relative quantification in a qPCR system. Values are the means ± standard error of six culture wells. The asterisk (*) on the bar graph indicates a significant difference ($p < 0.05$, Steel's test) between day one and day seven. The double asterisk (**) on the bar graph indicates a significant difference ($p < 0.05$, Mann–Whitney U-test) between cells cultured with and without MDZ.

2.3. *Effect of MDZ on Mineralization Induction of the PPU-7 Cell Line*

To obtain additional information about the effect of MDZ on mineralization inducibility, we cultured PPU-7 cells in a mineralization-inducing culture medium (Figure 3). The nodule formation and mineralization capacities of the cells were assessed with both Alizarin Red S and von Kossa staining (Figure 3a). At seven days following mineralization induction, in contrast to that of the cells not subjected to mineralization induction, the plate of the cells cultured in mineralization-inducing culture medium clearly displayed precipitated nodules by both staining methods, regardless of the addition of MDZ.

We also quantitatively analyzed the calcium content in PPU-7 cells (Figure 3b). At five days following mineralization induction, relative to the control cells without MDZ (i.e., no MDZ), the cells administered with MDZ-only displayed a dramatically increased amount of calcium deposition (approximately 2.0-fold).

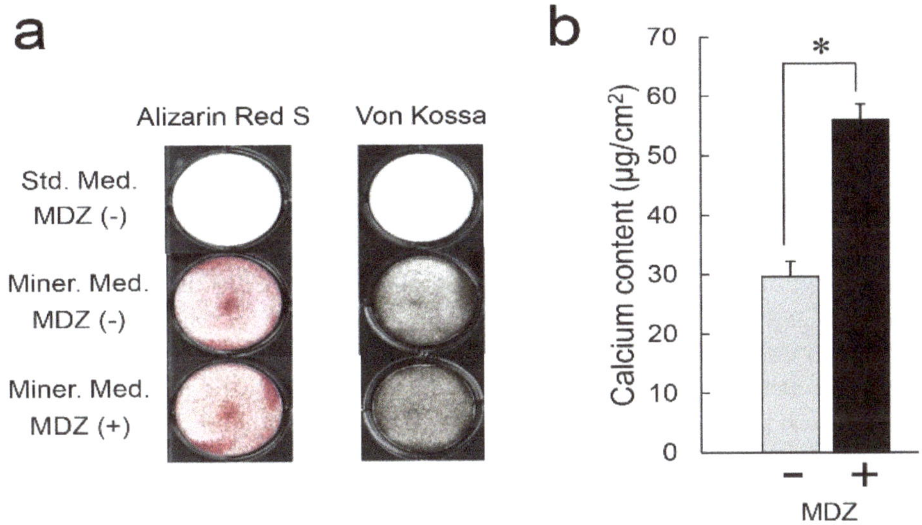

Figure 3. Effect of MDZ on nodule formation in the PPU-7 cell line. Nodule cultures were stained with (**a**) Alizarin Red S (left) and von Kossa (right) staining on day seven. In contrast to PPU-7 cells not subjected to mineralization induction, PPU-7 cells cultured in mineralization-inducing culture media clearly exhibited nodule formation regardless of the addition of MDZ. (**b**) Calcium contents in PPU-7 cells were determined on day five after the mineralization induction. Values are the means ± standard error of six culture wells. The asterisk (*) on the bar graph indicates a significant difference ($p < 0.05$, Mann–Whitney U-test) between the cells incubated with and without MDZ. Std. Med.: Standard culture medium, Miner. Med.: Mineralization-inducing culture medium.

2.4. *Detection of DPP in Precipitated Nodules from PPU-7 Cells*

We attempted to detect a dentin-specific protein, dentin phosphoprotein (DPP), in precipitated nodules induced by MDZ treatment in the PPU-7 cell line at the protein level. The precipitated nodules in PPU-7 cells were subjected to a series of three extractions: With a tris-guanidine buffer (G1), with hydrochloric acid–formic acid solution (HF), and with tris-guanidine buffer again (G2). These extractions yielded three fractions, the G1, HF, and G2 extracts, which were analyzed by SDS-polyacrylamide gel electrophoresis (SDS-PAGE) stained with SimplyBlue SafeStain (Figure 4a) and Stains-all stain (Figure 4b). In the G2 fraction obtained from PPU-7 cells incubated in mineralization-inducing culture medium, Stains-all-positive DPP doublet bands were observed at approximately 100 kDa by SDS-PAGE (Figure 4b, lanes 8 and 9). The addition of MDZ increased the intensity of the DPP doublets bands (Figure 4b, lane 8), whereas no DPP bands were detected in the extracts from PPU-7 cells cultured with the standard medium (Figure 4b, lane 7).

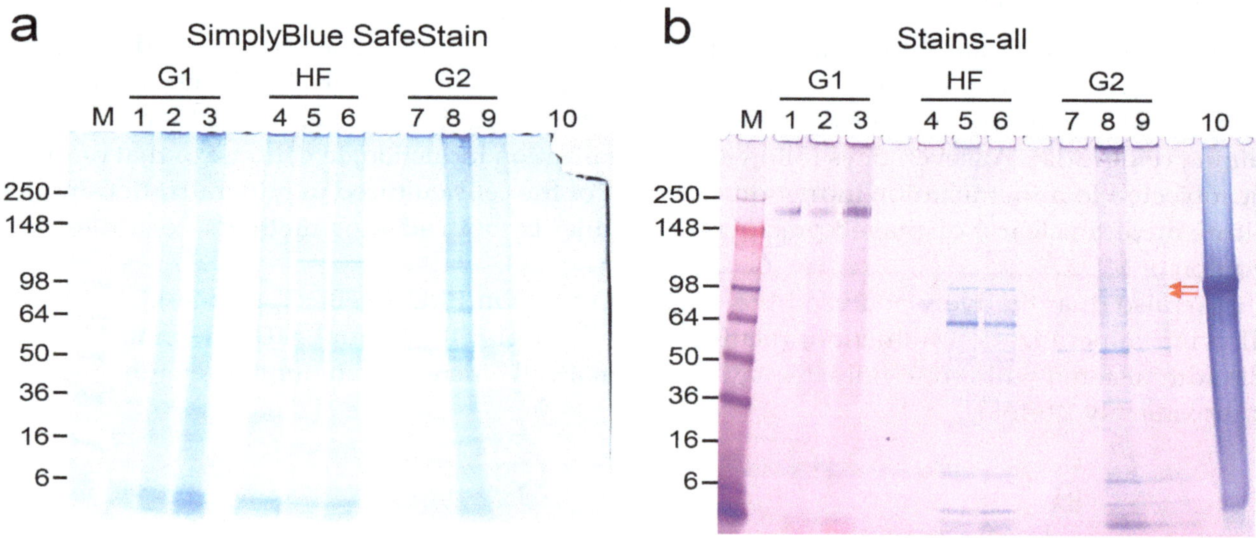

Figure 4. Sequential extraction of proteins from precipitated nodules induced by PPU-7 cells. Precipitated nodules formed in PPU-7 cells cultured in mineralization-inducing culture medium with (MDZ(+)) or without (MDZ(−)) MDZ were sequentially extracted by tris-guanidine (G1 extraction), formic acid–HCl (HF extraction) and tris-guanidine again (G2 extraction). The PPU-7 cells cultured with only standard medium were also extracted as a control. Analysis of the G1, HF, and G2 extracts by 5–20% gradient SDS-PAGE were stained with (**a**) SimplyBlue SafeStain and (**b**) Stains-all stain. Dentin phosphoprotein (DPP) doublet bands in lanes 5, 6, 8, 9, and 10 detected by Stains-all staining are indicated with a red arrow. Lanes 1, 4 and 7: Control; lanes 2, 5 and 8: MDZ(+); lanes 3, 6 and 9: MDZ(-); lane 10: DPP purified from porcine dentin. M: Molecular weight marker (SeeBlue Plus2 Pre-Stained standard).

2.5. X-ray Diffraction (XRD) Patterns of Precipitated Nodules

Based on all the above results, we further characterized the precipitated nodules from PPU-7 cells at the crystal engineering level. Figure 5a shows microbeam XRD patterns for samples grown with (magenta curve) and without (blue curve) MDZ in the culture solution. The pattern for a cell sheet (green curve) is shown only for reference. The cell sheet exhibited a broad intense peak at approximately $2\theta = 10°$, which tailed to higher 2θ values. Peaks attributed to the precipitates appeared at $2\theta = 26.0$, 28.7, and 32.0° (black circles); they were independent of the presence or absence of MDZ. The entire XRD pattern of the precipitates from the solution with MDZ was the same as that of the precipitates from the solution without MDZ, signifying that MDZ did not affect the kind of phase precipitated. The peak widths in the precipitate patterns were broad, indicating low crystallinity and/or small crystallites. Figure 5b–e shows ideal XRD patterns for dicalcium phosphate dihydrate ($CaHPO_4{\cdot}2H_2O$; DCPD) (b), octacalcium phosphate ($Ca_8(HPO_4)_2(PO_4)_4{\cdot}5H_2O$; OCP) (c), β-tricalcium phosphate (β-$Ca_3(PO_4)_2$; β-TCP) (d), and hydroxyapatite ($Ca_{10}(PO_4)_6(OH)_2$; HAP) (e), which were derived using the 2θ versus diffraction–intensity relationships in the corresponding Joint Committee on Powder Diffraction Standards (JCPDS) cards. The asterisks indicate the particular peaks used to identify each calcium phosphate phase. The XRD patterns of the precipitates did not show these particular peaks; however, the profile from $2\theta = 25$ to 35° resembled those for OCP and HAP.

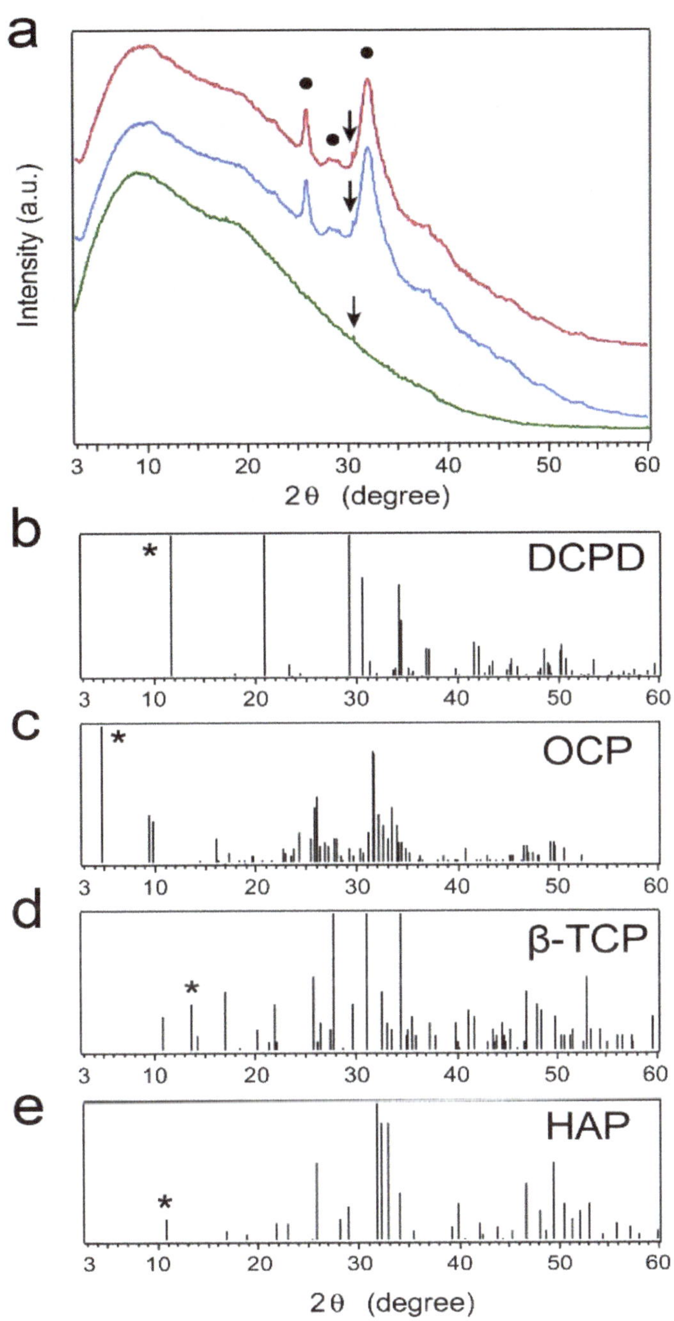

Figure 5. (**a**) Microbeam XRD patterns for samples grown with (magenta curve) and without (blue curve) MDZ in culture solution and for a cell sheet (green curve) for reference. Peaks attributed to the precipitates are indicated by black circles; spike peaks attributed to damage to the imaging plate are indicated by arrows. Ideal XRD patterns for (**b**) dicalcium phosphate dihydrate (DCPD), (**c**) octacalcium phosphate (OCP), (**d**) β-tricalcium phosphate (β-TCP), and (**e**) hydroxyapatite (HAP) derived using 2θ versus diffraction–intensity relationships in the corresponding JCPDS cards. The peaks used to identify each calcium phosphate phase are indicated by asterisks.

2.6. Scanning Electron Microscopy (SEM) Observations of Precipitated Nodules

A macroscopic SEM image of a cross-sectional sample (Figure 6a) showed that the morphology of the precipitates was not uniform. Both irregularly (white arrow) and regularly shaped precipitates (i.e., µm-scale precipitates with a ball-like appearance, yellow arrows) were observed. A magnified image of a region with these ball-like precipitates (Figure 6b) showed that they consisted of aggregated nanoparticles. The size of each nanoparticle was approximately 50 nm or less. The isotropic morphology of the elementary particles made it difficult to ascertain the phase of the calcium phosphate, so the precipitates were observed using TEM.

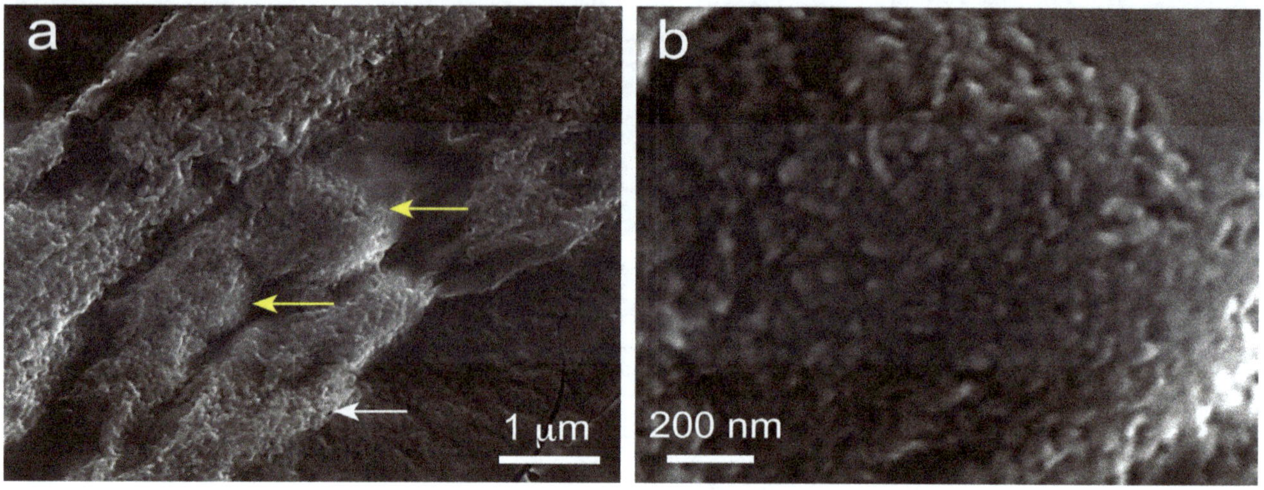

Figure 6. SEM images of a cross-sectional sample. (**a**) Low-magnification image showing irregularly shaped precipitates (white arrow) and ball-like ones (yellow arrows). (**b**) High-magnification images of ball-like precipitate showing nanoparticles sized approximately 50 nm.

2.7. Transmission Electron Microscopy (TEM) Observation and Selected-Area Electron Diffraction (SAED) Measurement of Precipitated Nodules in a Wide Area

A macroscopic TEM image of a microtome-cut section (Figure 7a) showed an irregularly shaped powder-like precipitate. A higher magnification image (Figure 7b) of the precipitate revealed that it consisted of nanorods (light blue arrows) and bulky materials (black arrows). These nanorods were not observed in the SEM image, probably because of their limited width (less than 10 nm).

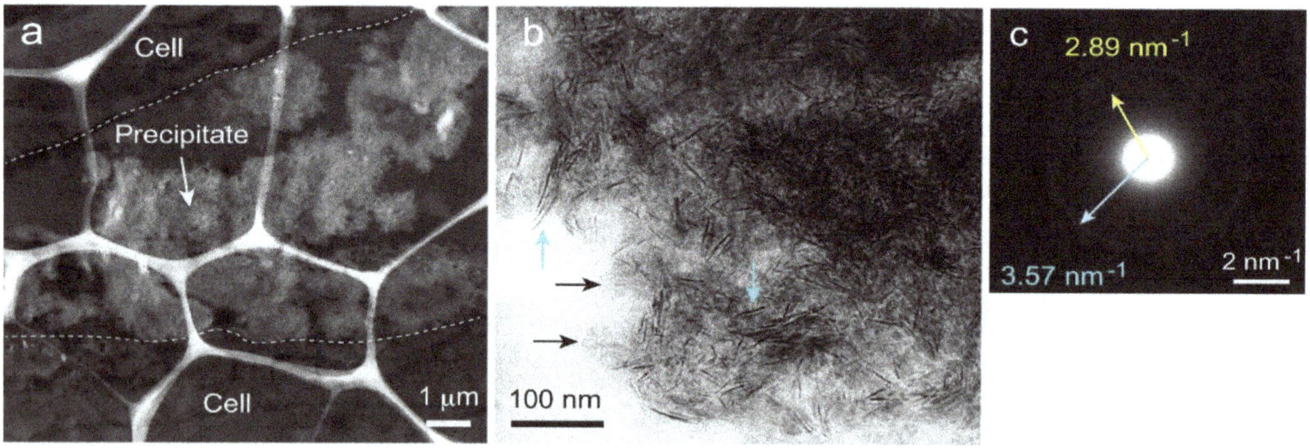

Figure 7. Wide-area TEM images of precipitates. (**a**) Low-magnification image of a microtome-cut sample. The dotted line shows the boundary between the cell sheet and precipitate region. (**b**) High-magnification image of precipitates. Many nanorods (light blue arrows) and bulky materials (black arrows) were observed. (**c**) Selected-Area Electron Diffraction (SAED) pattern measured at 800 nm ϕ. Two Debye rings (low and high intensities) were observed.

The Selected-Area Electron Diffraction (SAED) pattern of the precipitates measured at 800 nm ϕ showed two Debye rings (Figure 7c), indicating that the crystals in the precipitates were randomly oriented. The rings were 2.89 nm^{-1} (low-intensity ring) and 3.57 nm^{-1} (high-intensity ring) from the center. These characteristic distances were converted to interplanar distances, d, of 0.346 and 0.280 nm, respectively. For HAP, the diffraction plane corresponding to d = 0.346 nm (with a margin of error of <1.5%) was {002}. For OCP, there were several corresponding planes, such as {121} and $\{5\bar{2}0\}$. β-TCP also had several corresponding planes, including {1010} and $\{01\overline{10}\}$. DCPD, however, had no diffraction plane corresponding to a *d* of 0.346 nm.

The *d* of 0.280 nm corresponded to the {211}, {121}, and {112} diffraction planes for HAP, {511}, $\{7\bar{1}0\}$, etc. for OCP, and {002} for the DCPD. β-TCP had no diffraction plane corresponding to a *d* of 0.280 nm.

The relative intensity of the diffraction plane in each calcium phosphate crystal provided important information for identifying the calcium phosphate phase when the orientations of the crystals were random. The relative intensities of the {002}, {211}, {121}, and {112} diffraction planes of HAP were 49, 100, 43, and 70%, respectively. The diffraction intensities of each plane of the OCP corresponding to $d = 0.346$ or 0.280 nm were all less than 35%. Similarly, low diffraction intensities were also observed for the plane corresponding to $d = 0.346$ nm for β-TCP and the plane corresponding to $d = 0.280$ nm for DCPD. This result strongly suggests that the precipitates were HAP.

Since high-resolution TEM (HR-TEM) observation of the precipitates was difficult due to the overlapping crystals, a lattice image of each crystal in the precipitates was observed using a crushed sample.

2.8. High-Resolution TEM (HR-TEM) Observation and Fast Fourier Transform (FFT) Image Analysis of Precipitated Nodules in a Narrow Area

Figure 8a shows a magnified image of nanorods, a major component of the precipitates. Randomly oriented nanorods (white arrows) with a width less than 10 nm were identified, and lattice images were observed for each rod.

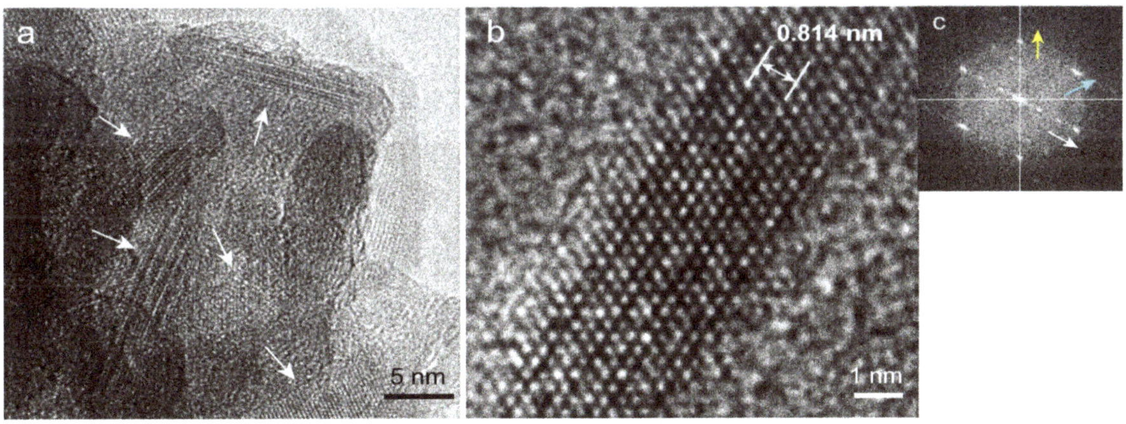

Figure 8. Narrow-area TEM images of nanorods. (**a**) Aggregation of nanorods. The orientation of each rod was random, and lattice fringes were observed in the rods. (**b**) HR-TEM image of a rod. The lattice image of the rod is visible. (**c**) FFT image of a rod. Three directions of the crystal planes are indicated by white, blue, and yellow arrows. The interplanar distance corresponding to the direction of the white arrow (0.814 nm) is superimposed in (**b**).

HR-TEM observation of a nanorod (Figure 8b) revealed a lattice pattern corresponding to the atomic arrangement. An FFT image of a nanorod (Figure 8c) revealed three periodic directions corresponding to $d = 0.814$, 0.277, and 0.276 nm (white, blue, and yellow arrows, respectively). The *d* of 0.814 nm corresponded to the {26} plane for HAP and the {012}, $\{10\bar{2}\}$, and $\{1\bar{1}2\}$ planes for β-TCP with a margin of error of <1.5%. In contrast, OCP and DCPD had no planes corresponding to $d = 0.814$ nm. The *d* values of 0.277 and 0.276 nm corresponded with many diffraction planes for HAP, β-TCP, OCP, and DCPD. For HAP, the corresponding planes were {112}, $\{2\bar{1}2\}$, and $\{\bar{2}12\}$; for β-TCP, {128}, $\{3\bar{2}8\}$, etc.; for OCP, {601}, $\{\bar{2}22\}$, etc., and for DCPD, the *d* of 0.277 nm corresponded to {002}.

The angle of intersection between the directions of the white and blue arrow was 59.0°, and between the directions of the white and yellow arrows was 120.3°. Although the *d*-value analysis indicated the possibility that the nanorod was HAP or β-TCP, comparison of the measured intersection angles with theoretical ones indicated that the nanorod was HAP (Table S3) The measured d values and intersection angles were consistent with the theoretical values with a margin of error of <1.5%. The directions of the white, blue, and yellow arrows corresponded to [100], [112], and $[\bar{2}12]$ for HAP. The image in Figure 8b therefore shows the HAP lattice viewed from the $[02\bar{1}]$ zone axis.

We performed similar observations and analyses for ten different nanorods in several areas and found that all of them were HAP.

Figure 9a shows a high-magnification TEM image corresponding to the bulky materials observed in Figure 7b. They consisted of nanoparticles (white arrows) with a diameter less than approximately 10 nm. This observation means that the cell-induced precipitates consisted of a mixture of nanorods and nanoparticles. The 50 nm particles observed by SEM (Figure 6) therefore were secondary particles consisting of smaller nanoparticles.

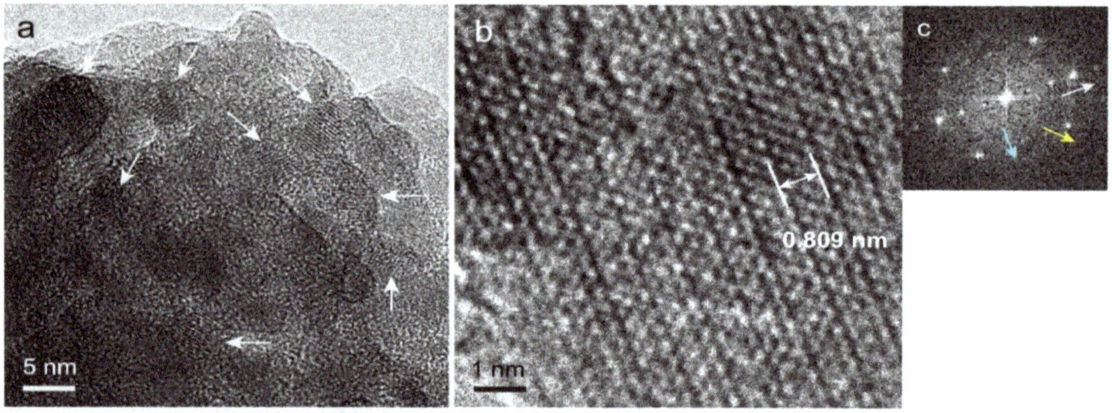

Figure 9. Narrow-area TEM images of bulky precipitates. (**a**) The precipitates consisted of nanoparticles sized less than approximately10 nm. (**b**) HR-TEM image of a nanoparticle. (**c**) FFT image of a nanoparticle. Three directions of crystal planes are indicated by white, blue, and yellow arrows. The interplanar distance corresponding to the direction of the white arrow (0.809 nm) is superimposed in (**b**).

A HR-TEM image of a nanoparticle (Figure 9b) revealed a lattice arrangement, and a FFT image of nanoparticles (Figure 9c) revealed at least three periodic directions. The d values corresponding to each direction (indicated by white, blue, and yellow arrows) were 0.809, 0.385, and 0.285 nm, respectively. The d of 0.809 nm corresponded to [26] for HAP, {012}, $\{10\bar{2}\}$, and $\{1\bar{1}2\}$ for β-TCP with a margin of error of <1.5%. OCP and DCPD had no planes corresponding to d = 0.809. The d of 0.385 nm corresponded to $\{1\bar{2}1\}$, {111}, and $\{\bar{2}11\}$ for HAP with a margin of error of <1.5%. OCP corresponded to several planes, such as $\{12\bar{1}\}$ and $\{22\bar{1}\}$. β-TCP and DCPD had no corresponding planes. The d of 0.281 nm corresponded to many planes for both HAP and OCP: $\{3\bar{2}1\}$, $\{21\bar{1}\}$, etc. for HAP, and {130}, {420}, etc. for OCP. DCPD corresponded to {002}, whereas β-TCP had no corresponding plane. The d-value analysis indicated that only HAP had planes corresponding to three directions. The intersection angle between the directions of the white (d = 0.809 nm) and blue (d = 0.385 nm) arrows was 90.7°, and between the directions of the white and yellow (d = 0.281 nm) arrows was 46.9°. These angles corresponded to those between [100] and $[1\bar{2}1]$ and between [100] and $[3\bar{2}1]$ for HAP, respectively. The measured d values and intersection angles between each plane were consistent with the theoretical values (with a margin of error <1.5%; see Table S3). The image in Figure 9b therefore corresponded to the HAP lattice viewed from the [012] zone axis. We performed similar observations and analyses for ten different nanoparticles in several areas and found that all of them were HAP.

2.9. Element Content in Precipitated Nodules Measured Using Scanning TEM Energy-Dispersive X-ray Spectroscopy (STEM-EDS)

Figure 10 shows a low-magnification (approximately 12 μm square) TEM image (a) and two-dimensional elemental mappings of Ca (b), P (c), and N (d) in the area in (a). Ca and P were observed in only the precipitates, and N was mostly observed in the cell region. A small amount of N was detected in the precipitate region; it was probably due to cell contamination. The energy-dispersive X-ray spectroscopy (EDS) spectrum (Figure 10e, magenta curve) corresponded to the region in Figure 10a where the average Ca/P atomic % ratio was 1.41 ± 0.01. This Ca/P ratio increased slightly with a decrease in the area size and reached equilibrium when the area size was less than a few μm. The blue and green curves show the spectra measured for 1.5 μm and 200 nm squares, the corresponding Ca/P ratios of which were 1.44 ± 0.01 and 1.45 ± 0.01. The detected elements (except C, O, N, and Cu) and their contents for the 200 nm square are shown in Table S4.

We performed EDS measurements on five different areas in the 1.5 μm square and determined that the average Ca/P atomic % ratio was 1.45 with a deviation of ± 0.02.

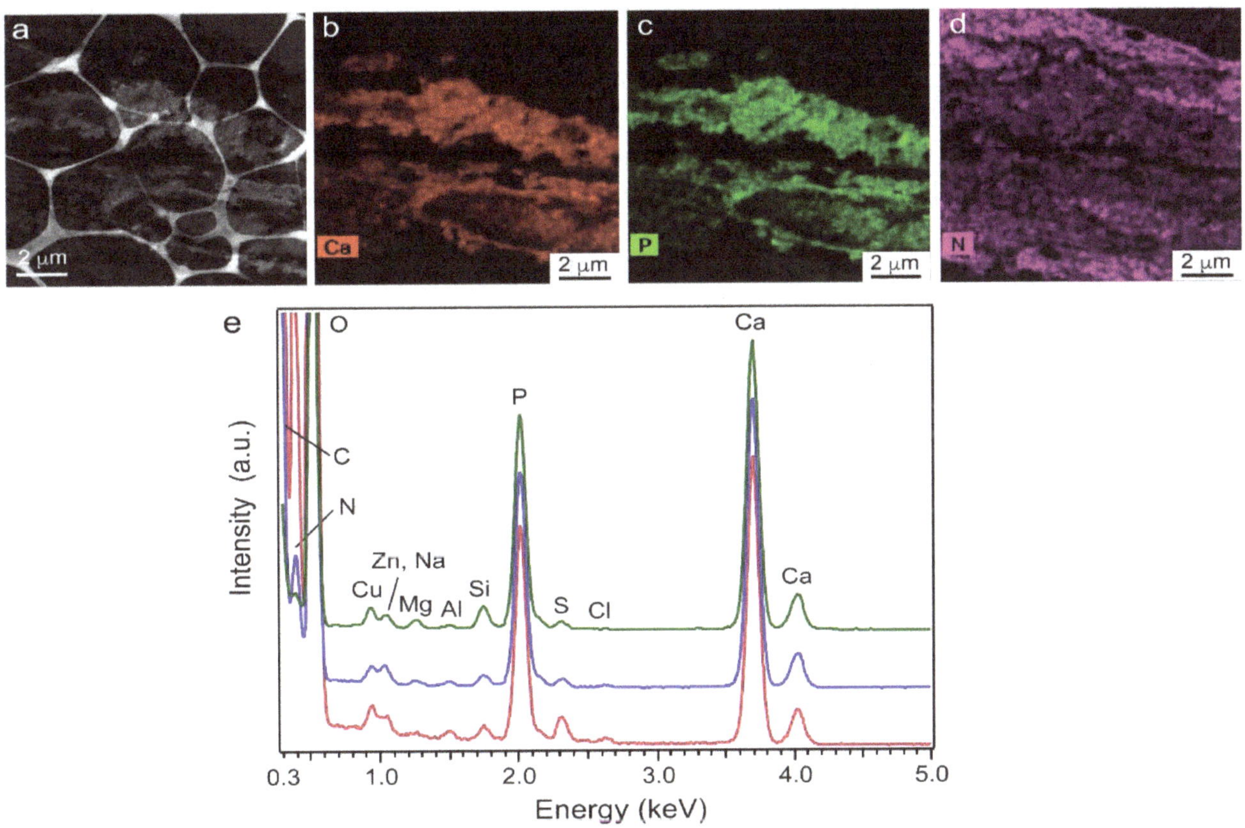

Figure 10. Scanning TEM energy-dispersive X-ray spectroscopy (STEM-EDS) analysis results for precipitates. (**a**) Low-magnification TEM image for energy-dispersive X-ray spectroscopy (EDS) analysis. Two-dimensional elemental mappings of (**b**) Ca, (**c**) P, and (**d**) N. (**e**) STEM-EDS spectra for three measured areas: approximately 12 μm, 1.5 μm, and 200 nm (magenta, blue, and green curves, respectively). Cu is attributed to the TEM grid, and Al is equipment specific. Each spectrum was normalized by the intensity of Ca at 3.7 keV.

3. Discussions

Cytokines such as BMP and TGF-β play important roles in the regulation of odontoblast differentiation [14,15,27,28]. When we established the PPU-7 cell line, we demonstrated that both BMP2 and TGF-β1 significantly affected cell proliferation, cell population doubling time, mRNA expression of dentin sialophosphoprotein (DSPP), which is one of the differentiation marker for odontoblasts, and ALP activity in the PPU-7 cell line. These findings are in agreement with the reports described above. In addition, considering the inherent ALP activity in the PPU-7 cell line, our data suggest that some level of ALP activity is required for the induction of the differentiation of PPU-7 cells into hard tissue-forming cells by BMP2 and/or TGF-β1.

In vitro study using human mesenchymal stem cells (hMSCs) shows that MDZ inhibits ALP activity and calcium deposition in hMSCs, suggesting a suppressive effect on osteogenic differentiation [23]. However, little was known about the effect of MDZ on the properties of dental pulp tissues. We therefore hypothesized that MDZ affects odontoblastic differentiation rather than the osteogenic differentiation of dental pulp stem cells. We demonstrated that the addition of MDZ-only to PPU-7 cells dramatically enhanced ALP activity and mineralization induction. This finding suggests that MDZ possesses the ability to induce the differentiation of PPU-7 cells into hard tissue-forming cells. Moreover, the results led us to investigate the combination of MDZ and cytokines, namely, BMP2 and TGF-β1.

In general, many drugs express their drug efficacy through a receptor. MDZ controls the GABA, which is the main inhibitory neurotransmitter. The GABAA receptor is a multi-subunit chloride channel that mediates the fastest inhibitory synaptic transmission in the central nervous system. The benzodiazepine class, which includes MDZ, enhances the effect of the neurotransmitter GABA at the GABAA receptor [17]. The GABAA receptor has at least 19 different subunits and shows different susceptibility to drugs depending on the combination of units [29,30]. The GABAA receptor beta 1 subunit (GABRB1) is strongly expressed in the human coronal pulp and permanent predentin/odontoblasts [31,32]. Although we demonstrated that MDZ-only treatment enhanced ALP activity and mineralization induction, combinations of MDZ with BMP2 or TGF-β1 tended to decrease both of them. Our findings suggest that the pharmacological interaction of the combination of MDZ with BMP2 or TGF-β1 reduces the susceptibility and/or reactivity of GABRB1.

Dental pulp stem cells possess a pluripotency for various types of specialized cells, such as neuron, cardiomyocytes, chondrocytes, odontoblasts, osteoblasts, and liver cells [33,34]. The starting population of these cells and their differentiated progeny are evaluated by analyzing the expression of specific gene markers. DSPP is an important marker of odontoblastic differentiation. We previously generated two amplification products from the full-length *DSPP* (*DSPP-v1*) and the DSP-only (*DSPP-v2*) transcripts and found that both the *DSPP-v1* and *DSPP-v2* products were predominantly observed in odontoblasts, whereas only trace expression of the *DSPP-v1* transcript was detected in dental pulp [35]. Our previous study showed that in addition to these two DSPP splice variants, matrix metalloproteases such as *MMP2* and *MMP20* can become odontoblast differentiation markers [36]. We demonstrated that the mRNA levels of *DSPP-v1*, *DSPP-v2* and *MMP2* were dramatically enhanced by MDZ at day seven. In contrast, mRNA expression levels of the osteoblastic differentiation markers OC and *RUNX2*, and the chondrogenic differentiation markers Col II and *ACAN* decreased over time regardless of the presence or absence of MDZ. These findings suggest that MDZ promotes the differentiation of PPU-7 cells into odontoblasts.

Alizarin Red S staining has been widely used to evaluate calcium deposits in cell culture [37], whereas von Kossa staining has generally been used to detect both phosphates and carbonates in calcium deposits [38]. We demonstrated that the formation of precipitated nodules in a mineralization-inducing culture medium in the presence or absence of MDZ was evident on the plate by both staining methods and that the MDZ-only treatment showed the highest ability to induce calcification. These findings suggest that the precipitated nodules possess calcium carbonate-based or calcium phosphate-based components and that the use of MDZ-only is the most effective in inducing mineralization in the PPU-7 cell line.

DPP is a highly phosphorylated protein in dentin with an isoelectric point near 1.1. Due to the biased amino acid composition and extensive acidity (35–40% phosphoserine and 40–50% aspartic acid) [39], DPP stains very strongly with Stains-all but does not stain with Coomassie Brilliant Blue. Genetic studies have shown that for porcine DPP, the length variations in the DPP code are closely correlated with the length variations observed at the protein level [40]. Therefore, DPP samples separately isolated from 22 pigs appear as single or doublet bands migrating between 96 kDa and 100 kDa on SDS-PAGE [40]. Our previous study showed that full-length *DSPP* containing DPP is an odontoblast-predominant transcript and that little DPP is present in porcine dental pulp, suggesting that DPP is a dentin-specific protein [35]. In this study, we demonstrated that DPP doublet bands were present in the precipitated nodules in PPU-7 cells cultured with a mineralization-inducing culture medium and that the addition of MDZ increased the intensity of the DPP doublet bands. Our data suggest that the precipitated nodules possessed dentin-like characteristics.

The HR-TEM observations and FFT analyses indicated that the nanorods and nanoparticles were HAP. To support this conclusion, SAED simulation of a HAP crystal viewed from a particular zone axis was performed using the ReciPro application. Figure S4 shows the SAED patterns of a HAP crystal viewed from $\{02\bar{1}\}$ (Figure S4a) and {012} (Figure S4b). The pattern corresponding to the $\{02\bar{1}\}$ direction (dotted hexagon) was essentially the same as the FFT image in Figure 8c. The diffraction spots corresponding to {012} and $\{\bar{1}12\}$ were not clearly visible in the FFT image, probably due to the width of the nanorods in those directions not having sufficient periodicity in the image. The simulated SAED corresponding to the {012} direction was consistent with the FFT image in Figure 9c, indicating that the nanorods and nanoparticles were indeed HAP. The two Debye rings observed in the wide-area SAED pattern (Figure 7c) revealed the most likely *d* values in randomly oriented HAP, and the XRD pattern of the precipitates showed peaks corresponding to those of HAP. These findings indicated that the precipitates consisted of a single phase of low-crystalline HAP. The STEM-EDS results showed that the HAP in the precipitates was calcium deficient.

In our previous study, an enamel-like HAP nanorod array was constructed on an amorphous calcium phosphate (ACP) substrate consisting of nanoparticles (<80 nm diameter) that had been compression molded [41]. When the substrate was immersed in a calcium phosphate solution without cells under pseudo-physiological conditions, ACP nanoparticles close to the substrate surface quickly transformed into HAP ones and grew perpendicularly as rods due to geometric selection. During this reaction, ACP nanoparticles located in the middle to deep regions of the substrate were transformed into low-crystalline HAP. We found that the macroscopic and microscopic morphologies of cell-induced HAP closely resembled those of HAP transformed from ACP nanoparticles. Figure S5 in Supplementary shows the TEM images, SAED patterns, and STEM-EDS spectra for both types of HAP crystal. The macroscopic morphology of the grown material was fibrous for both types (Figure S5a,c) and consisted of a mixture of nanorods and nanoparticles (Figure S5b,d). Regarding the morphology in elemental crystals and their aggregates, the two types of HAP crystal were similar. The SAED patterns for the grown materials measured at 800 nm ϕ were also similar (Figure S5e). The average Ca/P atomic % ratio of cell-induced HAP (Ca/P = 1.45) was slightly less than that of HAP transformed from ACP nanoparticles (Ca/P = 1.50) (Figure S5f) and that of human dentin [42]. One reason for this difference is the substitution of several cations, such as Zn and Mg, at Ca-ion sites in the cell-induced HAP, which occurred due to the complex composition of the initial growing fluid. Based on the content of each element shown in Table S2, the Ca/(Zn + Na + Mg + Si) atomic % ratio was approximately 7.48, meaning that the x component in $Ca_{10-x}(Zn, Na, Mg, Si)_x(PO_4)_6(OH)_2$ was approximately 1.18. Therefore, the calculated Ca/P molar ratio of the cell-induced HAP was 1.47, which was close to the measured ratio for the precipitates.

The morphological, structural, and chemical similarities between the cell-induced HAP and the ACP-transformed HAP strongly suggest that the cells, which had high ALP activity, produced locally concentrated phosphate ions, which nucleated ACP nanoparticles in the initial reaction stage. These particles subsequently transformed into low-crystalline HAP. Biological analysis after HAP precipitation showed that the initial pulpal cells differentiated into odontoblast cells and that the present system simulated the dentin matrix formation process, suggesting that the HAP in tooth dentin is formed by phase transformation from ACP nanoparticles. Indeed, a TEM image of human molar dentin (Figure S6) showed that it consisted of nanorods and nanoparticles, the same as for the images in Figure S5a,c.

4. Materials and Methods

These studies have received approval from the Institutional Ethics Review Committee of the Tsurumi University School of Dental Medicine (Project identification code #1318, 1 December 2015). Additionally, all animal experiments were approved by the Institutional Animal Care Committee and the Recombination DNA Experiment and Biosafety Committee of the Tsurumi University School of Dental Medicine. We have confirmed that all experiments were performed in accordance with relevant guidelines and regulations.

4.1. Alkaline Phosphatase (ALP) Activity Assay of the PPU-7 Cell Line

The PPU-7 cell line was established from porcine dental pulp cells by our group (see Figures S1–S3). We measured ALP activity in each well as described previously [43]. The cells were plated on a 96-well plate at a density of 3.16×10^4 cells/cm^2 and were cultured in the standard medium for 24 h. The medium was changed to growth medium supplemented with 0, 2.5, 5, or 10 μM of MDZ with 500 ng/mL of rhBMP2 (R&D Systems, Minneapolis, MN, USA) or with 1 ng/mL of rhTGF-β1 (Cell Signaling Technology, Danvers, MA, USA). After 72 additional hours of incubation, the cells were washed once with PBS, and ALP activity was assayed using 10 mM p-nitrophenylphosphate as the substrate in 100 mM 2-amino-2-methyl-1,3-propanediol-HCl buffer (pH 10.0) containing 5 mM $MgCl_2$ and incubated for 10 min at 37 °C. Adding 0.2 M NaOH quenched the reaction, and the absorbance at 405 nm was read on a plate reader.

4.2. Alkaline Phosphatase Staining

The cells were spread on a 24-well plate at density of 3.16×10^4 cells/cm^2. After incubation for 2 days, the cells were rinsed twice with PBS, fixed with 10% formaldehyde for 30 min, stained with 0.1 mg/mL of naphthol AS-MX phosphate (Sigma-Aldrich, St. Louis, MO, USA), 0.5% N,N-dimethylformamide, Fast Blue BB salt (Sigma-Aldrich), and 2 mM $MgCl_2$ in 0.1 M Tris–HCl buffer (pH 8.5) for 30 min at room temperature, and then washed with dH_2O and photographed.

4.3. Gene Expression of the PPU-7 Cell Line

The cells were extracted with an RNA extraction reagent (Isogen, Nippon Gene Co., Ltd., Tokyo, Japan). The purified total RNA (2 μg) was reverse transcribed; the reaction mixture consisted of SYBR Green PCR master mix (Roche), supplemented with 0.5 μM forward and reverse primers and 2 μL of cDNA as template. The specific primer sets were designed using Primer-BLAST software (URL: http://www.ncbi.nlm.nih.gov/tools/primer-blast). The specific primer sets and running conditions are shown in Table S1. *GAPDH* was used as the reference gene. Each ratio was normalized the relative quantification data of *DSPP-v1*, *DSPP-v2*, *MMP2*, OC, *RUNX2*, Col II and *ACAN* in comparison to a reference gene (*GAPDH*), generated on the basis of a mathematical model for relative quantification in qPCR system. All values were represented as means ± standard error. Statistical significance (*) was determined using a Steel's test, whereas (**) was determined using a Mann–Whitney U-test. In all cases, $p < 0.05$ was regarded as statistically significant.

4.4. Detection of Precipitated Nodules in PPU-7 Cells

PPU-7 cells were grown on a 12-well plate at an initial density of 3.16×10^4 cells/cm^2. After incubation for 24 h, the medium was changed to a mineralization-inducing medium containing 10 mM β-glycerophosphate and 50 μM ascorbic acid. The cells were cultured for up to 7 days. Mineralization was visualized by Alizarin Red S and von Kossa staining. After fixation with 4% paraformaldehyde neutral buffer solution for 30 min, the cells were stained with 1% Alizarin Red S (Sigma-Aldrich) solution for 10 min, then washed with distilled water and photographed. Alternatively, silver staining was performed using a von Kossa staining kit (Polysciences, Inc., Warrington, PA, USA) according to the manufacturer's instructions.

PPU-7 cells were grown on a 24-well plate at an initial density of 3.16×10^4 cells/cm^2. After incubation for 24 h, the medium was changed to a mineralization-inducing medium. The cells were cultured for up to 5 days. Each well on the plates was rinsed with PBS, and the calcium was dissolved in 0.5 mL of 0.5 N HCl by gentle rocking for 1 h. The calcium concentration in the eluate was spectrophotometrically determined at 570 nm by following the color development with a calcium assay kit (Calcium C-test Wako, Wako Pure Chemical Industries, Ltd.). All values were normalized against the cultivation area.

4.5. Statistical Analysis

For ALP assays and qPCR and calcium analyses, all values are presented as the mean $\pm$ standard error. Statistical significance (*) was determined using the Mann–Whitney U-test for qPCR analysis and a nonparametric Steel's test for the ALP assay and calcium analysis. $p < 0.05$ was regarded as statistically significant for Steel's test, and $p < 0.01$ or $p < 0.05$ was regarded as statistically significant for the Mann–Whitney U-test.

4.6. Characterization of Proteins in the Precipitated Nodules from PPU-7 Cells

The PPU-7 cell line was grown in standard medium or in mineralization-inducing culture medium on the 6 cm culture dish at an initial density of 3.16×10^4 cells/cm^2 for 14 days, and the cell sheet was scraped off with a cell scraper. The cell sample was suspended with 50 mM Tris–HCl/4M guanidine buffer (pH 7.4) containing Protease Inhibitor Cocktail Set III [1 mM 4-(2-aminoethyl) benzenesulfonyl fluoride hydrochloride (AEBSF), 0.8 mM aprotinin, 50 mM bestatin, 15 mM E-64, 20 mM leupeptin, and 10 mM pepstatin (Calbiochem EMD Chemicals Inc., Gibbstown, NJ, USA)] and 1 mM 1,10-phenanthroline (Sigma-Aldrich), and was homogenized using a Polytron (Capitol Scientific, Inc., Austin, TX, USA) homogenizer for 30 s at half speed. Insoluble material was pelleted by centrifugation (15,900g) and the supernatant (G1 extract) was stored at −80 °C. The guanidine-insoluble material was extracted against 0.17 N HCl and 0.95% formic acid containing 10 mM benzamidine (Sigma-Aldrich), 1 mM PMSF, and 1 mM 1,10-phenanthroline using the homogenizer. Following centrifugation, the acid-soluble supernatant (HF extract) was stored at −80 °C. The pellet was extracted with 50 mM Tris–HCl/4M guanidine buffer (pH 7.4) containing Protease Inhibitor Cocktail Set III and centrifuged, and the supernatant (G2 extract) was stored at −80 °C. The G1, HF, and G2 extracts were desalted with an Amicon Ultra centrifugal filter (0.5 mL, MW = 3000 cut off) (Merck Millipore, Darmstadt, Germany). Following the quantitative analysis of total protein in each extract using a Pierce 660 nm Protein Assay Reagent (Thermo Fisher Scientific, Waltham, MA, USA), the amount of total protein was normalized by dividing the amount of total protein in control (i.e., PPU-7 cell line was cultured in the standard medium), and characterized by sodium dodecyl sulfate–polyacrylamide gel electrophoresis (SDS-PAGE).

SDS-PAGE was performed using a 15% e-PAGEL mini gel (ATTO Corporation, Tokyo, Japan). The gel was stained with SimplyBlue SafeStain (Invitrogen) or Stains-all stain (Sigma-Aldrich). The apparent molecular weights of the protein bands were estimated by comparison with the SeeBlue Plus2 Pre-Stained standard (Life Technologies/Invitrogen).

4.7. Degree of Supersaturation with Respect to Each Calcium Phosphate Phase

The calcium phosphate phases that form under physiological conditions are DCPD, OCP, β-TCP, and HAP. We calculated the degree of supersaturation, σ, of the initial culture fluid with respect to each phase using:

$$\sigma = (IP/K_{sp})^{1/n} - 1 \text{ (n = 2, 16, 5, and 18 for DCPD, OCP, } \beta\text{-TCP, and HAP, respectively)} \quad (1)$$

where IP is the ionic activity of the solution and K_{sp} is the solubility product constant of the material at 37 °C [44]. The concentration of each ion in the fluid and the degree of supersaturation are given in Table S2.

4.8. XRD

Microbeam XRD (RAPID, Rigaku) with monochromated Cu-Kα radiation was used to characterize the precipitates at 50 kV and 30 mA. The incident beam was focused to a diameter of approximately 100 μm and irradiated perpendicular to the surface of the cell sheet. The diffraction was recorded on an imaging plate, and the digital data on the plate were converted to the intensity versus 2θ relationship using DISPLAY software (Rigaku). The diffraction peak positions were referenced to those of different calcium phosphate phases in the JCPDS cards (DCPD: Card 11–293, OCP: Card 26–1056, β-TCP: Card 9–169, HAP: Card 9–432).

4.9. SEM

Field-emission scanning electron microscopy (FE-SEM, JSM-7000F, JEOL, Ltd.) with an acceleration voltage of 5 kV was used to observe cross-sectional samples. The samples were coated with an osmium film (approximately 3 nm thick) before observation.

4.10. TEM Observation and Elemental Analysis Using STEM-EDS

Two types of samples were prepared for TEM observations. Ultramicrotome-cut samples were prepared by embedding cell sheets with precipitates in epoxy resin and placing them in a dark room for 48 h at room temperature. After the resin completely filled the gaps (precipitate regions) between cell sheets, the resin was solidified using ultraviolet irradiation. The solidified block was then sliced using a diamond knife into samples with a thickness of 70–100 nm. The samples were placed on a TEM grid with a Cu mesh for observation. Samples crushed in an agate mortar were dispersed in 99.5% ethanol solution, which was ultrasonically stirred for 5 min at 40 kHz. An aliquot of the stirred solution was placed on a TEM grid with a Cu mesh and allowed to dry naturally in air. An analytical TEM (Tecnai Osiris, FEI Co.) with an acceleration voltage of 200 kV was used to observe the samples. SAED measurement with a typical area of 800 nm or 200 nm ϕ was simultaneously performed to characterize the material.

Two-dimensional elemental mapping and quantitative analysis of the content of each element were performed using a Super-X EDS system in the TEM. The probe diameter used for analysis was approximately 0.5 nm, and the amplitude was approximately 0.55 nA. The beam residence time at each measurement position was 10 μs, and the analysis was completed within 5 min. The relative content of each element was calculated from the energy-dispersive spectra by using peak deconvolution.

5. Conclusions

Drug repositioning is the process of discovering, validating, and marketing previously approved drugs for new indications. Due to the promise of reduced costs and expedited approval schedules, the research field of drug repositioning has been attracting attention [45]. To find candidates for drug repositioning, a standard database consisting of both approved and failed drugs has been developed as a web application [46]. Without using the database, the present study demonstrated that MDZ enhances the differentiation of PPU-7 cells to odontoblast and promotes the formation of dentin-like hydroxyapatite. Further studies are required to elucidate the pharmacokinetic and pharmacological efficacy of MDZ in animal experiments. In the dental field, these findings support the repositioning of MDZ to promote dentin regeneration for endodontic treatments, such as pulp capping. Moreover, these findings support advancing research from pig to human experimental models using human DPSCs to discover MDZ's potential, not only for future dental treatments, but also for organ regenerative medicine.

Author Contributions: Conceptualization, T.K., K.O. and Y.Y.; Formal Analysis, T.K., K.O., M.M.S., R.Y., T.C., R.C. and Y.H.; Investigation, T.K., K.O. and Y.Y.; Data Curation, T.K., K.O., R.Y., T.C., R.C., K.F.-A., H.K. and Y.Y.; Writing-Original Draft Preparation, T.K., K.O. and Y.Y.; Writing-Review & Editing, K.O. and Y.Y.

Acknowledgments: We thank Ichiro Saito from the Department of Pathology at the School of Dental Medicine, Tsurumi University, and Yoshinobu Asada from the Department of Pediatric Dentistry at the School of Dental Medicine, Tsurumi University for their support.

Abbreviations

mRNA	messenger ribonucleic acid
SDS	sodium dodecyl sulfate
kDa	kilodalton
Tris	2-amino-2-hydroxymethyl-propane-1,3-diol
PMSF	phenylmethylsulfonyl fluoride
PBS	phosphate buffered saline

References

1. Zafar, M.S.; Khurshid, Z.; Almas, K. Oral tissue engineering progress and challenges. *Tissue Eng. Regen. Med.* **2015**, *12*, 387–397. [CrossRef]
2. Hu, L.; Gao, Z.; Xu, J.; Zhu, Z.; Fan, Z.; Zhang, C.; Wang, J.; Wang, S. Decellularized Swine Dental Pulp as a Bioscaffold for Pulp Regeneration. *BioMed Res. Int.* **2017**, *2017*, 9342714. [CrossRef] [PubMed]
3. Yasui, T.; Mabuchi, Y.; Morikawa, S.; Onizawa, K.; Akazawa, C.; Nakagawa, T.; Okano, H.; Matsuzaki, Y. Isolation of dental pulp stem cells with high osteogenic potential. *Inflamm. Regen.* **2017**, *37*, 8. [CrossRef] [PubMed]
4. Hayashi, Y.; Imai, M.; Goto, Y.; Murakami, N. Pathological mineralization in a serially passaged cell line from rat pulp. *J. Oral Pathol. Med.* **1993**, *22*, 175–179. [CrossRef] [PubMed]
5. Nagata, T.; Yokota, M.; Ohishi, K.; Nishikawa, S.; Shinohara, H.; Wakano, Y.; Ishida, H. 1α,25-dihydroxyvitamin D_3 stimulation of osteopontin expression in rat clonal dental pulp cells. *Arch. Oral Biol.* **1994**, *39*, 775–782. [CrossRef]
6. MacDougall, M.; Selden, J.K.; Nydegger, J.R.; Carnes, D.L. Immortalized mouse odontoblast cell line MO6-G3 application for in vitro biocompatibility testing. *Am. J. Dent.* **1998**, *11*, S11–S16. [PubMed]
7. Thonemann, B.; Schmalz, G. Bovine dental papilla-derived cells immortalized with HPV 18 E6/E7. *Eur. J. Oral Sci.* **2000**, *108*, 432–441. [CrossRef] [PubMed]
8. Iwata, T.; Yamakoshi, Y.; Simmer, J.P.; Ishikawa, I.; Hu, J.C. Establishment of porcine pulp-derived cell lines and expression of recombinant dentin sialoprotein and recombinant dentin matrix protein-1. *Eur. J. Oral Sci.* **2007**, *115*, 48–56. [CrossRef]
9. Kamata, N.; Fujimoto, R.; Tomonari, M.; Taki, M.; Nagayama, M.; Yasumoto, S. Immortalization of human dental papilla, dental pulp, periodontal ligament cells and gingival fibroblasts by telomerase reverse transcriptase. *J. Oral Pathol. Med.* **2004**, *33*, 417–423. [CrossRef]
10. Galler, K.M.; Schweikl, H.; Thonemann, B.; D'Souza, R.N.; Schmalz, G. Human pulp-derived cells immortalized with Simian Virus 40 T-antigen. *Eur. J. Oral Sci.* **2006**, *114*, 138–146. [CrossRef]
11. Yang, X.; van der Kraan, P.M.; van den Dolder, J.; Walboomers, X.F.; Bian, Z.; Fan, M.; Jansen, J.A. STRO-1 selected rat dental pulp stem cells transfected with adenoviral-mediated human bone morphogenetic protein 2 gene show enhanced odontogenic differentiation. *Tissue Eng.* **2007**, *13*, 2803–2812. [CrossRef] [PubMed]
12. Ohazama, A.; Tucker, A.; Sharpe, P.T. Organized tooth-specific cellular differentiation stimulated by BMP4. *J. Dent. Res.* **2005**, *84*, 603–606. [CrossRef] [PubMed]

13. Shimabukuro, Y.; Ueda, M.; Ozasa, M.; Anzai, J.; Takedachi, M.; Yanagita, M.; Ito, M.; Hashikawa, T.; Yamada, S.; Murakami, S. Fibroblast growth factor-2 regulates the cell function of human dental pulp cells. *J. Endod.* **2009**, *35*, 1529–1535. [CrossRef] [PubMed]
14. Tjaderhane, L.; Koivumaki, S.; Paakkonen, V.; Ilvesaro, J.; Soini, Y.; Salo, T.; Metsikko, K.; Tuukkanen, J. Polarity of mature human odontoblasts. *J. Dent. Res.* **2013**, *92*, 1011–1016. [CrossRef]
15. Li, Y.; Lu, X.; Sun, X.; Bai, S.; Li, S.; Shi, J. Odontoblast-like cell differentiation and dentin formation induced with TGF-β1. *Arch. Oral Biol.* **2011**, *56*, 1221–1229. [CrossRef]
16. Neves, V.C.; Babb, R.; Chandrasekaran, D.; Sharpe, P.T. Promotion of natural tooth repair by small molecule GSK3 antagonists. *Sci. Rep.* **2017**, *7*, 39654. [CrossRef]
17. Olkkola, K.T.; Ahonen, J. Midazolam and other benzodiazepines. In *Modern Anesthetics. Handbook of Experimental Pharmacology*; Schuttler, J., Schwilden, H., Eds.; Springer: Berlin, Germany, 2008; Volume 182, pp. 335–360.
18. Smith, R.; Brown, J. Midazolam for status epilepticus. *Aust. Prescr.* **2017**, *40*, 23–25. [CrossRef]
19. So, E.C.; Chen, Y.C.; Wang, S.C.; Wu, C.C.; Huang, M.C.; Lai, M.S.; Pan, B.S.; Kang, F.C.; Huang, B.M. Midazolam regulated caspase pathway, endoplasmic reticulum stress, autophagy, and cell cycle to induce apoptosis in MA-10 mouse Leydig tumor cells. *OncoTargets Ther.* **2016**, *9*, 2519–2533.
20. Ohno, S.; Kobayashi, K.; Uchida, S.; Amano, O.; Sakagami, H.; Nagasaka, H. Cytotoxicity and type of cell death induced by midazolam in human oral normal and tumor cells. *Anticancer Res.* **2012**, *32*, 4737–4747. [PubMed]
21. Stevens, M.F.; Werdehausen, R.; Gaza, N.; Hermanns, H.; Kremer, D.; Bauer, I.; Kury, P.; Hollmann, M.W.; Braun, S. Midazolam activates the intrinsic pathway of apoptosis independent of benzodiazepine and death receptor signaling. *Reg. Anesth. Pain Med.* **2011**, *36*, 343–349. [CrossRef]
22. Mishra, S.K.; Kang, J.H.; Lee, C.W.; Oh, S.H.; Ryu, J.S.; Bae, Y.S.; Kim, H.M. Midazolam induces cellular apoptosis in human cancer cells and inhibits tumor growth in xenograft mice. *Mol. Cells* **2013**, *36*, 219–226. [CrossRef] [PubMed]
23. Zhang, T.; Shao, H.; Xu, K.Q.; Kuang, L.T.; Chen, R.F.; Xiu, H.H. Midazolam suppresses osteogenic differentiation of human bone marrow-derived mesenchymal stem cells. *Eur. Rev. Med. Pharmacol. Sci.* **2014**, *18*, 1411–1418. [PubMed]
24. Sloan, A.J.; Rutherford, R.B.; Smith, A.J. Stimulation of the rat dentine-pulp complex by bone morphogenetic protein-7 in vitro. *Arch. Oral Biol.* **2000**, *45*, 173–177. [CrossRef]
25. Chen, S.; Gu, T.T.; Sreenath, T.; Kulkarni, A.B.; Karsenty, G.; MacDougall, M. Spatial expression of Cbfa1/Runx2 isoforms in teeth and characterization of binding sites in the dspp gene. *Connect. Tissue Res.* **2002**, *43*, 338–344. [CrossRef] [PubMed]
26. 1000 Genomes Project Consortium. A map of human genome variation from population-scale sequencing. *Nature* **2010**, *467*, 1061–1073. [CrossRef] [PubMed]
27. Qin, W.; Yang, F.; Deng, R.; Li, D.; Song, Z.; Tian, Y.; Wang, R.; Ling, J.; Lin, Z. Smad 1/5 is involved in bone morphogenetic protein-2-induced odontoblastic differentiation in human dental pulp cells. *J. Endod.* **2012**, *38*, 66–71. [CrossRef] [PubMed]
28. Li, J.; Huang, X.; Xu, X.; Mayo, J.; Bringas, P., Jr.; Jiang, R.; Wang, S.; Chai, Y. SMAD4-mediated WNT signaling controls the fate of cranial neural crest cells during tooth morphogenesis. *Development* **2011**, *138*, 1977–1989. [CrossRef]
29. Cope, D.W.; Hughes, S.W.; Crunelli, V. $GABA_A$ receptor-mediated tonic inhibition in thalamic neurons. *J. Neurosci.* **2005**, *25*, 11553–11563. [CrossRef]
30. Bormann, J. The 'ABC' of GABA receptors. *Trends Pharmacol. Sci.* **2000**, *21*, 16–19. [CrossRef]
31. Kim, J.H.; Jeon, M.; Song, J.S.; Lee, J.H.; Choi, B.J.; Jung, H.S.; Moon, S.J.; DenBesten, P.K.; Kim, S.O. Distinctive genetic activity pattern of the human dental pulp between deciduous and permanent teeth. *PLoS ONE* **2014**, *9*, e102893. [CrossRef]
32. Kim, S.H.; Kim, S.; Shin, Y.; Lee, H.S.; Jeon, M.; Kim, S.O.; Cho, S.W.; Ruparel, N.B.; Song, J.S. Comparative Gene Expression Analysis of the Coronal Pulp and Apical Pulp Complex in Human Immature Teeth. *J. Endod.* **2016**, *42*, 752–759. [CrossRef] [PubMed]
33. Potdar, P.D.; Jethmalani, Y.D. Human dental pulp stem cells: Applications in future regenerative medicine. *World J. Stem Cells* **2015**, *7*, 839–851. [CrossRef] [PubMed]

34. Shi, S.; Gronthos, S. Perivascular niche of postnatal mesenchymal stem cells in human bone marrow and dental pulp. *J. Bone Miner. Res.* **2003**, *18*, 696–704. [CrossRef] [PubMed]
35. Yamamoto, R.; Oida, S.; Yamakoshi, Y. Dentin Sialophosphoprotein-derived Proteins in the Dental Pulp. *J. Dent. Res.* **2015**, *94*, 1120–1127. [CrossRef] [PubMed]
36. Niwa, T.; Yamakoshi, Y.; Yamazaki, H.; Karakida, T.; Chiba, R.; Hu, J.C.; Nagano, T.; Yamamoto, R.; Simmer, J.P.; Margolis, H.C.; et al. The dynamics of TGF-β in dental pulp, odontoblasts and dentin. *Sci. Rep.* **2018**, *8*, 4450. [CrossRef]
37. Puchtler, H.; Meloan, S.N.; Terry, M.S. On the history and mechanism of alizarin and alizarin red S stains for calcium. *J. Histochem. Cytochem.* **1969**, *17*, 110–124. [CrossRef]
38. Puchtler, H.; Meloan, S.N. Demonstration of phosphates in calcium deposits: a modification of von Kossa's reaction. *Histochemistry* **1978**, *56*, 177–185. [CrossRef]
39. Saito, T.; Toyooka, H.; Ito, S.; Crenshaw, M.A. In vitro study of remineralization of dentin: effects of ions on mineral induction by decalcified dentin matrix. *Caries Res.* **2003**, *37*, 445–449. [CrossRef]
40. Yamakoshi, Y.; Lu, Y.; Hu, J.C.; Kim, J.W.; Iwata, T.; Kobayashi, K.; Nagano, T.; Yamakoshi, F.; Hu, Y.; Fukae, M.; et al. Porcine dentin sialophosphoprotein: length polymorphisms, glycosylation, phosphorylation, and stability. *J. Biol. Chem.* **2008**, *283*, 14835–14844. [CrossRef]
41. Onuma, K.; Iijima, M. Artificial enamel induced by phase transformation of amorphous nanoparticles. *Sci. Rep.* **2017**, *7*, 2711. [CrossRef]
42. Teruel Jde, D.; Alcolea, A.; Hernandez, A.; Ruiz, A.J. Comparison of chemical composition of enamel and dentine in human, bovine, porcine and ovine teeth. *Arch. Oral Biol.* **2015**, *60*, 768–775. [CrossRef] [PubMed]
43. Nagano, T.; Oida, S.; Suzuki, S.; Iwata, T.; Yamakoshi, Y.; Ogata, Y.; Gomi, K.; Arai, T.; Fukae, M. Porcine Enamel Protein Fractions Contain Transforming Growth Factor-β1. *J. Periodontol.* **2006**, *77*, 1688–1694. [CrossRef] [PubMed]
44. Wang, L.; Nancollas, G.H. Calcium orthophosphates: crystallization and dissolution. *Chem. Rev.* **2008**, *108*, 4628–4669. [CrossRef] [PubMed]
45. Rodriguez-Esteban, R. A Drug-Centric View of Drug Development: How Drugs Spread from Disease to Disease. *PLoS Comput. Biol.* **2016**, *12*, e1004852. [CrossRef] [PubMed]
46. Brown, A.S.; Patel, C.J. A standard database for drug repositioning. *Sci. Data* **2017**, *4*, 170029. [CrossRef] [PubMed]

11

Tuning Nano-Amorphous Calcium Phosphate Content in Novel Rechargeable Antibacterial Dental Sealant

Maria Salem Ibrahim [1,2], Faisal D. AlQarni [3], Yousif A. Al-Dulaijan [3], Michael D. Weir [4], Thomas W. Oates [4], Hockin H. K. Xu [4,5,6] and Mary Anne S. Melo [4,*]

1 Program in Dental Biomedical Sciences, University of Maryland School of Dentistry, Baltimore, MD 21201, USA; msyibrahim@gmail.com

2 Department of Preventive Dental Sciences, College of Dentistry, Imam Abdulrahman bin Faisal University, Dammam 34212, Saudi Arabia

3 Department of Substitutive Dental Sciences, College of Dentistry, Imam Abdulrahman bin Faisal University, Dammam 34212, Saudi Arabia; falqarni@icloud.com (F.D.A.); yaldulaijan@gmail.com (Y.A.A-D.)

4 Department of Advanced Oral Sciences and Therapeutics, University of Maryland School of Dentistry, Baltimore, MD 21201, USA; MWeir@umaryland.edu (M.D.W.); TOates@umaryland.edu (T.W.O.); HXu@umaryland.edu (H.H.K.X.)

5 Center for Stem Cell Biology & Regenerative Medicine, University of Maryland School of Medicine, Baltimore, MD 21201, USA

6 Marlene and Stewart Greenebaum Cancer Center, University of Maryland School of Medicine, Baltimore, MD 21201, USA

* Correspondence: mmelo@umaryland.edu

Abstract: Dental sealants with antibacterial and remineralizing properties are promising for caries prevention among children and adolescents. The application of nanotechnology and polymer development have enabled nanoparticles of amorphous calcium phosphate (NACP) and dimethylaminohexadecyl methacrylate (DMAHDM) to emerge as anti-caries strategies via resin-based dental materials. Our objectives in this study were to (1) incorporate different mass fractions of NACP into a parental rechargeable and antibacterial sealant; (2) investigate the effects on mechanical performance, and (3) assess how the variations in NACP concentration would affect the calcium (Ca) and phosphate (PO_4) ion release and re-chargeability over time. NACP were synthesized using a spray-drying technique and incorporated at mass fractions of 0, 10, 20 and 30%. Flexural strength, flexural modulus, and flowability were assessed for mechanical and physical performance. Ca and PO_4 ion release were measured over 70 days, and three ion recharging cycles were performed for re-chargeability. The impact of the loading percentage of NACP upon the sealant's performance was evaluated, and the optimized formulation was eventually selected. The experimental sealant at 20% NACP had flexural strength and flexural modulus of 79.5 ± 8.4 MPa and 4.2 ± 0.4 GPa, respectively, while the flexural strength and flexural modulus of a commercial sealant control were 70.7 ± 5.5 MPa ($p > 0.05$) and 3.3 ± 0.5 GPa ($p < 0.05$), respectively. A significant reduction in flow was observed in the experimental sealant at 30% NACP ($p < 0.05$). Increasing the NACP mass fraction increased the ion release. The sealant formulation with NACP at 20% displayed desirable mechanical performance and ideal flow and handling properties, and also showed high levels of long-term Ca and PO_4 ion release and excellent recharge capabilities. The findings provide fundamental data for the development of a new generation of antibacterial and rechargeable Ca and PO_4 dental sealants to promote remineralization and inhibit caries.

Keywords: dental sealant; resin sealant; calcium phosphate nanoparticles; long-term ion release; remineralization; ion recharge

1. Introduction

Dental caries is still a highly prevalent oral disease worldwide despite the various approaches that have been used to prevent it [1,2]. These approaches include fluoride exposure, sugar intake control, brushing and dental sealants [3]. Dental sealants help prevent caries in pits and fissures of primary and permanent teeth, acting as a physical barrier for food accumulation and bacterial growth [4]. Accumulative evidence from epidemiologic findings has shown positive outcomes for caries prevention when the teeth are sealed, in comparison to non-sealed teeth in children and adolescents [4,5]. It was found that sealants on permanent molars may reduce dental caries for up to 24–48 months when compared to that of no sealant application [3,4]. In terms of sealants' retention, resin-based sealants are the materials with a higher success rate [6]. Even so, findings have shown an increase in dental resin-based sealants failures due to bacterial colonization under the restored fissures, thereby, initiating and progressing the carious lesion beneath the sealant [4].

Caries lesions at the sealed occlusal surfaces were initiated when the balance between the remineralization and demineralization of the tooth structure was adversely affected, and demineralization exceeded the remineralization abilities, resulting in the dissolution of hydroxyapatite crystals [7]. To allow the remineralization process to occur, adequate levels of calcium (Ca) and phosphate (PO_4) ions must be available [8]. Antibacterial and remineralizing resin-based sealants could be one of the most desirable approaches for management of dental caries in children and adolescents due to the potential of reduced bacteria and provide localized ion release near the tooth surface.

Recently, new fundamental research findings have highlighted the application of nanotechnology and polymer development in dental materials, enabling nanoparticles of amorphous calcium phosphate (NACP) and quaternary ammonium methacrylate such as dimethylaminohexadecyl methacrylate (DMAHDM) to emerge as anti-caries strategies via resin-based materials [9,10]. Amorphous calcium phosphate ($Ca_3[PO_4]_2$), as a precursor of the final crystalline hydroxyapatite, has been investigated as a suitable remineralizing agent. There is a growing body of evidence suggesting that NACP could enhance the remineralizing capacity due to a greater surface area-to-volume ratio [11,12]. NACP had a relatively high specific surface area of 17.76 m^2/g, compared to about 0.5 m^2/g of traditional micron-sized calcium phosphate particles used in dental resins [13,14]. Supported by the high performance of Ca and PO_4 ion release provided by a nanostructured compound, NACP has led to new possibilities for combating enamel demineralization [15].

Resin-based sealants with the ability to release Ca and PO_4 ions are expected to suppress the demineralization process and prevent dental caries. However, ion-depletion effect with loss of bioactivity over time (short-term ion release) has been a major drawback for calcium phosphate-containing resins [6,16]. Recently, significant levels of Ca and PO_4 ions were released from NACP-containing resins that were sustainable over long periods of time and with rechargeable capacity [17,18]. The rechargeable capability of NACP-containing dental materials have opened new horizons and are expected to lead to relevant changes in remineralizing approaches [19]. The repeatable recharge process to re-release Ca and PO_4 ions can lead to supersaturation into the surrounding microenvironments under acidic attacks, such as enamel areas located within deep occlusal pits and fissures with difficult access to brush. These ions can play a vital role in the precipitation of crystallites. This capability is highly desirable in a resin-based formulation for sealing the occlusal pits and fissures where high rates of demineralization happen and result in almost 50% of all caries in school children [2,4].

Many of the innovative bioactive strategies and technologies require new dental materials with new combinations of properties to meet the basic properties of the conventional polymeric materials [13]. This is true for resin-based formulations that are needed for dental sealant applications. For example, regarding the chemical and physical characteristics, the resin-based sealants must possess a high degree of wettability, and flow and viscosity that allow the penetration between the occlusal fissures and grooves of the teeth [5]. Another important characteristic is the resistance to abrasion and fracture, which would demonstrate the adequate mechanical performance of the material [6]. This is a challenging combination of characteristics when developing new resin-based formulations. Frequently, the incorporation of new agents in the resin-based system decreases the strength or bioactivity.

The present study reports the development of new antibacterial resin-based sealants that include NACP for Ca and PO_4 ion release and recharge properties. Our objectives were to (1) incorporate different mass fractions of NACP into parental rechargeable antibacterial sealant; (2) investigate the effects on mechanical performance; and (3) assess how the variations in NACP concentration would affect the Ca and PO_4 ions release and re-chargeability over time. It was hypothesized that adding an increased percentage of NACP would have acceptable mechanical and physical performances, while producing substantial initial ion release and a long-term repeated recharge capability.

2. Results

Illustration of the rechargeable NACP approach to dealing with the dissolution-diffusion process of enamel demineralization around dental sealants is shown schematically in Figure 1. The ion recharge cycle diagram displayed the ion re-release from the exhausted and recharged NACP-containing resin-based sealants in Figure 1A. Three recharge/re-release cycles were performed, and each re-release was measured for 14 days. The ion re-release increased with increasing the NACP filler level. Figure 1B shows the TEM image of NACP synthesized using the spray-drying technique having sizes of about 100–300 nm. The structural model of amorphous calcium phosphate is exemplified in this image, and the potential application for sealing the occlusal surface of the posterior teeth is illustrated.

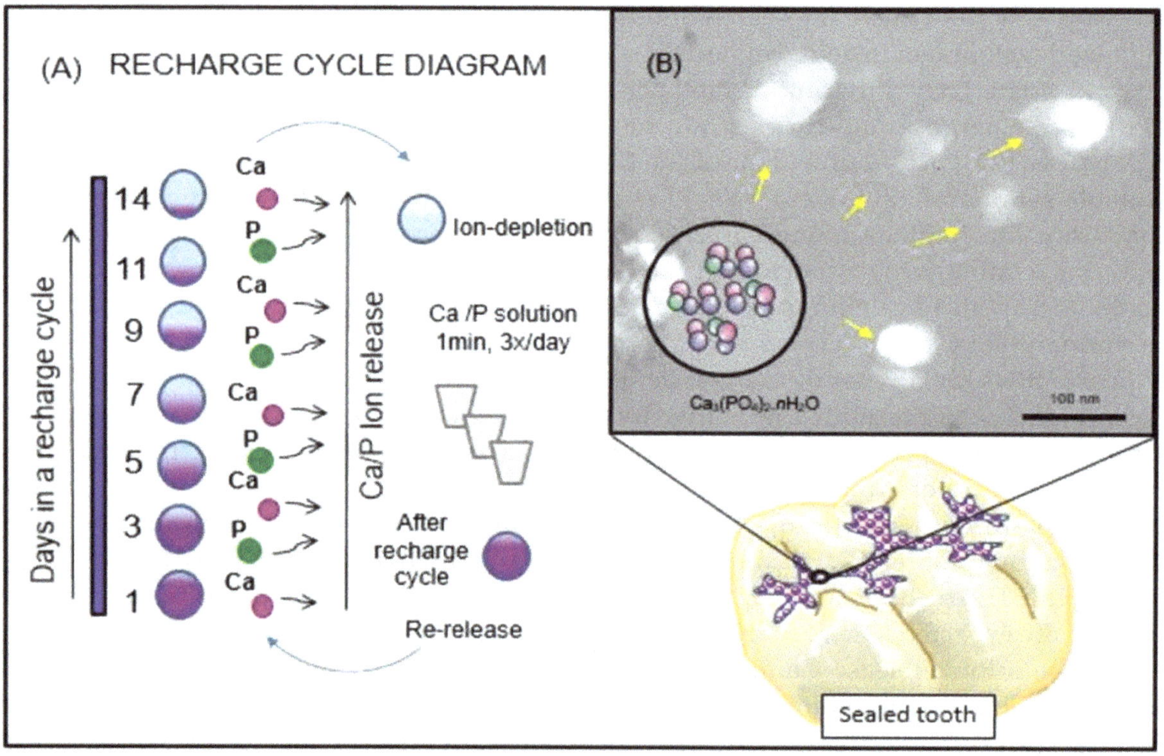

Figure 1. Schematic diagram of the rechargeable nanoparticles of amorphous calcium phosphate (NACP) sealant approach to deal with enamel demineralization around dental sealants: In (**A**), the recharge cycle diagram illustrates the re-release from the exhausted and recharged NACP sealants. Three recharge/re-release cycles were performed, and each re-release was measured for 14 days. The ion re-release increased with increasing the NACP filler level. In (**B**), the TEM image of NACP from the spray-drying technique having sizes of about 100–300 nm.

Figure 2 describes the flexural strength and modulus of the antibacterial and rechargeable resin-based sealants (Mean ± SD; $n = 8$). In Figure 2A, the flexural strength showed a decreasing trend with increasing NACP percentage, because the glass filler level was decreasing from 50% to 20%. The experimental sealant at 20% NACP had the flexural strength and flexural modulus of 79.5 ± 8.4 MPa and 4.2 ± 0.4 GPa, respectively. The commercial high viscosity sealant control showed flexural strength and flexural modulus of 70.7 ± 5.5 MPa ($p > 0.05$) and 3.3 ± 0.5 GPa ($p < 0.05$). These results demonstrated that the rechargeable antibacterial sealant at 20% mass fraction of NACP had mechanical properties similar to or higher than that of the commercial sealant/flowable composite control. Only the sealant with 30% NACP had a significantly lower strength that those other groups ($p < 0.05$).

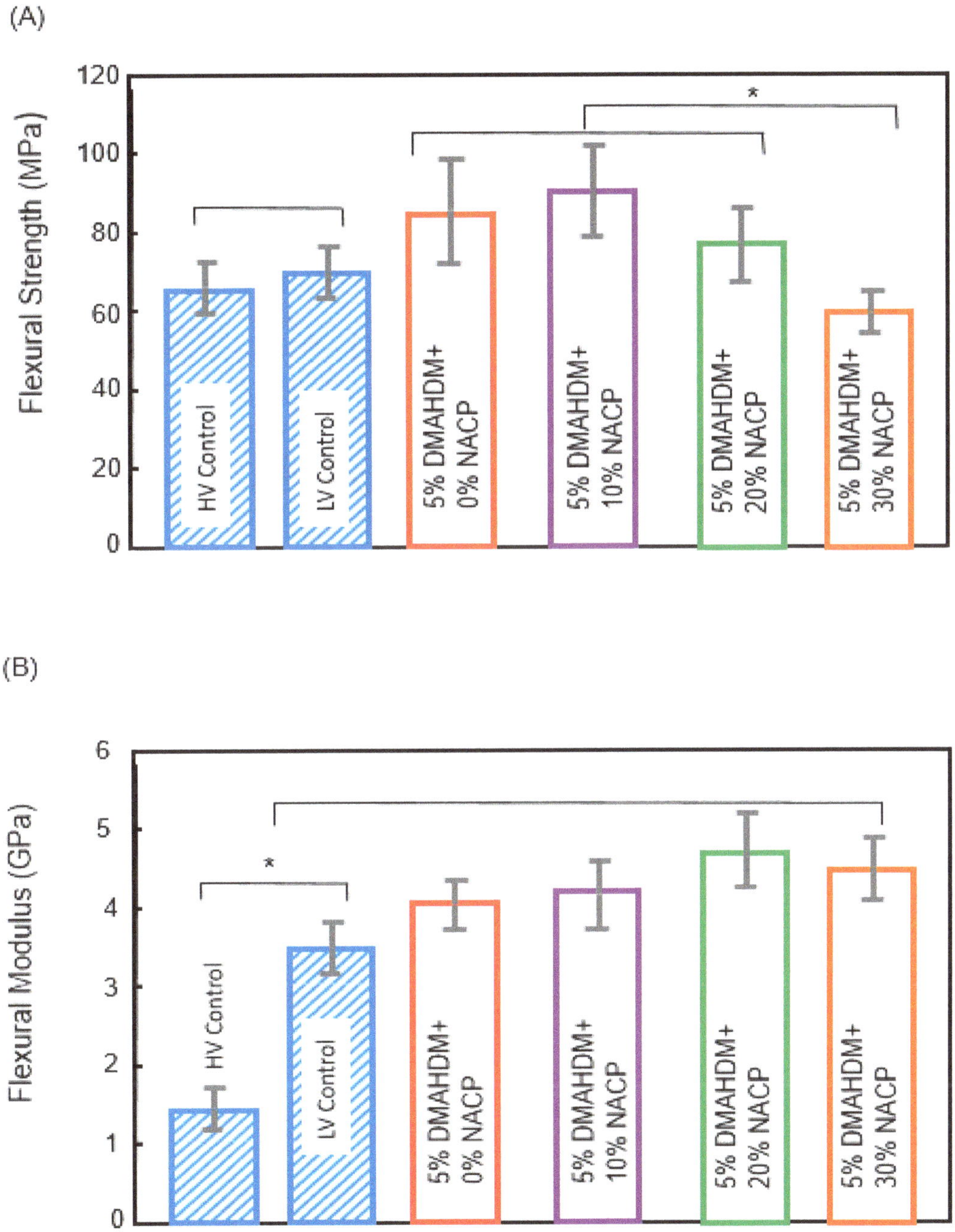

Figure 2. Bar graphs of (**A**) flexural strength and (**B**) flexural modulus (Mean ± SD; $n = 8$) of resin-based sealants. The asterisk means that there was a statistically significant difference between the groups.

The flow results for the experimental and control resin-based sealants (Mean ± SD; $n = 6$) are plotted in Figure 3. NACP at a mass fraction of 30% compromised the flow of the sealant ($p < 0.05$). Experimental sealant with a mass fraction of 20% NACP had a flow that was not significantly different from the control ($p > 0.05$).

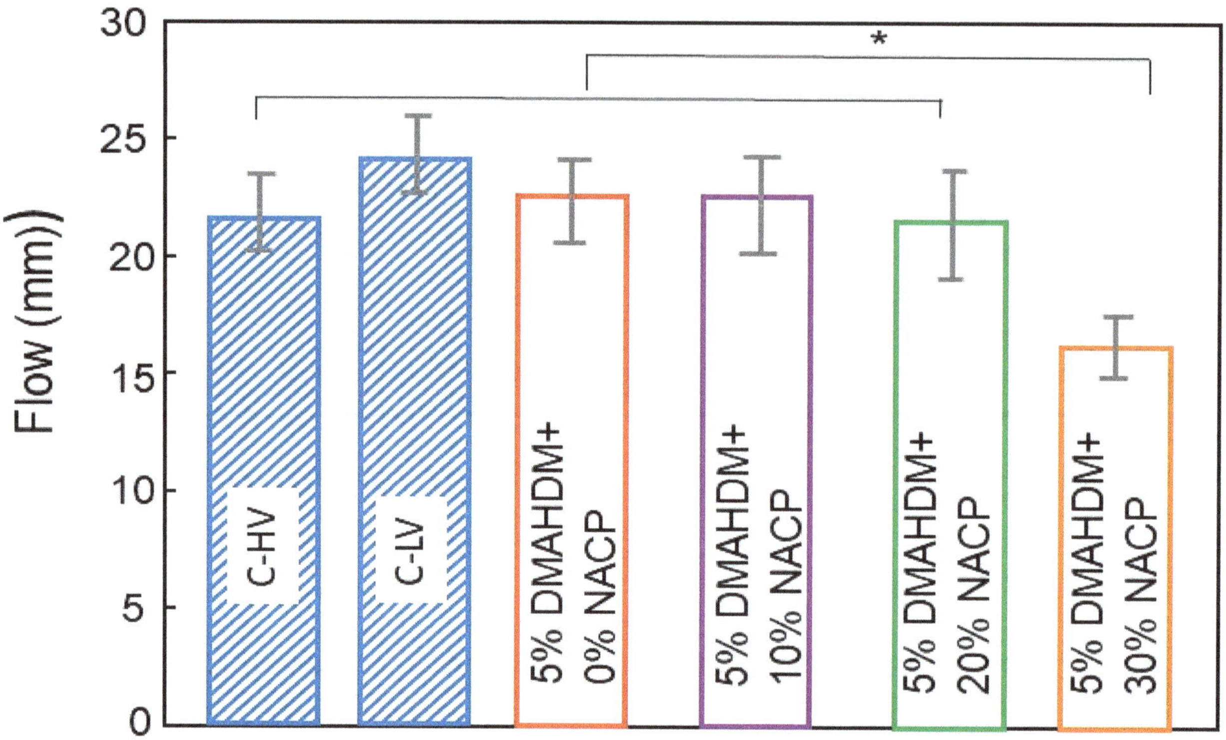

Figure 3. Means ± SD of flow analysis of the resin-based sealant formulations ($n = 6$). The asterisk means that there was a statistically significant difference between the groups.

Figure 4 plots the Ca and PO_4 initial ion release over time (Mean ± SD; $n = 6$). After 70 days of ion release, 30% NACP + 5% DMAHDM sealant had higher Ca ion release of 4.70 ± 0.95 mmol/L. This amount was significantly different from 20% NACP + 5% DMAHDM sealant that released 3.64 ± 0.11 mmol/L ($p < 0.05$). The PO_4 ion release had similar release behavior. The 30% NACP + 5% DMAHDM sealant showed 4.25 ± 0.12 mmol/L of PO_4 ion release, followed by the 20% NACP + 5% DMAHDM with 3.41 ± 0.10 mmol/L of PO_4 ion release ($p < 0.05$). During the 70 days, the pH increased from approximately 4.5 to 6.5 for the groups of the formulations containing 20% and 30% NACP. These changes represent the neutralizing capabilities of calcium and phosphate ion release.

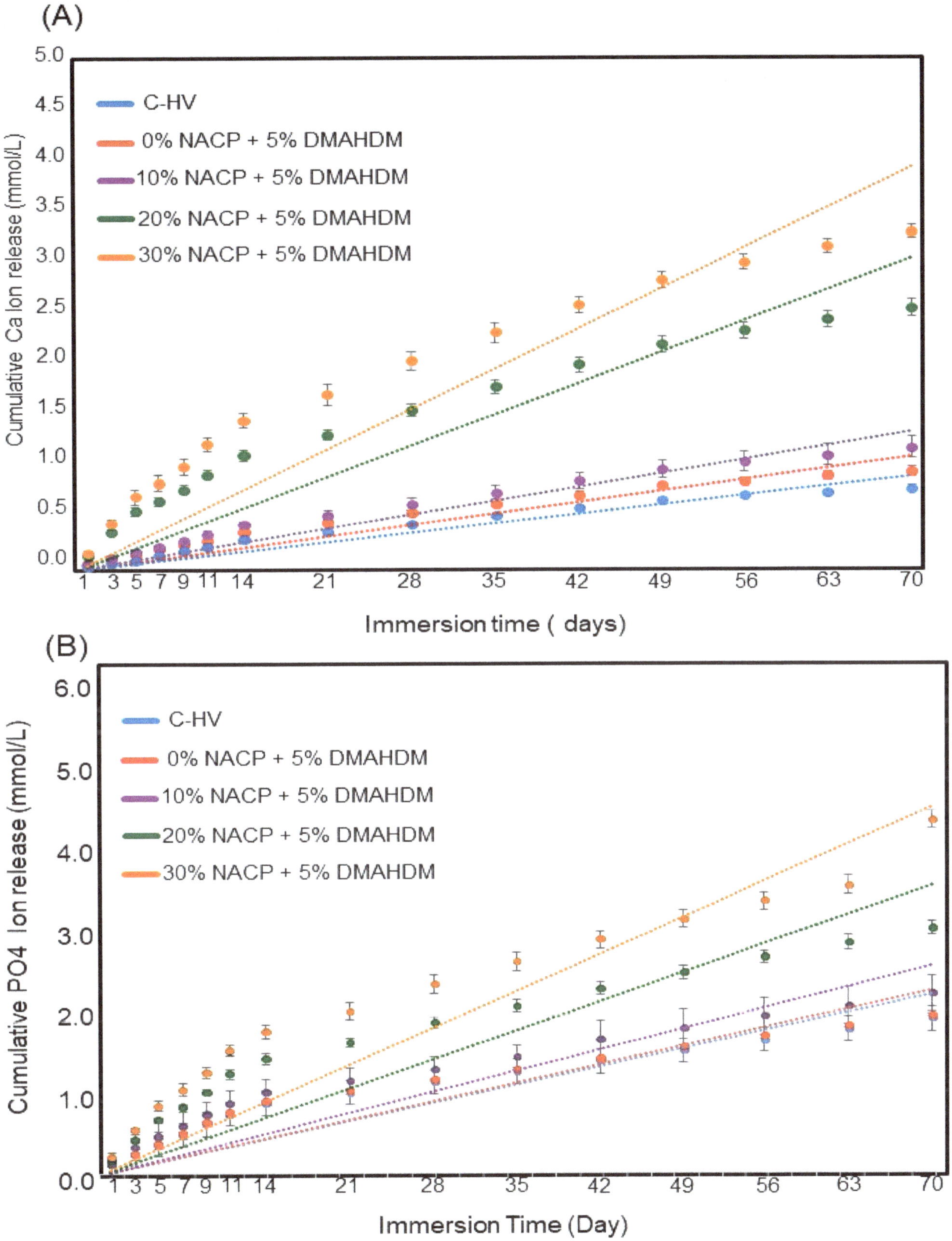

Figure 4. Cumulative initial ions release from sealants (Mean ± SD; $n = 6$). In (**A**), Calcium (Ca) ion and in (**B**) Phosphate ions. The dots for each group show the exact data and the dotted line is its approximate linear trend for each formulation.

The results of the three cycles of ion recharge and re-release are presented in Figure 5. The Ca ion re-releases after the first cycle were 0.46 ± 0.03, 0.73 ± 0.03, and 0.94 ± 0.04 for the experimental sealants with 10%, 20% and 30% NACP, respectively ($p < 0.05$ between the three groups). On the other hand, the PO_4 ion re-release after the first cycle were 1.10 ± 0.01, 1.22 ± 0.02, and 1.25 ± 0.03 for the experimental sealants with 10%, 20% and 30% NACP, respectively ($p > 0.05$ between the 20% and 30% NACP groups). All the experimental sealants showed good Ca and PO_4 ion recharging abilities in the three cycles tested.

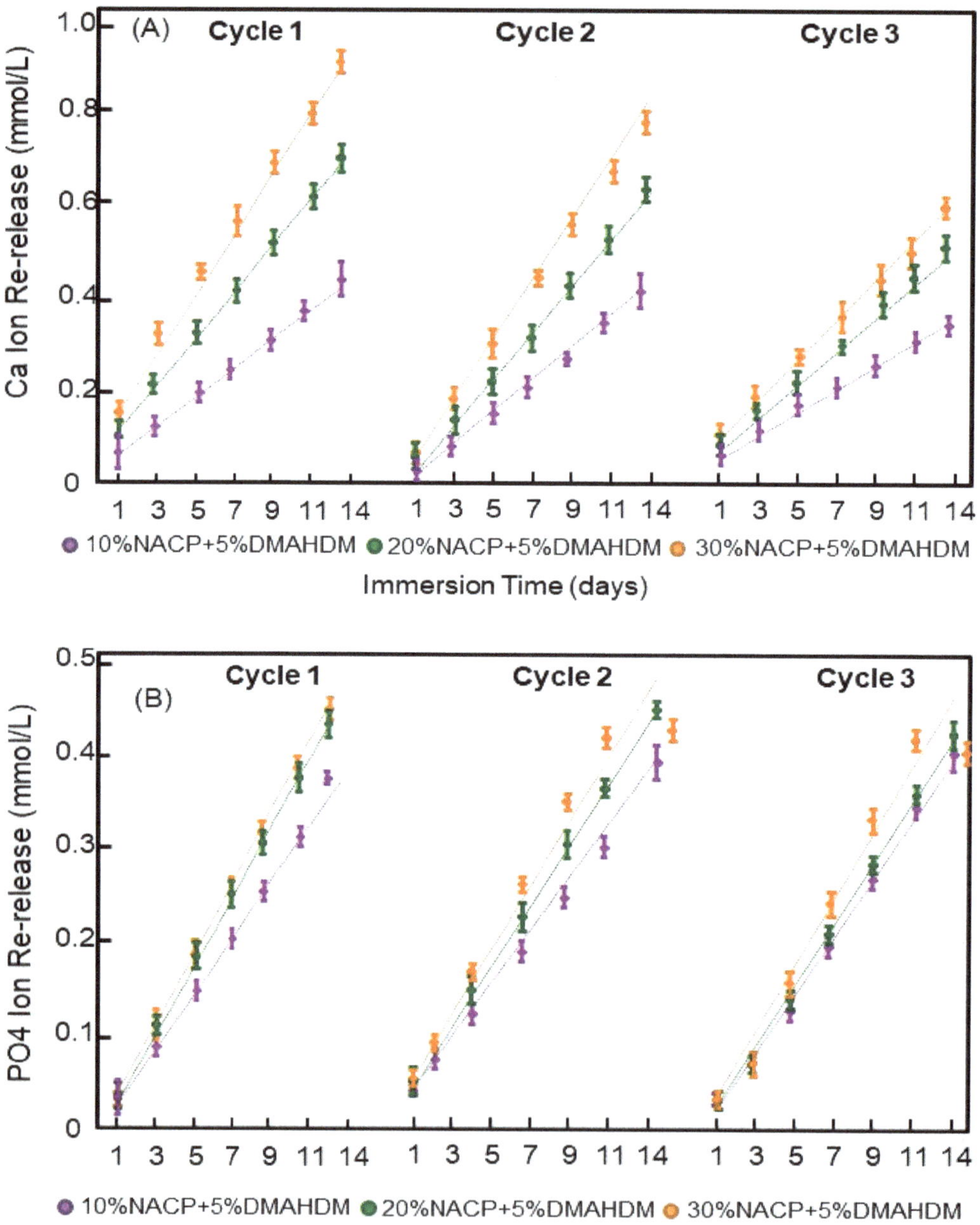

Figure 5. Cumulative ions re-release from the recharged resin dental sealants (Mean $\pm$ SD; $n = 3$) after three cycles of ions recharge and re-release. The dots for each group show the exact data and the dotted line is its approximate linear trend for each formulation. In (**A**), Calcium ion and in (**B**) Phosphate ions. There was no decrease in the ion re-release amounts with increasing the number of recharge and re-release cycles.

3. Discussion

Recent studies have developed rechargeable NACP resin-based materials for long-term Ca and PO_4 ion release to combat tooth decay [17,19], but the effects of NACP filler level on antibacterial sealant properties had not been reported. Developing a new dental material for sealant applications must meet the basic property requirements of clinicians. Thus, in the present study, an antibacterial and rechargeable Ca and PO_4 releasing sealant was developed for the first time. The effects of NACP mass fraction on mechanical and physical performance and Ca and PO_4 ions initial release and re-release were determined to allow the development of ideal formulation with bioavailable ions for potential enamel remineralization of occlusal pits and fissures.

In the case of the enlarged pit and fissure sealing, the mechanical properties of the material become more important since the material can be placed onto areas that encounter mechanical stresses during clenching [6]. In that situation, it appears clearly from the results that flowable resin composites have by far better flexural moduli than the pit and fissure sealants tested. Here, we assessed the flexural strength, flexural modulus and flow of different formulations and compared them to the commercial resin-based sealant and flowable composite that did not contain NACP. The percentage load of the glass filler ranged from 50% in 5% DMAHDM + 0% NACP sealant to 20% in 5% DMAHDM + 30% NACP formulation. Previous studies also revealed that the incorporation of a high content mass fraction of nanoparticles, such as 40% might have a negative impact on material properties [20,21]. Therefore, only three different mass fractions of NACP were used in this study: 5% DMAHDM + 10% NACP, 5% DMAHDM + 20% NACP, and 5% DMAHDM + 30% NACP. However, the results obtained in this study revealed a significant interference of the NACP at the 30% mass fraction with the flow of the experimental sealant. In deep fissures and grooves, the flow of the material is an important characteristic to help seal the total surface [4]. It is expected that the sealant's flow ability could be compromised when the experimental sealant incorporates the highest amount of NACP. Our findings suggest that the new formulation with 20% NACP did not negatively affect the mechanical and physical properties, while providing substantial Ca and PO_4 ions to inhibit caries.

Adding different caries-preventive measures and strategies to the sealant may increase its effect on caries prevention [5]. In previous studies, antibacterial resins containing quaternary ammonium methacrylates with an alkyl chain length of 16 (DMAHDM) were synthesized and assessed with a higher antibacterial potency against oral bacteria as an outcome. The mechanism of positively charged quaternary amine disrupting the negatively charged bacterial membranes supported the decrease in bacterial coverage nearly 90% for resin formulations at 5% DMAHDM [17,19]. The long-term antibacterial activity of DMAHDM was demonstrated by Zhang et al. [20] and attributed to the fact that the antibacterial monomer was copolymerized with the resin by forming a covalent bonding with the polymer network. Thus, the development of a resin-based dental sealant that also holds remineralizing properties could be essential to improve the function of the resin-based dental sealant on posterior teeth fissures and grooves for caries prevention.

Regarding recharge ability, this study builds upon the methodology provided by Zhang et al. [21]. Their report confirmed that the recharge of calcium and phosphate ions from resin-based formulations was achievable, while also establishing some of the variables important for ion release and recharge such as chemical composition of resin matrix and number of suitable cycles for recharge of the specimens. For the tested formulations, the 20% NACP sealant showed a release of 3.64 ± 0.11 mmol/L ($p < 0.05$) of Ca ions and 3.41 ± 0.10 mmol/L of PO_4 ions during the 70-day period. The effect of the NACP percentage loading within the resin-based antibacterial formulation containing 5% DMAHDM on the rate of Ca and PO_4 is reported in Figure 4A,B. When comparing the 20% NACP formulation and 10% NACP formulation, an approximate three times increase in Ca and PO_4 ions released was observed. However, as the NACP percentage load increased, the rate of diffusion of ions from the sealants increased approximately 5%. It appears that an increase in the NACP concentration by a factor of 1.5 does not provide the same corresponding increase in Ca and PO_4 ion concentration over 70 days, which makes the 20%NACP formulations suitable for the proposed application.

Referring to previous studies from our group, this release concentration of Ca and PO_4 ions was similar to release and recharge rates previously observed in a 30% NACP parental formulation with high inorganic filler content for reinforcement [17]. This variation could be attributed to the differences in the filler level in each formulation since in order for these ions to be available for remineralization, they must diffuse through the resin matrix, in this case, 50% PEHB.

The chemical composition of the formulation has a unique role for rechargeability. Since one of our objectives in this study was to develop ion-rechargeable resin-based sealants, PEHB resin matrix was chosen. The PEHB resin had shown high ion-recharging abilities in previous reports [19,22,23]. In the present study, the sealant showed promising ion recharging abilities because of the great amount of re-released Ca and PO_4 ions after each cycle of ion-recharge. This is likely due to the acidic adhesive monomer PMGDM [18], which consists of a large part of the parental resin matrix PEHB. The suggested recharge mechanism of NACP is based on the ability of PMGDM chelate with the recharging Ca ions during the recharging process, and release the ions when it is exposed to the acidic environment, such as pH 4. Further study is needed to investigate Ca and P ion recharge and re-release mechanisms in solutions that mimic the oral environment, such as artificial saliva.

4. Materials and Methods

4.1. Development of Dental Resin Sealants

The resin matrix consisted of 44.5% of pyromellitic glycerol dimethacrylate (PMGDM) (Hampford, Stratford, CT, USA), 39.5% of ethoxylated bisphenol a dimethacrylate (EBPADMA) (Sigma-Aldrich, St. Louis, MO, USA), 10% of 2-hydroxyethyl methacrylate (HEMA) (Esstech, Essington, PA, USA), and 5% of bisphenol a glycidyl dimethacrylate (Esstech) [17]. 1% of phenylbis (2,4,6-trimethylbenzoyl)-phosphine oxide (BAPO) (Sigma-Aldrich) was added as a photo-initiator. This resin matrix is referred to as PEHB. To formulate a sealant with antibacterial properties, dimethylaminohexadecyl methacrylate (DMAHDM) was synthesized via a modified Menschutkin reaction using a method as described previously [22].

NACP was synthesized by a spray-drying technique according to previous methodology [21]. Briefly, calcium carbonate and dicalcium phosphate were dissolved in acetic acid to produce Ca ions with a concentration of 8 mmol/L and PO_4 ions with a concentration of 5.3 mmol/L, then this solution was sprayed in a heated chamber using a spray-drying machine. An electrostatic precipitator was used to harvest the NACP with a particle size of average $\pm$ 116 nm. The silanized barium boroaluminosilicate glass particles were added for reinforcement purposes and had an average size of 1.4 μm (Caulk/Dentsply, Milford, DE, USA). The fillers were incorporated into the resin matrix at a filler level of 50%. Two main types of resin-based materials were available as pit and fissure sealants: filled flowable composite and unfilled resin-based sealants, both were used as commercial controls in this study. Hence, the following six sealants were tested.

1. Commercial Low-viscosity Sealant control termed "C-LV." (FluroShield, Dentsply Caulk, Milford, DE, USA)".
2. Commercial High-viscosity Sealant/Flowable Composite control termed "C-HV." (Virtuoso, Den-Mat Holdings, Lompoc, CA, USA).
3. Experimental Sealant termed "5% DMAHDM + 0% NACP" (45% PEHB + 5% DMAHDM + 50% Glass + 0% NACP).
4. Experimental Sealant termed "5% DMAHDM + 10% NACP" (45% PEHB + 5% DMAHDM + 40% Glass + 10% NACP).
5. Experimental Sealant termed "5% DMAHDM + 20% NACP" (45% PEHB + 5% DMAHDM + 30% Glass + 20% NACP).

6. Experimental Sealant termed "5% DMAHDM + 30% NACP" (45% PEHB + 5% DMAHDM + 20% Glass + 30% NACP).

4.2. Flexural Strength and Flexural Modulus

Samples for flexural strength and flexural modulus testing were prepared using 2 × 2 × 25 mm stainless steel molds. Each paste was placed into the mold which was covered with Mylar strips and glass slides from both open sides of the mold then light-cured (500 mW/cm^2, 60 s, Triad 2000, Dentsply, York, PA, USA) for on each open side. Samples were stored at 37 °C for 24 h. Flexural strength and flexural modulus were measured using three-point flexure with a 10 mm span at a crosshead-speed of 1 mm/min on a computer-controlled universal testing machine (MTS 5500R, Cary, NC, USA) [24].

Flexural strength (F) was calculated by using the following formula:

$F = (3LS)/(2WH^2)$, where L is the maximum load; S is the span; W is the width of the specimen and H is the height.

Flexural Modulus (M) was determined as:

$M = (LS^3 3)/(4WH^3 3d)$, where L is the maximum load; S is the span; W is the width of the specimen, H is the height of the specimen, and d is the defluxion corresponding to the load L.

4.3. Flow Analysis

The recommendations of the ISO 6876/2012 and ANSI/ADA2000 standards were followed [25]. Briefly, two glass plates of 40 mm × 40 mm and approximately 5 mm thickness were used. The weight of one glass plate was approximately 20 g. The paste of each sealant was placed in the center of one of the glass plates using a graduated syringe. The amount of sealant was approximately 0.05 mL. The second glass plate was placed on top of the sealant; then a 100 g weight was used to make a total weight of approximately 120 g. After 10 minutes, the weight was removed, and the largest and smallest diameters of the discs formed by the compressed sealants were measured with the aid of a digital caliber (Mitutoyo MTI Corp., Huntersville, NC, USA) [26]. Six tests were done for each sealant.

4.4. Measurement of Initial Calcium and Phosphate Ions Release from NACP

Three specimens of approximately 2 × 2 × 12 mm were immersed in 50 mL of sodium chloride (NaCl) solution (133 mmol/L). The NaCl solution was previously buffered to pH 4 with 50 mmol/L of lactic acid to simulate a cariogenic low pH condition [27]. The specimen volume per solution ratio was almost 2.9 mm^3/mL following previous study [22]. The tubes ($n = 6$) were kept in a 37 °C incubator during the experiment. Aliquots were collected at 1, 3, 5, 7, 9, 11, 14, 21, 28, 35, 42, 49, 56, 63 and 70 days. The Ca and PO_4 ions concentrations from collected aliquots were analyzed using SpectraMax® M Series Multi-Mode Microplate Reader from Molecular Devices [28]. The absorbance was measured using known standards and calibration curves. After each collection, the NaCl solution was replaced by a fresh solution. All the groups were tested for the initial Ca and PO_4 ions release [29].

4.5. Calcium and Phosphate Ions Recharge and Re-Release

After the calcium and phosphate ions released for 70 days, the specimens were stored for almost 6 months before starting the ion recharging experiment to exhaust the ions in all the specimen and ensure there is no additional ion release. The pH of the immersion solutions was assessed by the same period of time. Then, these ion-exhausted specimens were used for the ion recharging experiment. The Ca ion recharging solution was made of 100 mmol/L $CaCl_2$ and 50 mmol/L HEPES buffer [18]. The PO_4 ion recharge solution was made of 60 mmol/L $KHPO_4$ and 50 mmol/L HEPES buffer. Both solutions were adjusted to pH 7 by the use of 1 mol/L KOH [19]. Three specimens of approx. 2 × 2 × 12 mm were immersed in 5 mL of the calcium ion or phosphate ion recharging solution and gently vortexed for 1 min using Analog Vortex Mixer, (Fisher Scientific, Waltham, MA, USA) to simulate the action of using mouthwash [30]. Specimens were immersed three times for 1 minute each time. This is for a total of 3 min of ion recharge. After that, the recharged specimens were immersed in a

50 mL NaCl solution, which was adjusted to pH 4 as described in Section 4.4. This immersion was to measure the Ca and PO_4 ion re-release on day 1, 2, 3, 5, 9, 11 and 14. After 14 days, the specimens were recharged again, and then the ion re-release was measured for 14 days at day 1, 2, 3, 5, 7, 9, 11 and 14 [31]. The same cycle or recharge and release were repeated for three times as described in Figure 1. The Ca and PO_4 ion measurements were assessed in the same way as mentioned in Section 4.4.

4.6. Statistical Analysis

Kolmogorov-Smirnov test and Levene test were performed to confirm the normality and equal variance of data. The results of flexural strength, flexural modulus, flow and Ca and PO_4 ion release and re-release were analyzed using one-way analysis of variance (ANOVA). Multiple comparisons between the different groups were conducted using Bonferroni's multiple comparison tests. All the statistical analyses were performed by SPSS 22.0 software (SPSS, Chicago, IL, USA) at an alpha of 0.05.

5. Conclusions

The effects of different percentage loading of the remineralizing agent, NACP in new dental material formulations have been studied in a thorough and systematic approach. Considering the clinically relevant properties for dental sealants, the formulation containing 20% of NACP was selected as the optimal composition. The material flow was highly related to the mass fraction of the filler in the resin. At 20% NACP, the PEHB-based resin sealant provides high levels of Ca and PO_4 ions release and durable repeated recharge capability, with no negative effect on the mechanical and physical properties of the sealant. Therefore, this is a promising approach to provide long-term ion release to promote remineralization and inhibit dental caries in occlusal surfaces of teeth in children and adolescents.

Author Contributions: Conceptualization, H.H.K.X., and M.A.S.M.; Methodology, H.H.K.X. and M.A.S.M.; Investigation, M.S.I., F.D.A., Y.A.A.-D.; Writing—M.S.I. and M.A.S.M.; Writing—Review & Editing, H.H.K.X.; Funding Acquisition, H.H.K.X., and M.A.S.M.; Resources, M.D.W., T.W.O.; Supervision, M.D.W. and T.W.O.; Project Administration, M.A.S.M. and M.D.W.

Acknowledgments: We thank Pei Feng, Associate Dean of Research, UMB School of Dentistry, and Nancy Lin, National Institute of Standards and Technology for comments that greatly improved the manuscript.

References

1. GBD 2015 Disease and Injury Incidence and Prevalence Collaborators. Global, regional, and national incidence, prevalence, and years lived with disability for 310 diseases and injuries, 1990–2015: A systematic analysis for the Global Burden of Disease Study 2015. *Lancet* **2017**, *388*, 1545–1602.
2. Benzian, H.; Hobdell, M.; Mackay, J. Putting teeth into chronic diseases. *Lancet* **2011**, *377*, 464. [CrossRef]
3. Skeie, M.S.; Klock, K.S. Dental caries prevention strategies among children and adolescents with immigrant-or low socioeconomic backgrounds- do they work? A systematic review. *BMC Oral Health* **2018**, *18*, 20. [CrossRef] [PubMed]
4. Ahovuo-Saloranta, A.; Forss, H.; Walsh, T.; Nordblad, A.; Mäkelä, M.; Worthington, H.V. Pit and fissure sealants for preventing dental decay in permanent teeth. *Cochrane Database Syst. Rev.* **2017**, *7*, 1–167. [CrossRef] [PubMed]
5. Beauchamp, J.; Caufield, P.W.; Crall, J.J.; Donly, K.; Feigal, R.; Gooch, B.; Ismail, A.; Kohn, W.; Siegal, M.; Simonsen, R. Evidence-based clinical recommendations for the use of pit-and-fissure sealants: A report of the American Dental Association Council on Scientific Affairs. *J. Am. Dent. Assoc.* **2008**, *139*, 257–268. [CrossRef] [PubMed]
6. Poulsen, S.; Beiruti, N.; Sadat, N. A comparison of retention and the effect on caries of fissure sealing with a glass-ionomer and a resin-based sealant. *Community Dent. Oral Epidemiol.* **2001**, *29*, 298–301. [CrossRef] [PubMed]

7. Cury, J.A.; Tenuta, L.M.A. Enamel remineralization: Controlling the caries disease or treating early caries lesions? *Braz. Oral Res.* **2009**, *23*, 23–30. [CrossRef] [PubMed]
8. Tenuta, L.M.; Del Bel Cury, A.A.; Bortolin, M.C.; Vogel, G.L.; Cury, J.A. Ca, Pi, and F in the fluid of biofilm formed under sucrose. *J. Dent. Res.* **2006**, *85*, 834–838. [CrossRef] [PubMed]
9. Melo, M.A.; Orrego, S.; Weir, M.D.; Xu, H.H.; Arola, D.D. Designing multi-agent dental materials for enhanced resistance to biofilm damage at the bonded interface. *ACS Appl. Mater. Interfaces* **2016**, *8*, 11779–11787. [CrossRef] [PubMed]
10. Feng, X.; Zhang, N.; Xu, H.H.; Weir, M.; Melo, M.A.; Bai, Y.; Zhang, K. Novel orthodontic cement containing dimethylaminohexadecyl methacrylate with strong antibacterial capability. *Dent. Mater. J.* **2017**, *36*, 669–676. [CrossRef] [PubMed]
11. Weir, M.D.; Chow, L.C.; Xu, H.H.K. Remineralization of demineralized enamel via calcium phosphate nanocomposite. *J. Dent. Res.* **2012**, *91*, 979–984. [CrossRef] [PubMed]
12. Melo, M.A.S.; Weir, M.D.; Rodrigues, L.K.A.; Xu, H.H.K. Novel calcium phosphate nanocomposite with caries-inhibition in a human in situ model. *Dent. Mater.* **2013**, *29*, 231–240. [CrossRef] [PubMed]
13. Melo, M.A.S.; Guedes, S.F.F.; Xu, H.H.K.; Rodrigues, L.K.A. Nanotechnology-based restorative materials for dental caries management. *Trends Biotechnol.* **2013**, *31*, 459–467. [CrossRef] [PubMed]
14. Cheng, L.; Zhang, K.; Weir, M.D.; Melo, M.A.; Zhou, X.; Xu, H.H. Nanotechnology strategies for antibacterial and remineralizing composites and adhesives to tackle dental caries. *Nanomedicine* **2015**, *10*, 627–641. [CrossRef] [PubMed]
15. Chole, D.; Lokhande, P.; Shashank, K.; Bakle, S.; Devagirkar, A.; Dhore, P. Comparative Evaluation of the Fluoride Release and Recharge through Four Different Types of Pit and Fissure Sealants: An In Vitro Study. *Int. J. Adv. Heal Sci.* **2015**, *2*, 1–6.
16. Melo, M.A.S.; Powers, M.; Passos, V.F.; Weir, M.D.; Xu, H.H. Ph-activated nano-amorphous calcium phosphate-based cement to reduce dental enamel demineralization. *Artif. Cells Nanomed. Biotechnol.* **2017**, *45*, 1778–1785. [CrossRef] [PubMed]
17. Al-Dulaijan, Y.A.; Cheng, L.; Weir, M.D.; Melo, M.A.S.; Liu, H.; Oates, T.W.; Wang, L.; Xu, H.H.K. Novel rechargeable calcium phosphate nanocomposite with antibacterial activity to suppress biofilm acids and dental caries. *J. Dent.* **2018**, *72*, 44–52. [CrossRef] [PubMed]
18. Melo, M.A.; Cheng, L.; Weir, M.D.; Hsia, R.C.; Rodrigues, L.K.; Xu, H.H. Novel dental adhesive containing antibacterial agents and calcium phosphate nanoparticles. *J. Biomed. Mater. Res. B Appl. Biomater.* **2013**, *101*, 620–629. [CrossRef] [PubMed]
19. Li, F.; Weir, M.D.; Chen, J.; Xu, H.H.K. Effect of charge density of bonding agent containing a new quaternary ammonium methacrylate on antibacterial and bonding properties. *Dent. Mater.* **2014**, *30*, 433–441. [CrossRef] [PubMed]
20. Zhang, K.; Cheng, L.; Wu, E.J.; Weir, M.D.; Bai, Y.; Xu, H.H. Effect of water-ageing on dentine bond strength and anti-biofilm activity of bonding agent containing new monomer dimethylaminododecyl methacrylate. *J. Dent.* **2013**, *41*, 504–513. [CrossRef] [PubMed]
21. Zhang, L.; Weir, M.D.; Chow, L.C.; Antonucci, J.M.; Chen, J.; Xu, H.H.K. Novel rechargeable calcium phosphate dental nanocomposite. *Dent. Mater.* **2016**, *32*, 285–293. [CrossRef] [PubMed]
22. Wu, J.; Zhou, H.; Weir, M.D.; Melo, M.A.; Levine, E.D.; Xu, H.H. Effect of the dimethylaminohexadecyl methacrylate mass fraction on fracture toughness and antibacterial properties of CaP nanocomposite. *J. Dent.* **2015**, *43*, 1539–1546. [CrossRef] [PubMed]
23. Zhang, N.; Melo, M.A.; Chen, C.; Liu, J.; Weir, M.D.; Bai, Y.; Xu, H.H. Development of a multifunctional adhesive system for prevention of root caries and secondary caries. *Dent. Mater.* **2015**, *31*, 1119–1131. [CrossRef] [PubMed]
24. Xie, X.J.; Xing, D.; Wang, L.; Zhou, H.; Weir, M.D.; Bai, Y.X.; Xu, H.H. Novel rechargeable calcium phosphate nanoparticle-containing orthodontic cement. *Int. J. Oral Sci.* **2017**, *9*, 24–32. [CrossRef] [PubMed]
25. Melo, M.A.; Wu, J.; Weir, M.D.; Xu, H.H. Novel antibacterial orthodontic cement containing quaternary ammonium monomer dimethylaminododecyl methacrylate. *J. Dent.* **2014**, *42*, 1193–1201. [CrossRef] [PubMed]
26. Zhang, N.; Melo, M.A.; Antonucci, J.; Lin, N.; Lin-Gibson, S.; Bai, Y.; Xu, H.H. Novel dental cement to combat biofilms and reduce acids for orthodontic applications to avoid enamel demineralization. *Materials* **2016**, *9*, 413. [CrossRef] [PubMed]

27. Zhang, N.; Weir, M.D.; Chen, C.; Melo, M.A.; Bai, Y.; Xu, H.H. Orthodontic cement with protein-repellent and antibacterial properties and the release of calcium and phosphate ions. *J. Dent.* **2016**, *50*, 51–59. [CrossRef] [PubMed]
28. *ISO 6876:2012. Dentistry–Root Canal Sealing Materials*; International Organization for Standardization: Geneva, Switzerland, 2012.
29. Xie, X.; Wang, L.; Xing, D.; Arola, D.D.; Weir, M.D.; Bai, Y.; Xu, H.H. Protein-repellent and antibacterial functions of a calcium phosphate rechargeable nanocomposite. *J. Dent.* **2016**, *52*, 15–22. [CrossRef] [PubMed]
30. Melo, M.A.; Cheng, L.; Zhang, K.; Weir, M.D.; Rodrigues, L.K.; Xu, H.H. Novel dental adhesives containing nanoparticles of silver and amorphous calcium phosphate. *Dent. Mater.* **2013**, *29*, 199–210. [CrossRef] [PubMed]
31. Zhang, L.; Weir, M.D.; Chow, L.C.; Reynolds, M.A.; Xu, H.H.K. Rechargeable calcium phosphate orthodontic cement with sustained ion release and re-release. *Sci. Rep.* **2016**, *6*, 36476. [CrossRef] [PubMed]

12

The Retentive Strength of Laser-Sintered Cobalt-Chromium-Based Crowns after Pretreatment with a Desensitizing Paste Containing 8% Arginine and Calcium Carbonate

Raphael Pilo, Sharon Agar-Zoizner, Shaul Gelbard and Shifra Levartovsky *

Department of Oral Rehabilitation, The Maurice and Gabriela Goldschleger School of Dental Medicine, Tel- Aviv University, Tel -Aviv 6997801, Israel; rafipilo@gmail.com (R.P.); sharon.agar@gmail.com (S.A.-Z.); s1gelbard@gmail.com (S.G.)

* Correspondence: shifralevartov@gmail.com

Abstract: The retention of laser-sintered cobalt-chromium (Co-Cr)-based crowns were examined after dentin pretreatment with desensitizing paste containing 8% arginine and calcium carbonate (DP-ACC). Forty lower first molars were prepared using a standardized protocol. The Co-Cr crowns were produced using selective laser melting. The teeth were either pretreated with the desensitizing paste or not pretreated. After one week, each group was cemented with glass ionomer cement (GIC) or zinc phosphate cement (ZPC). Surface areas of the teeth were measured before cementation. After aging, a universal testing machine was used to test the retentive strength of the cemented crown-tooth assemblies. The debonded surfaces of the teeth and crowns were examined at 2.7× magnification. Pretreating the dentin surfaces with the desensitizing paste before cementation with GIC or ZPC did not affect the retention of the Co-Cr crowns. The retention of the GIC group (6.04 ± 1.10 MPa) was significantly higher than that of the ZPC group (2.75 ± 1.25 MPa). The predominant failure mode for the ZPC and the nontreated GIC group was adhesive cement-dentin failure; for the treated GIC group, it was adhesive cement-crown failure. The desensitizing paste can be safely used to reduce post-cementation sensitivity without reducing the retentive strength of Co-Cr crowns cemented with GIC or ZPC.

Keywords: desensitizing paste; dentin; retention; cements; cobalt-chromium

---

1. Introduction

Dentin hypersensitivity following tooth preparation and cementation of fixed partial dentures (FPDs) has been a common phenomenon [1]. Post-cementation complaints from patients are received for 20 to 30% of crowns inserted [2], and this rate remains at 6% and 3% after two and three years, respectively [3]. There are several explanations for this postoperative sensitivity. One outcome of aggressive tooth preparation is an increased number of opened and expanded dentinal tubules [4,5]. This condition is further aggravated by inadequate provisional restorations and removal of the smear layer due to acid etching induced by the cements [6]. Porcelain fused to metal (PFM) restorations, for example, are most commonly luted with zinc phosphate or glass ionomer cements (GICs), which are acidic in nature [7].

In an effort to control postoperative sensitivity, various desensitizing agents have been used to seal dentinal tubules before crown cementation; however, the literature is inconsistent regarding the effects of these agents on the retentive strength of FPDs. Sailer et al. [8,9] and Stawarczyk et al. [10,11] showed that glutaraldehyde/HEMA pretreatment and resin sealing of dentin following tooth preparation had a beneficial effect on the shear bond strength of self-adhesive resin cement. Other studies have reported that dentin desensitizing by means of glutaraldehyde-containing primers or dentin sealing by means of bonding agents did not affect the bond strength of the cements tested [12,13]. On the other hand, several studies have demonstrated that these agents decrease crown retention to some extent [14,15]. Aranha et al. [16] showed that specimens treated with dentin desensitizers (except Gluma) yielded significantly lower mean bond strengths than nontreated control specimens.

Recently, a new in-office Colgate Sensitive Pro-Relief Desensitizing Paste containing 8% arginine and calcium carbonate (DP-ACC) was shown to provide immediate and lasting relief from dentin hypersensitivity [17–21]. No significant difference in the bonding strength of composites to enamel or dentin pretreated with this desensitizing paste has been reported [22–24]. In addition, pretreating dentin surfaces with DP-ACC prior to cementation did not affect the retention of complete cast metal crowns luted with a glass ionomer cement (GIC) [25] or the retention of zirconium oxide crowns luted with a resin-modified GIC or a self-adhesive resin cement [26].

Recently, a new additive manufacturing technology operated by computer-aided design and computer-aided manufacturing (CAD/CAM), referred to as selective laser melting (SLM) technology, has been introduced for fabricating cobalt-chromium (Co-Cr) frameworks for PFM crowns. Co-Cr crowns produced with SLM exhibit a marginal and internal accuracy that is comparable to that of conventional production procedures but save time and facilitate laboratory procedures [27–29].

No information has been found in the literature concerning the influence of pretreating dentin with DP-ACC on the retentive strength of Co-Cr crowns produced by the SLM technology and cemented by zinc phosphate cement (ZPC) and glass ionomer cement (GIC), which are the most frequently used cements for luting metal-based restorations.

The aim of this in vitro study was to evaluate the effect of the pretreatment of dentin with DP-ACC on the retentive strength of SLM Co-Cr copings cemented by ZPC and GIC. The null hypotheses were as follows: (1) the retentive strength of the SLM Co-Cr copings cemented by ZPC and GIC to human extracted teeth is not affected by DP-ACC, and (2) the retentive strength of the two cements is similar.

2. Results

The retentive strength (mean, SD) of the treated and untreated cementation groups are presented in Table 1. Pretreating the dentin surfaces with DP-ACC prior to cementation with either GIC or ZPC did not affect the retentive strength of the Co-Cr copings ($p = 0.780$). The retention obtained with Fuji I capsules (GIC) was significantly ($p = 0.001$) higher than that obtained with Harvard Cement OptiCaps (ZPC). The interaction between cement and dentin treatment was not significant ($p = 0.208$).

Table 1. Mean (SD) retentive strength (MPa) of the cobalt-chromium-based crown for all cementation groups.

Cement Type	Treatment	Sample No.	Mean Retentive Value (MPa)	Standard Deviation
GIC	1	10	6.39	1.06
	2	10	5.73	1.10
	Total	20	6.04	1.10
ZPC	1	10	2.39	0.99
	2	10	3.10	1.44
	Total	20	2.75	1.25
Total	1	20	4.29	2.27
	2	20	4.41	1.83
	Total	40	4.36	2.03

Treatment: 1, Without pretreatment with DP-ACC (control); 2, With pretreatment with DP-ACC.

Examination by magnifying glasses of the failure mode after the dislodgment of the crown revealed that for ZPC, the predominant failure mode was adhesive cement-dentin failure. In 85% of the surfaces, all (53%) or part (32%) of the surface of the crown was covered with cement, and the rest were detected on the dentin (Figure 1). This mode of failure was consistent regardless of whether the dentin was pretreated with DP-ACC or not. In the GIC group, the predominant failure mode was adhesive cement-crown failure. In 62% of the surfaces, all (40%) or part (22%) of the surface of the dentin was covered with cement, and the rest were detected on the crown (Figure 1). This failure mode was inconsistent between the groups. In the nontreated group, more surfaces exhibited the adhesive cement-dentin mode of failure; in the treated group, more surfaces exhibited the adhesive cement-crown mode of failure (Figure 1). Cohesive cement failure was barely seen in all groups, while cohesive dentin failure did not occur.

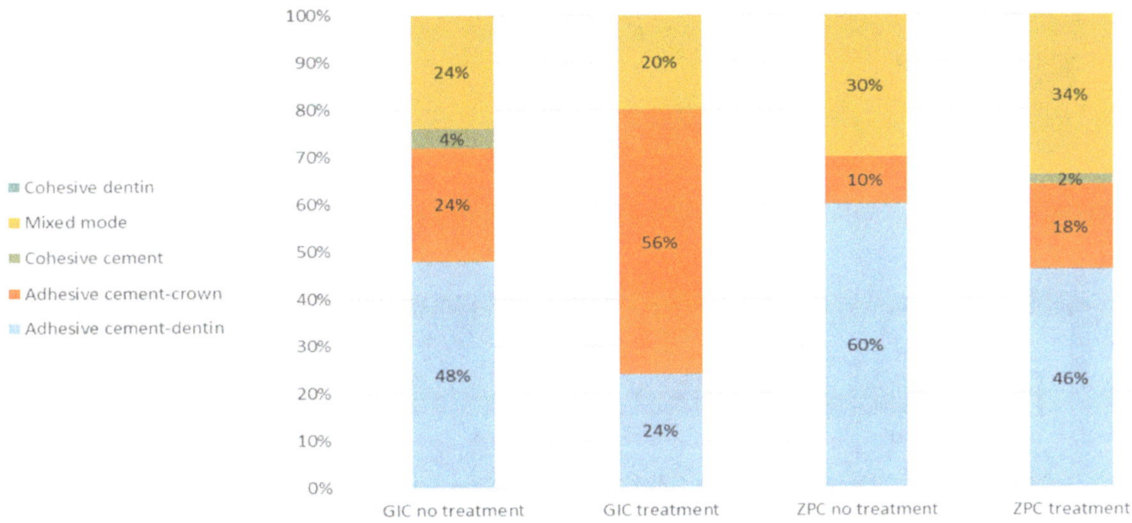

Figure 1. Distribution of failure modes (number of surfaces) for each cementation group.

Scanning electron microscopy (SEM) images of the dentin surfaces illustrating the various modes of failure are presented for the ZPC (Figure 2a–c) and GIC (Figure 3a,b) groups. Figure 2a–c illustrates the mixed mode of failure, whereas most of the dentin surface exhibits longitudinal striations of the bur, with a small part covered with the ZPC. This type of failure was consistent in the untreated (A,B), as well as the treated (C) ZPC groups.

Figure 3a,b illustrates the adhesive crown cement mode of failure, with most of the dentin surface covered with cement. This mode of failure was typical of the treated GIC group.

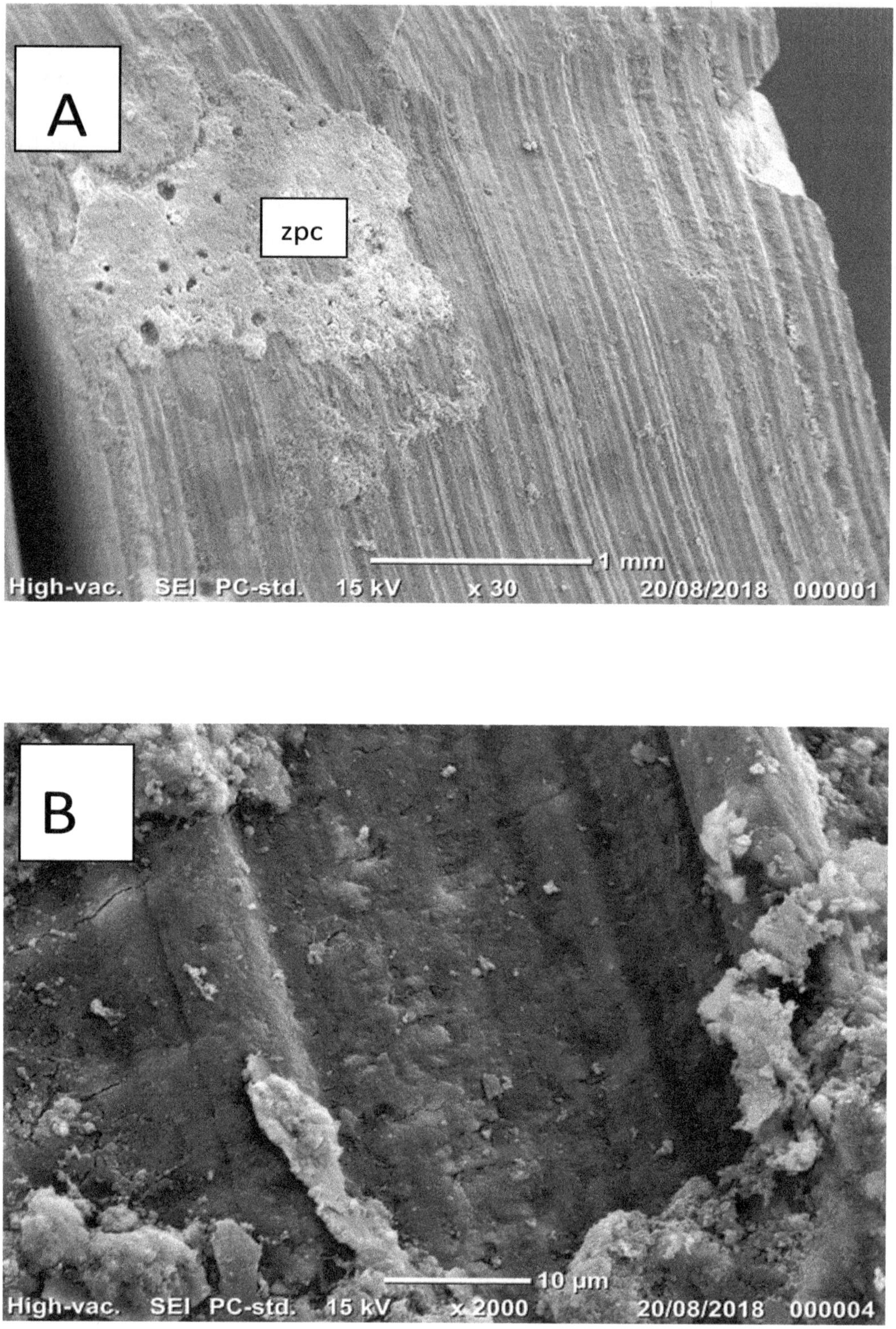

Figure 2. *Cont.*

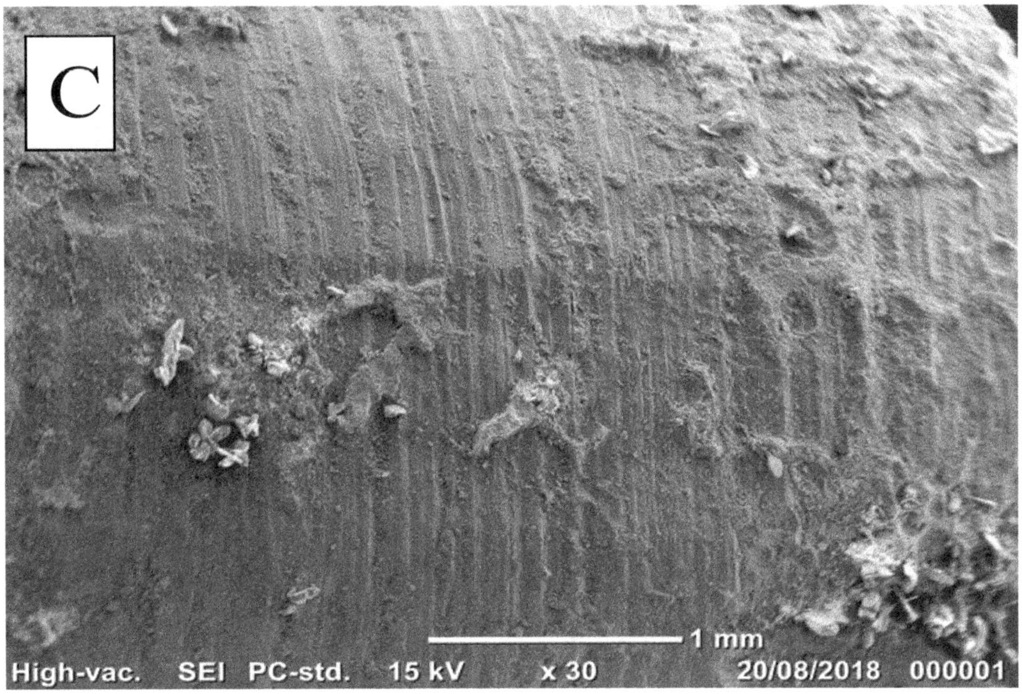

Figure 2. A–C (ZPC group). Scanning electron microscopy image of the untreated (**A**,**B**) and treated (**C**) dentin surfaces after failure illustrating the mixed mode of failure; the majority exhibited adhesive cement-dentin failure, while most of the dentin surface exhibited longitudinal striations of the bur, with only a small part covered with cement (ZPC). This type of predominantly adhesive cement-dentin failure was typical of the ZPC group.

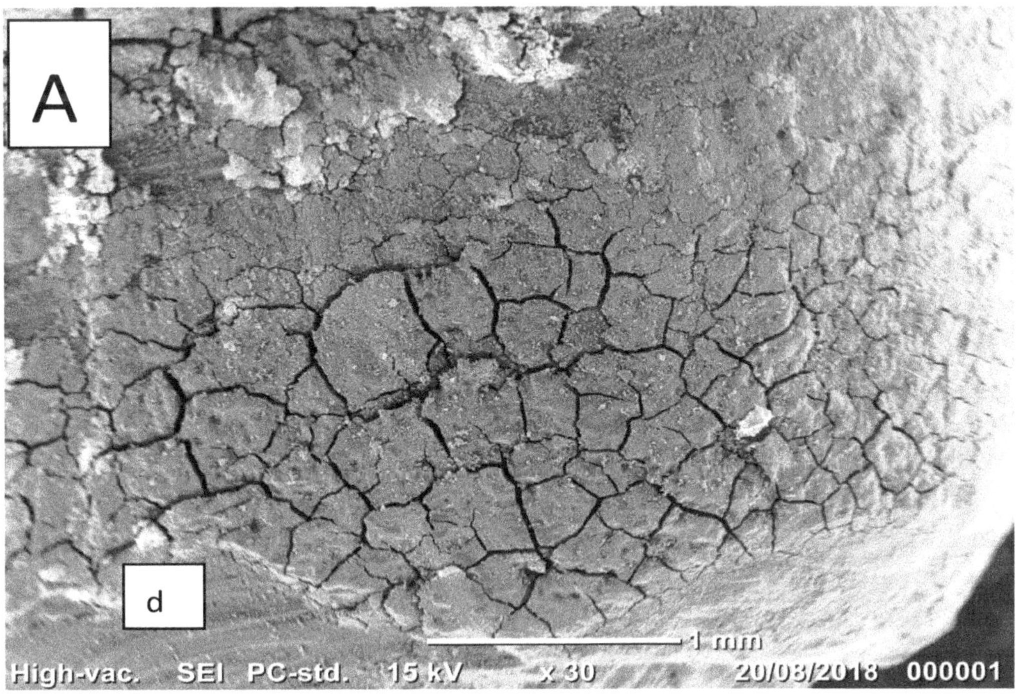

Figure 3. *Cont.*

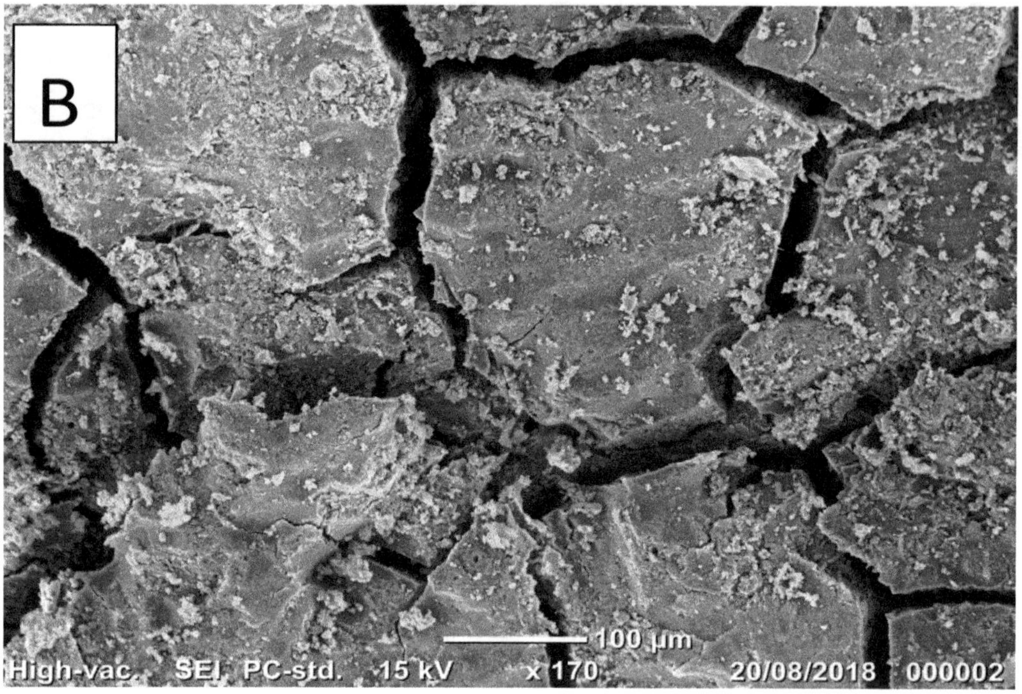

Figure 3. A,B (GIC group). Scanning electron microscopy images of the treated dentin surface after failure. (**A**) Most of the dentin surface is covered with cement (30×), and only a small part of the dentin is exposed (d), demonstrating the striations of the bur. (**B**) At greater magnification (170×), craze lines in the cement layer caused by the dehydration process are evident.

3. Discussion

Colgate Sensitive Pro-Relief Desensitizing Paste contains arginine, bicarbonate, and calcium carbonate and is highly effective in occluding dentin tubules, as was previously demonstrated by confocal laser scanning microscopy (CLSM) and SEM [30]. This paste has been shown to physically plug and seal exposed dentin tubules and to effectively provide dentin hypersensitivity relief [31], which has been reported to last for up to 28 days and to reduce the post-preparation and post-cementation sensitivity of vital teeth that serve as abutments for FPDs; however, this treatment may be advocated only if retentive strength is not affected [20].

In the current study, the retention of cobalt-chromium-based (Co-Cr) copings was tested one week after dentin pretreatment with DP-ACC in order to resemble a period of reevaluation prior to final cementation. The luting agents used in this study were GIC and ZPC. Both cements are acid-base materials associated with post-cementation sensitivity, which can last for a week [32]. GIC and ZPC are popular choices for luting metal-based restorations. GIC relies on both the mechanical retention to surface irregularities and the chelation to calcium in the tooth structure, while ZPC relies only on mechanical retention to both dentin and crown surfaces [33,34]. GICs are naturally adhesive to dentin; initially due to the presence of polyacrylic acid, forming hydrogen bonds between the free carboxyl groups and the strongly bound water layers residing on the surface of the dentin. Subsequently they are gradually replaced by ionic bonds involving mainly calcium in the mineral phase at the surface of the dentin and carboxylate groups in the cement. Imaging of dentin surfaces treated with DP-ACC reveals surface coverage including the tubule orifices. This surface coverage may thus interfere with the interaction of the cement with the mineral phase of the surface dentin as well as block the longitudinal striations of the bur and, thus, impair both the micromechanical and chemical mode of action of the cements, affecting the bond strength/retention.

The current results support the first null hypothesis of the study, implying that pretreatment with DP-ACC would have no effect on the retentive strength of SLM Co-Cr crown copings cemented to human extracted teeth with GIC or ZPC. Our results are in agreement with those of another study that demonstrated that pretreating dentin surfaces with DP-ACC prior to cementation did not affect the retention of complete cast metal crowns luted with GIC [25]. Moreover, in the aforementioned study, pretreatment with DP-ACC showed the best retention of complete cast metal crowns compared to all other dentin desensitizers tested. Pilo et al. [26] showed the same results with zirconium oxide (Y-TZP) crowns luted with either resin-modified glass ionomer cement (RMGIC) or self-adhesive resin cement (SARC).

Our second null hypothesis was rejected because the retentive strength of GIC was significantly higher than that of ZPC. This conclusion is in accordance with a previous study of Wiskott et al. [35] demonstrating that crowns luted with resin composite cement and GIC were more resistant to dynamic lateral loading than those luted using ZPC. On the other hand, Gorodovsky et al. [36] reported no significant difference between the retention of zinc phosphate and that of glass ionomer. A review of the research of different cements did not reveal a consistent conclusion about the retentive strength of GIC in comparison with that of ZPC. Some studies showed a higher retentive strength for ZPC, and others reported a higher retentive strength for GIC; some showed no significant difference between the two cements [33]. However, it should be noted that all the aforementioned ZPC studies used the classic Harvard Cement normal setting, whereas in the current study, the newer Harvard Cement OptiCaps was used. The latter is the capsulated version intended to overcome mistakes in mixing and dosing. It has been shown that Vickers hardness increases with more powder with a rise in mean values following an exponential curve ranging between 34 and 66 MPa [37]. Comparison studies between hand-mixed and capsulated ZPC have not been reported yet.

The lack of effect on the retentive strength of ZPC from DP-ACC was also verified by an absence of change in failure mode, which was mainly adhesive cement-dentin failure. This finding implies that all or most of the crown was covered by ZPC, probably due to surface irregularities of the intaglio of the Co-Cr copings. In the GIC group, the predominant failure mode was adhesive cement-crown failure. This finding implies that all or most of the dentin was covered by GIC, probably due to the chemical interaction between the calcium in the mineral phase at the surface of the dentin and carboxylate groups in the cement, implying that in spite of the surface coverage by the DP-ACC, many calcium ions are still available for bonding. Although the DP-ACC did not affect the retentive strength, the failure mode varied between the groups; in the nontreated group, most of the cement remained on the crown, while in the treated group, most of the dentin was covered with cement. These differences might be explained by chelation between the polyalkenoic chains in GIC also with the calcium carbonate contained in the DP-ACC, which physically plugs and seals exposed dentin tubules.

This is an in vitro study, hence, the subjective desensitizing effect of the DP-ACC on vital teeth prepared for FPD must be validated in clinical studies before being recommended for use.

4. Materials and Methods

The study sample comprised forty freshly extracted, caries-free, intact lower first molars that were extracted for periodontal reasons (age range 40–60). Approval from the Ethics Committee of Tel Aviv University was obtained (#21-08-16), and all individuals signed an informed consent.

The teeth were stored in a germ-free 0.1% thymol tap water solution at room temperature for a maximum of two weeks until experimentation. Each tooth was suspended in the middle of an aluminum ring and was mounted 2 mm apical to the cementoenamel junction (CEJ) in poly(methyl methacrylate) resin (Quick resin, Ivoclar, Schaan, Liechtenstein) after notching the roots for retention purposes. The mounted teeth were stored in tap water at room temperature at all times.

A standardized protocol yielding an axial height of 5 mm and a 10° taper was followed for preparation. The occlusal surface was sectioned perpendicular to the long axis with a water-cooled precision saw (Isomet Plus, Buehler, IL, USA). A 0.4-mm, 360° chamfer finish line located 1 mm above the CEJ with a 10° taper preparation was obtained by a rigidly secured, high-speed handpiece equipped with a diamond bur (C1-Strauss, Ra'anana, Israel) mounted on a custom-designed, surveyor-like apparatus. A new diamond bur was used for each tooth.

The prepared teeth were digitally scanned by a laboratory scanner (Series 7, Dental Wing, Letourneux, Montreal, Canada) operated by blue light and equipped with five axes of rotation, and STL files were obtained. Forty Co-Cr copings were produced using an SLM system (Eosint M 280, EOS, Krailling, Germany) at a commercial dental laboratory (MS Systems, Or Yehuda, Israel). The CAD-CAM Co-Cr cores were 1.0 mm thick with a 50 μm virtual cement spacer layer. To facilitate tensile loading, an occlusal loop (4-mm outer diameter and 2-mm inner diameter) was designed extending coronally from the occlusal surface [38]. The teeth were randomly assigned to two groups (2 × 20). In one group, the dentin surfaces were pretreated with DP-ACC using prophy cups under light pressure according to the manufacturer's recommendations. In the second group (the control group), the dentin surfaces were not pretreated. After placing the Co-Cr copings on each tooth, they were stored at 37 °C under 100% humidity for one week, resembling a period of reevaluation prior to final cementation. Two luting cements were evaluated (2 × 10) in each group: a GIC (GC Fuji I Capsule, GC, Tokyo, Japan) and a ZPC (Harvard Cem OptiCaps, Harvard Dental International, GmbH). The areas of the axial and occlusal surfaces of each prepared tooth were measured prior to cementation, as previously described [38]. The cements were used according to the manufacturer's recommendations. Cementing each crown to its tooth was conducted in a standardized manner under a constant load of 50 N (Force gauge, FG 20, Lutron, Taiwan) for 10 min and then allowed to set for 24 h.

The cemented crown-tooth assemblies were stored in tap water at 37 °C for two weeks, followed by thermal cycling between water temperatures of 5 and 55 °C for 5000 cycles with a 10 s dwell time (Y. Manes, Tel-Aviv, Israel). After thermal cycling, the crown-tooth assemblies were subjected to dislodgment forces through a 1.2-mm diameter metal cable entangled through the occlusal loop along the apico-occlusal axis using a universal testing machine (Instron, Model 4502, Instron Corp., Buckinghamshire, UK) at a crosshead speed of 1 mm/min until failure. The force at dislodgment was recorded and divided by the total surface area of each prepared sample to yield the retention value (Pa).

The debonded surfaces of the teeth and crowns were examined with magnifying glasses at 2.7× magnification (Orascoptic, Middleton, WI, USA). Each surface of the dentin-crown interface was analyzed separately (five surfaces per tooth). Failure was classified based on the criteria presented in Table 2.

Table 2. Classification of failure criteria.

Classification	Description	Criteria
1	Cement principally on crown surface	Adhesive cement-dentin
2	Cement principally on dentin surface	Adhesive cement-crown
3	Cement equally distributed on dentin & crown surfaces	Cohesive cement
4	Mixed mode	Adhesive & cohesive cement
5	Fracture of the tooth	Cohesive dentin

A separate analysis was performed for each matched Co-Cr tooth surface (buccal, lingual, mesial, distal, and occlusal). For each category, the number of surfaces was counted and presented as a percentage of all the surfaces for the specific cement.

To analyze the dentin surfaces, the debonded surfaces of some teeth representing different failure categories from each group were examined under an SEM (Quantum 2000) in high vacuum mode following gold sputter-coating. The acquisition conditions were as follows: 25 kV, 90 μA and 40–1000× magnification.

Statistical Analysis

Retentive strength was evaluated using two-way analysis of variance (ANOVA) with repeated measures; cement ($n = 2$) and pretreatment ($n = 2$) were the independent variables. The level of significance was 0.05.

5. Conclusions

An 8.0% arginine and calcium carbonate in-house desensitizing paste can be safely used on dentin to reduce post-cementation sensitivity without compromising the retention of SLM Co-Cr crowns cemented with either ZPC or GIC.

Author Contributions: Conceptualization: R.P., S.G. and S.L.; investigation: S.A.-Z.; methodology: R.P. and S.L.; supervision: S.L.; writing—original draft: R.P. and S.L.; writing—review and editing: R.P.

References

1. Rosenstiel, S.F.; Rashid, R.G. Postcementation hypersensitivity: Scientific data versus dentists' perceptions. *J. Prosthodont.* **2003**, *12*, 73–81. [CrossRef]
2. Johnson, G.H.; Powell, L.V.; DeRouen, T.A. Evaluation and control of post-cementation pulpal sensitivity: Zinc phosphate and glass ionomer luting cements. *J. Am. Dent. Assoc.* **1993**, *124*, 38–46. [CrossRef]
3. Thylstrup, A.; Bille, J.; Qvist, V. Radiographic and observed tissue changes in approximal carious lesions at the time of operative treatment. *Caries Res.* **1986**, *20*, 75–84. [CrossRef] [PubMed]
4. Bernier, J.L.; Knapp, M.J. A new pulpal response to high-speed dental instruments. *Oral Surg. Oral Med. Oral Pathol. Oral Radiol.* **1958**, *11*, 167–183. [CrossRef]
5. Richardson, D.; Tao, L.; Pashley, D.H. Dentin permeability: Effects of crown preparation. *Int. J. Prosthodont.* **1991**, *4*, 219–225.
6. Langeland, K.; Langeland, L.K. Pulp reactions to crown preparation, impression, temporary crown fixation, and permanent cementation. *J. Prosthet. Dent.* **1965**, *15*, 129–143. [CrossRef]
7. Zaimoglu, A.; Aydin, A.K. An evaluation of smear layer with various desensitizing agents after tooth preparation. *J. Prosthet. Dent.* **1992**, *68*, 450–457. [CrossRef]
8. Sailer, I.; Tettamanti, S.; Stawarczyk, B.; Fischer, J.; Hammerle, C.H. In vitro study of the influence of dentin desensitizing and sealing on the shear bond strength of two universal resin cements. *J. Adhes. Dent.* **2010**, *12*, 381–392. [CrossRef]
9. Sailer, I.; Oendra, A.E.; Stawarczyk, B.; Hammerle, C.H. The effects of desensitizing resin, resin sealing, and provisional cement on the bond strength of dentin luted with self-adhesive and conventional resincements. *J. Prosthet. Dent.* **2012**, *107*, 252–260. [CrossRef]
10. Stawarczyk, B.; Hartmann, R.; Hartmann, L.; Roos, M.; Ozcan, M.; Sailer, I.; Hammerle, C.H. The effect of dentin desensitizer on shear bond strength of conventional and self-adhesive resin luting cements after aging. *Oper. Dent.* **2011**, *36*, 492–501. [CrossRef]
11. Stawarczyk, B.; Hartmann, L.; Hartmann, R.; Roos, M.; Ender, A.; Ozcan, M.; Sailer, I.; Hammerle, C.H. Impact of gluma desensitizer on the tensile strength of zirconia crowns bonded to dentin: An in vitro study. *Clin. Oral Investig.* **2012**, *16*, 201–213. [CrossRef] [PubMed]
12. Cobb, D.S.; Reinhardt, J.W.; Vargas, M.A. Effect of HEMA-containing dentin desensitizers on shear bond strength of a resin cement. *Am. J. Dent.* **1997**, *10*, 62–65. [PubMed]
13. Soeno, K.; Taira, Y.; Matsumura, H.; Atsuta, M. Effect of desensitizers on bond strength of adhesive luting agents to dentin. *J. Oral Rehabil.* **2001**, *28*, 1122–1128. [CrossRef] [PubMed]
14. Yim, N.H.; Rueggeberg, F.A.; Caughman, W.F.; Gardner, F.M.; Pashley, D.H. Effect of dentin desensitizers and cementing agents on retention of full crowns using standardized crown preparations. *J. Prosthet. Dent.* **2000**, *83*, 459–465. [CrossRef]

15. Huh, J.B.; Kim, J.H.; Chung, M.K.; Lee, H.Y.; Choi, Y.G.; Shim, J.S. The effect of several dentin desensitizers on shear bond strength of adhesive resin luting cement using self-etching primer. *J. Dent.* **2008**, *36*, 1025–1032. [CrossRef] [PubMed]
16. Aranha, A.C.; Siqueira Junior Ade, S.; Cavalcante, L.M.; Pimenta, L.A.; Marchi, G.M. Microtensile bond strengths of composite to dentin treated with desensitizer products. *J. Adhes. Dent.* **2006**, *8*, 85–90. [PubMed]
17. Hamlin, D.; Williams, K.P.; Delgado, E.; Zhang, Y.P.; DeVizio, W.; Mateo, L.R. Clinical evaluation of the efficacy of a desensitizing paste containing 8% arginine and calcium carbonate for the in-office relief of dentin hypersensitivity associated with dental prophylaxis. *Am. J. Dent.* **2009**, *22*, 16A–20A.
18. Schiff, T.; Delgado, E.; Zhang, Y.P.; Cummins, D.; DeVizio, W.; Mateo, L.R. Clinical evaluation of the efficacy of an in-office desensitizing paste containing 8% arginine and calcium carbonate in providing instant and lasting relief of dentin hypersensitivity. *Am. J. Dent.* **2009**, *22*, 8A–15A.
19. Ayad, F.; Ayad, N.; Zhang, Y.P.; DeVizio, W.; Cummins, D.; Mateo, L.R. Comparing the efficacy in reducing dentin hypersensitivity of a new toothpaste containing 8.0% arginine, calcium carbonate, and 1450 ppm fluoride to a commercial sensitive toothpaste containing 2% potassium ion: An eight-week clinical study on Canadian adults. *J. Clin. Dent.* **2009**, *20*, 10–16.
20. Docimo, R.; Montesani, L.; Maturo, P.; Costacurta, M.; Bartolino, M.; DeVizio, W.; Zhang, Y.P.; Cummins, D.; Dibart, S.; Mateo, L.R. Comparing the efficacy in reducing dentin hypersensitivity of a new toothpaste containing 8.0% arginine, calcium carbonate, and 1450 ppm fluoride to a commercial sensitive toothpaste containing 2% potassium ion: An eight-week clinical study in Rome, Italy. *J. Clin. Dent.* **2009**, *20*, 17–22.
21. Nathoo, S.; Delgado, E.; Zhang, Y.P.; DeVizio, W.; Cummins, D.; Mateo, L.R. Comparing the efficacy in providing instant relief of dentin hypersensitivity of a new toothpaste containing 8.0% arginine, calcium carbonate, and 1450 ppm fluoride relative to a benchmark desensitizing toothpaste containing 2% potassium ion and 1450 ppm fluoride, and to a control toothpaste with 1450 ppm fluoride: A three-day clinical study in New Jersey, USA. *J. Clin. Dent.* **2009**, *20*, 123–130. [PubMed]
22. Garcia-Godoy, A.; Garcia-Godoy, F. Effect of an 8.0% arginine and calcium carbonate in-office desensitizing paste on the shear bond strength of composites to human dental enamel. *Am. J. Dent.* **2010**, *23*, 324–326. [PubMed]
23. Wang, Y.; Liu, S.; Pei, D.; Du, X.; Ouyang, X.; Huang, C. Effect of an 8.0% arginine and calcium carbonate in-office desensitizing paste on the microtensile bond strength of self-etching dental adhesives to human dentin. *Am. J. Dent.* **2012**, *25*, 281–286. [PubMed]
24. Canares, G.; Salgado, T.; Pines, M.S.; Wolff, M.S. Effect of an 8.0% arginine and calcium carbonate desensitizing toothpaste on shear dentin bond strength. *J. Clin. Dent.* **2012**, *23*, 68–70. [PubMed]
25. Chandavarkar, S.M.; Ram, S.M. A comparative evaluation of the effect of dentin desensitizers on the retention of complete cast metal crowns. *Contemp. Clin. Dent.* **2015**, *6*, S45–S50. [CrossRef] [PubMed]
26. Pilo, R.; Harel, N.; Nissan, J.; Levartovsky, S. The retentive strength of cemented zirconium oxide crowns after dentin pretreatment with desensitizing paste containing 8% arginine and calcium carbonate. *Int. J. Mol. Sci.* **2016**, *17*, 426. [CrossRef] [PubMed]
27. Quante, K.; Ludwig, K.; Kern, M. Marginal and internal fit of metal-ceramic crowns fabricated with a new laser melting technology. *Dent. Mater.* **2008**, *24*, 1311–1315. [CrossRef]
28. Ucar, Y.; Akova, T.; Akyil, M.S.; Brantley, W.A. Internal fit evaluation of crowns prepared using a new dental crown fabrication technique: Laser-sintered Co-Cr crowns. *J. Prosthet. Dent.* **2009**, *102*, 253–259. [CrossRef]
29. Tamac, E.; Toksavul, S.; Toman, M. Clinical marginal and internal adaptation of CAD/CAM milling, laser sintering, and cast metal ceramic crowns. *J. Prosthet. Dent.* **2014**, *112*, 909–913. [CrossRef]
30. Lavender, S.A.; Petrou, I.; Heu, R.; Stranick, M.A.; Cummins, D.; Kilpatrick-Liverman, L.; Sullivan, R.J.; Santarpia, R.P., III. Mode of action studies on a new desensitizing dentifrice containing 8.0% arginine, a high cleaning calcium carbonate system and 1450 ppm fluoride. *Am. J. Dent.* **2010**, *23*, 14A–19A.
31. Panagakos, F.; Schiff, T.; Guignon, A. Dentin hypersensitivity: Effective treatment with an in-office desensitizing paste containing 8% arginine and calcium carbonate. *Am. J. Dent.* **2009**, *22*, 3A–7A. [PubMed]
32. Shetty, R.M.; Bhat, S.; Mehta, D.; Srivatsa, G.; Shetty, Y.B. Comparative analysis of postcementation hypersensitivity with glass ionomer cement and a resin cement: An in vivo study. *J. Contemp. Dent. Pract.* **2012**, *13*, 327–331. [PubMed]
33. Rosenstiel, S.F.; Land, M.F.; Crispin, B.J. Dental luting agents: A review of the current literature. *J. Prosthet. Dent.* **1998**, *80*, 280–301. [CrossRef]

34. Pattanaik, B.K.; Nagda, S.J. An evaluation of retention and marginal seating of Ni-Cr alloy cast restorations using three different luting cements: An in vitro study. *Indian. J. Dent. Res.* **2012**, *23*, 20–25. [CrossRef] [PubMed]
35. Wiskott, H.W.; Nicholls, J.I.; Belser, U.C. The relationship between abutment taper and resistance of cemented crowns to dynamic loading. *Int. J. Prosthodont.* **1996**, *9*, 117–139. [PubMed]
36. Gorodovsky, S.; Zidan, O. Retentive strength, disintegration, and marginal quality of luting cements. *J. Prosthet. Dent.* **1992**, *68*, 269–274. [CrossRef]
37. Behr, M.; Rosentritt, M.; Loher, H.; Kolbeck, C.; Trempler, C.; Stemplinger, B.; Kopzon, V.; Handel, G. Changes of cement properties caused by mixing errors: The therapeutic range of different cement types. *Dent. Mater.* **2008**, *24*, 1187–1193. [CrossRef] [PubMed]
38. Pilo, R.; Lewinstein, I.; Ratzon, T.; Cardash, H.S.; Brosh, T. The influence of dentin and/or metal surface treatment on the retention of cemented crowns in teeth with an increased taper. *Dent. Mater.* **2008**, *24*, 1058–1064. [CrossRef] [PubMed]

13

Evaluation of Biological Response of STRO-1/c-Kit Enriched Human Dental Pulp Stem Cells to Titanium Surfaces Treated with Two Different Cleaning Systems

Enrico Conserva [1,2,†], Alessandra Pisciotta [1,†], Laura Bertoni [1], Giulia Bertani [1], Aida Meto [1], Bruna Colombari [1], Elisabetta Blasi [1], Pierantonio Bellini [1,2], Anto de Pol [1], Ugo Consolo [1,2] and Gianluca Carnevale [1,*]

1. Department of Surgery, Medicine, Dentistry and Morphological Sciences with interest in Transplant, Oncology and Regenerative Medicine, University of Modena and Reggio Emilia, 41125 Modena, Italy; enrico.conserva@unimore.it (E.C.); alessandra.pisciotta@unimore.it (A.P.); laura.bertoni@unimore.it (L.B.); giulia.bertani@unimore.it (G.B.); aida.meto@unimore.it (A.M.); bruna.colombari@unimore.it (B.C.); elisabetta.blasi@unimore.it (E.B.); pierantonio.bellini@unimore.it (P.B.); anto.depol@unimore.it (A.d.P.); ugo.consolo@unimore.it (U.C.)
2. Operative Unit of Dentistry and Maxillofacial Surgery, Department Integrated Activity-Specialist Surgeries, University-Hospital of Modena, 41125 Modena, Italy

* Correspondence: gianluca.carnevale@unimore.it

† These authors contributed equally to this work.

Abstract: Peri-implantitis—an infection caused by bacterial deposition of biofilm—is a common complication in dentistry which may lead to implant loss. Several decontamination procedures have been investigated to identify the optimal approach being capable to remove the bacterial biofilm without modifying the implant surface properties. Our study evaluated whether two different systems—Ni-Ti Brushes (Brush) and Air-Polishing with 40 μm bicarbonate powder (Bic40)—might alter the physical/chemical features of two different titanium surfaces—machined (MCH) and Ca^{++} nanostructured (NCA)—and whether these decontamination systems may affect the biological properties of human STRO-1^{+}/c-Kit^{+} dental pulp stem cells (hDPSCs) as well as the bacterial ability to produce biofilm. Cell morphology, proliferation and stemness markers were analysed in hDPSCs grown on both surfaces, before and after the decontamination treatments. Our findings highlighted that Bic40 treatment either maintained the surface characteristics of both implants and allowed hDPSCs to proliferate and preserve their stemness properties. Moreover, Bic40 treatment proved effective in removing bacterial biofilm from both titanium surfaces and consistently limited the biofilm re-growth. In conclusion, our data suggest that Bic40 treatment may operatively clean smooth and rough surfaces without altering their properties and, consequently, offer favourable conditions for reparative cells to hold their biological properties.

Keywords: human dental pulp stem cells; stemness properties; titanium surface properties

---

1. Introduction

The use of dental implants in daily clinical practice is currently widespread and in huge growth: the modern implant therapy allows in fact not only to offer a biological and functional advantage for many patients, compared with fixed or removable prosthetic solutions but also to obtain excellent long term results, as confirmed by previous studies reporting survival rates of 95.7% and 92.8% after 5 and 10 years, respectively [1]. However, despite these high survival rates, implant rehabilitation can fail. The most relevant troubles concerning osseointegrated implants are the peri-implant diseases, such as mucositis (reversible) and peri-implantitis (not reversible). Peri-implantitis has been defined as a disease with infectious pathogenesis characterized by a mucosal lesion often associated with bleeding, suppuration, increased probing depth always accompanied by marginal bone loss [2]. In this context, several factors affecting the systemic health status of the patients, that is, chronic diseases, autoimmune/inflammatory diseases, in combination with poor oral hygiene and smoking might influence the host-microbial interface very early in the healing phase following dental implant thus increasing the risk of peri-implant diseases [3].

The formation and organization of a bacterial biofilm on the implant portions exposed to the oral cavity is the initial cause of the peri-implant diseases and its removal is the goal to prevent or treat these diseases. Microbial biofilm commonly occurs in the oral cavity; it consists of a multispecies community, including Gram+ and Gram− bacteria as well as fungal cells, organized as sessile cells, tightly embedded in a matrix of polysaccharide origin. Biofilm formation and development is a process that begins with adhesion of initially planktonic microorganisms, followed by growth, extracellular polymeric matrix production, detachment and delocalization. Microbial biofilm occurs both in biotic and abiotic surfaces; once structured, biofilm-associated cells acquire enhanced resistance to cleaning treatment, antimicrobial drugs and host immune defences with respect to their planktonic counterparts [4]. To date, several methods have been developed with the aim of decontaminating implants: mechanical systems (Titanium brushes, Air-polishing systems, Ultra-Subsonic systems, Laser, Curettes) and chemical systems or antimicrobial solutions (Chlorhexidine in solution or in gel, Stannous fluoride, Tetracycline, Minocycline, Citric acid, Hydrogen peroxide and Gel etching with 35% phosphoric acid) [5–7]. Most of these decontaminating treatments might alter the chemical-physical properties of the implant surface [8–11]. Therefore, the ideal decontamination system is expected to be capable of breaking and removing the bacterial biofilm, without modifying the surface properties and thus maintaining the implant surface biologically favourable to adhesion and differentiation of the reparative cells grown onto the implant. It is well known indeed that the micro/nanotopography and the chemical composition of implant surfaces might influence the osseointegration process, by affecting and modifying the biological properties of the cells that interact with the surface [12–15]. Based on these considerations, among several decontamination techniques investigated, Nickel Titanium (Ni-Ti) brushes and Air Polishing systems have aroused interest. Ni-Ti is a resistant material with high flexibility when subjected to heating/cooling alternations. Moreover, the centrifugal force of the motor movement, the pressure exerted by the operator's hand and the heating/cooling alternations allow the brush to effectively reach even the most difficult spaces to clean. As a matter of fact, Ni-Ti brushes proved more effective in removing plaque than steel or plastic curettes, being, at the same time, less aggressive towards the implant surfaces [16–19]. Likewise, air-polishing devices based on the use of bicarbonate powder, which historically represents the first type of substance used in this approach, were shown to be highly effective in the mechanical removal of biofilm from different surface types, such as machined, SLA, sandblasted and TPS, with previous data showing that this approach provided better outcomes when compared to other instruments, such as plastic inserts of sonic devices [9,20,21].

Human DPSCs can be easily obtained from routine tooth extraction procedures and own self-renewal properties and a high regenerative potential [22]. Although dental pulp stem cells are a heterogeneous cell population, the immune selection against the stemness markers c-Kit and STRO-1 allows to isolate an adequate source of pre-osteoblast/odontoblast cells [23,24] which represent the ideal cell candidate in order to mimic in vitro the physiological processes of osseointegration and to investigate how different cleansing approaches might modify the cells-implants interactions.

The aim of this study was to investigate whether the use of two different mechanical decontamination systems, namely Ni-Ti Brushes and Air-Polishing System with 40 μm bicarbonate powder, might alter the roughness and chemical composition of two different implant surfaces (Machined and Ca^{++} Nano-incorporated) and whether the two decontamination systems may impact the biological and stemness features of DPSCs as well as the bacterial ability to produce biofilm.

2. Results

2.1. Titanium Surface Characterization

Scanning electron microscopy (SEM) analysis carried out on MCH surfaces from each experimental group is shown in Figure 1A. At lower magnifications, MCH control surface displayed concentric irregularities according to our previous findings [15]. The polishing treatment with Ni-Ti brush was characterized by grooves oriented in all the directions through the entire surface of the disks, as reported in either lower and higher magnifications. On the MCH titanium surfaces treated with Bic40, the presence of slight alterations of the whole surface was observed. Particularly, newly formed irregularities were detected on the entire treated disk (Figure 1A).

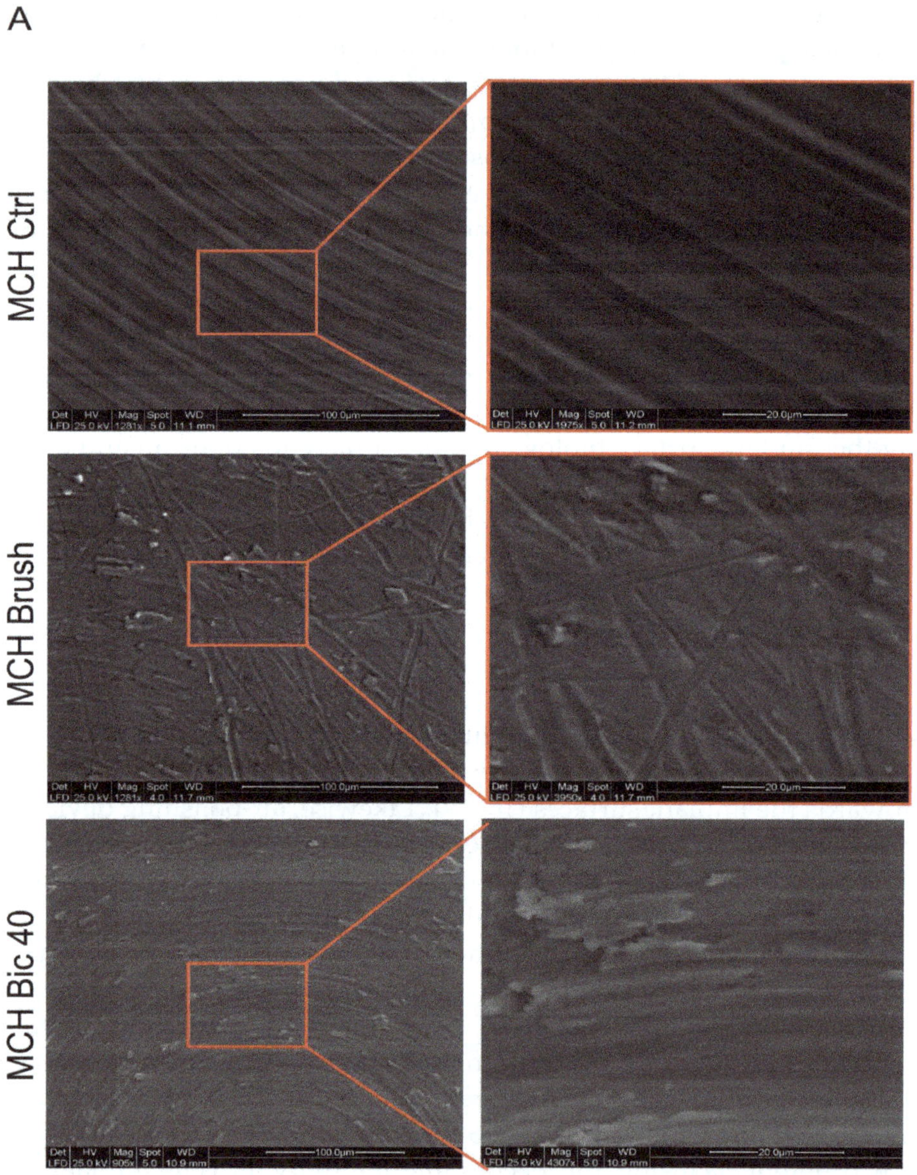

Figure 1. *Cont.*

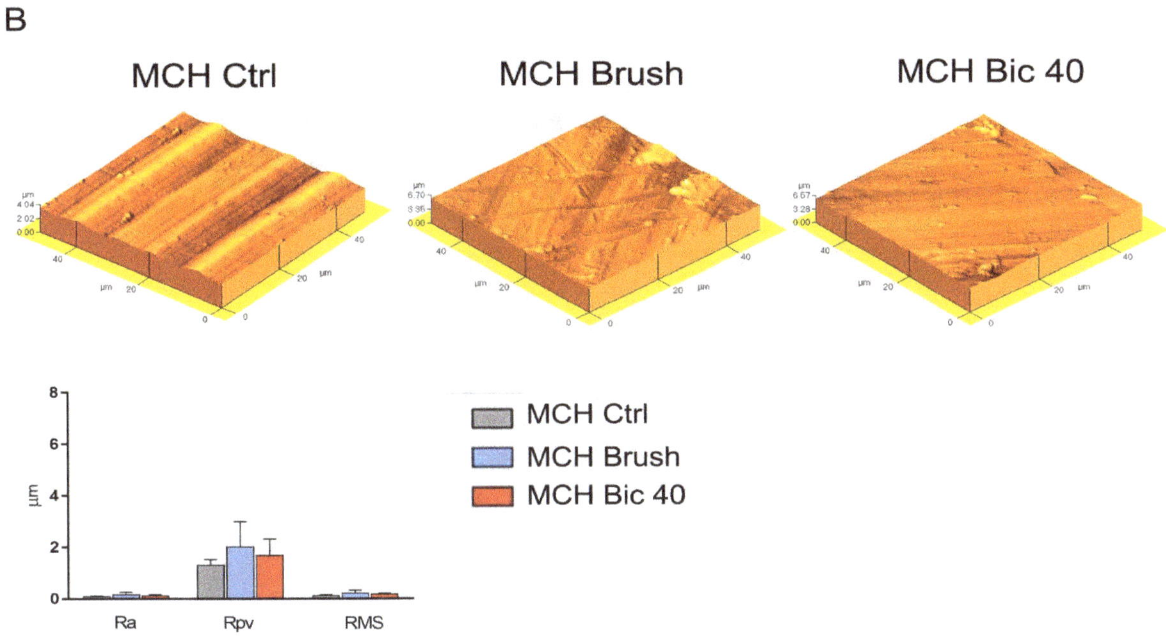

Figure 1. Machined (MCH) surfaces characterization after cleaning treatments. (**A**) Scanning electron microscopy (SEM) analysis at different magnifications was carried out on MCH titanium surfaces from the three experimental groups (Ctrl, Brush and Bic40, as indicated) in order to evaluate the surface topography. Scale bars: 100 µm (left) and 20 µm (magnifications on the right). (**B**) Atomic force microscopy (AFM) analysis of MCH surfaces. Histograms report the surface roughness expressed as Ra, Rpv and Rsm values. Values represent mean ± SD of three independent experiments; one-way ANOVA followed by Newman-Keuls post-hoc test.

Furthermore, atomic force microscopy (AFM) analysis was performed to evaluate the roughness of MCH disks following the different polishing treatments. In particular, as shown in Figure 1B, Ra, Rpv and Rsm were determined for each experimental group. With regard to Rpv parameter, higher values were recorded in MCH Brush group, in comparison to control MCH and MCH Bic40, although these differences were not statistically significant (Figure 1B). At the same time, SEM analysis was carried out on NCA surfaces from the three experimental groups. Data are reported in Figure 2A. According to previous data from our group [15], control NCA were characterized by homogeneous irregularities spread through the whole analysed area. The polishing treatment with Brush induced a notable modification of the surface: particularly, a flattening of the peaks typical of NCA surface was observed at lower and higher magnifications. Conversely, the air-polishing treatment with Bic40 did not induce any relevant alteration of the nanotopography of the surface. These observational data were not confirmed by AFM analyses, as a matter of fact, Ra, Rpv and Rms parameters did not differ among the three experimental groups. Likely, this evidence might be due to the AFM instrumental sensitivity (Figure 2B). Taken together, data on surface roughness of MCH and NCA surfaces treated with Bic40 did not show any significant difference, in terms of nanotopography, from both MCH and NCA controls.

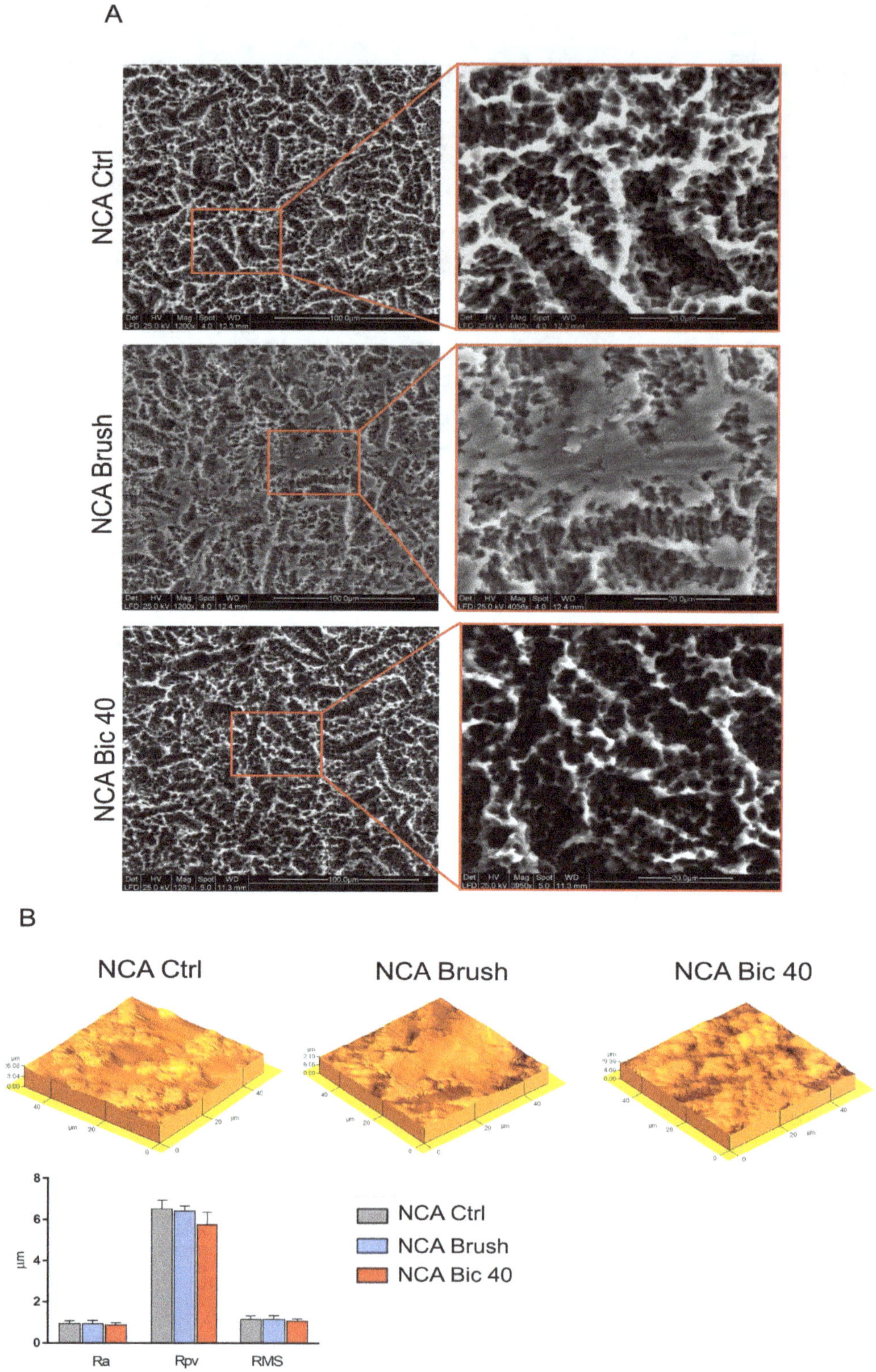

Figure 2. NCA surfaces characterization after cleansing treatments. (**A**) SEM analysis at different magnifications was carried out on NCA titanium surfaces from the three experimental groups (Ctrl, Brush and Bic40, as indicated) in order to evaluate the surface topography. Scale bars: 100 µm (left) and 20 µm (magnifications on the right). (**B**) AFM analysis of NCA surfaces. Histograms report the surface roughness expressed as Ra, Rpv and Rsm values. Values represent mean ± SD of three independent experiments. No statistically significant difference was detected among the groups; one-way ANOVA followed by the Newman-Keuls post-hoc test.

2.2. *Stem Cells Morphology and Proliferation on Titanium Surfaces after Polishing Treatments*

The hDPSCs morphology was evaluated by confocal microscopy, as shown in Figures 3 and 4. Cells were stained with phalloidin and DAPI. After 7 days of culture under standard conditions on MCH surfaces, hDPSCs displayed a fibroblast-like morphology with cells being arranged parallel to the surface grooves without showing significant differences following the Brush and Bic40 polishing treatments. With regard to the distribution of cells through the surface area, we noticed that hDPSCs cultured on MCH Brush oriented not only along the grooves due to the industrial fabrication but also along the scratches created after the Brush cleaning. No differences were observed in hDPSCs seeded on MCH Bic40 when compared to the control group (Figure 3A). Also, no differences in terms of proliferation rate were observed among the three experimental groups as indicated by histograms (Figure 3B).

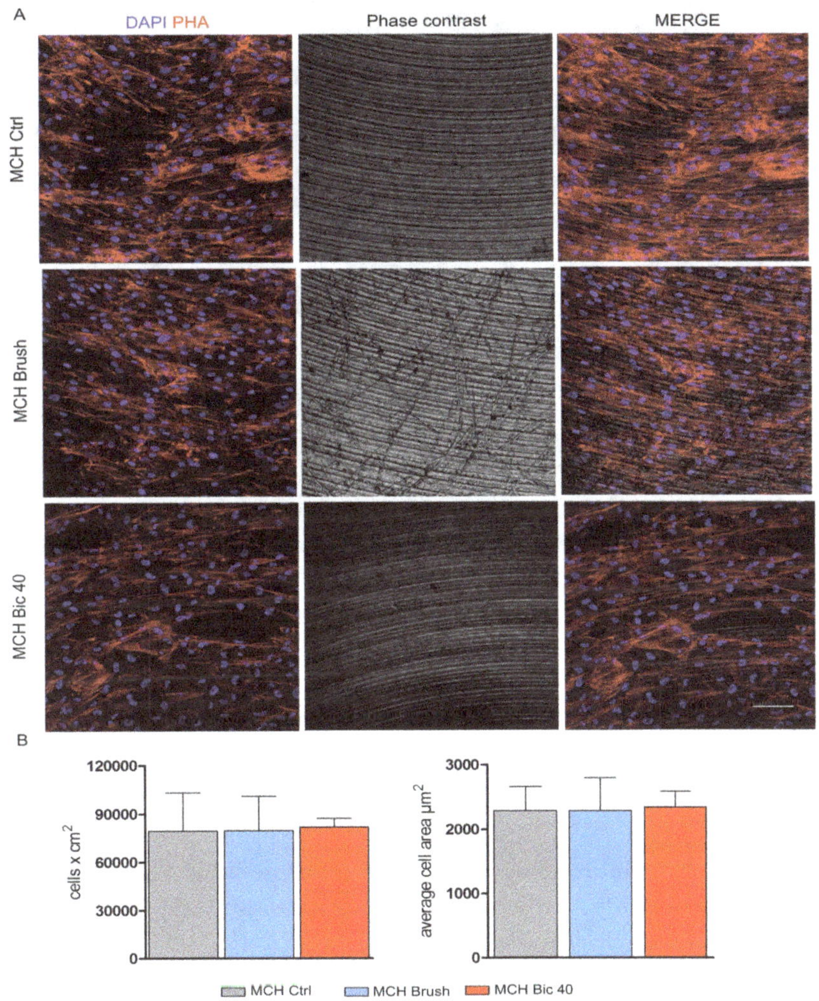

Figure 3. Evaluation of hDPSCs morphology and proliferation on MCH titanium surfaces. (**A**) hDPSCs morphology was assessed by confocal microscopy with phalloidin staining after 7 days of culture on MCH Ctrl, MCH Brush and MCH Bic40 surfaces. (**B**) Cell proliferation on titanium disks was measured by counting cell nuclei after DAPI staining. Histograms show cell numbers after 7 days of culture on titanium surfaces from the three experimental groups. Values represent mean ± SD. No statistically significant difference was detected among the groups; one-way ANOVA followed by the Newman-Keuls post-hoc test. Scale bar: 100 µm.

Figure 4 shows the morphology, distribution and proliferation of hDPSCs after 7 days of culture on NCA surfaces following Brush and Bic40 treatments. As formerly described, the culture on NCA disks induced a morphology alteration in hDPSCs. In particular, cells were homogeneously spread through the whole area and showed an irregular shape with reduction of the average cell area. The same features were observed in hDPSCs cultured on NCA Brush disks. Interestingly, when NCA disks were cleaned with Bic40 hDPSCs grew still homogeneously although recovering their typical fibroblast-like morphology, as reported when cultured on MCH disks. This shift in morphology was reflected also by an increased proliferation rate and by values of average cell area of hDPSCs cultured on NCA Bic40, with respect to NCA Ctrl and NCA Brush (* $p < 0.05$, Figure 4B).

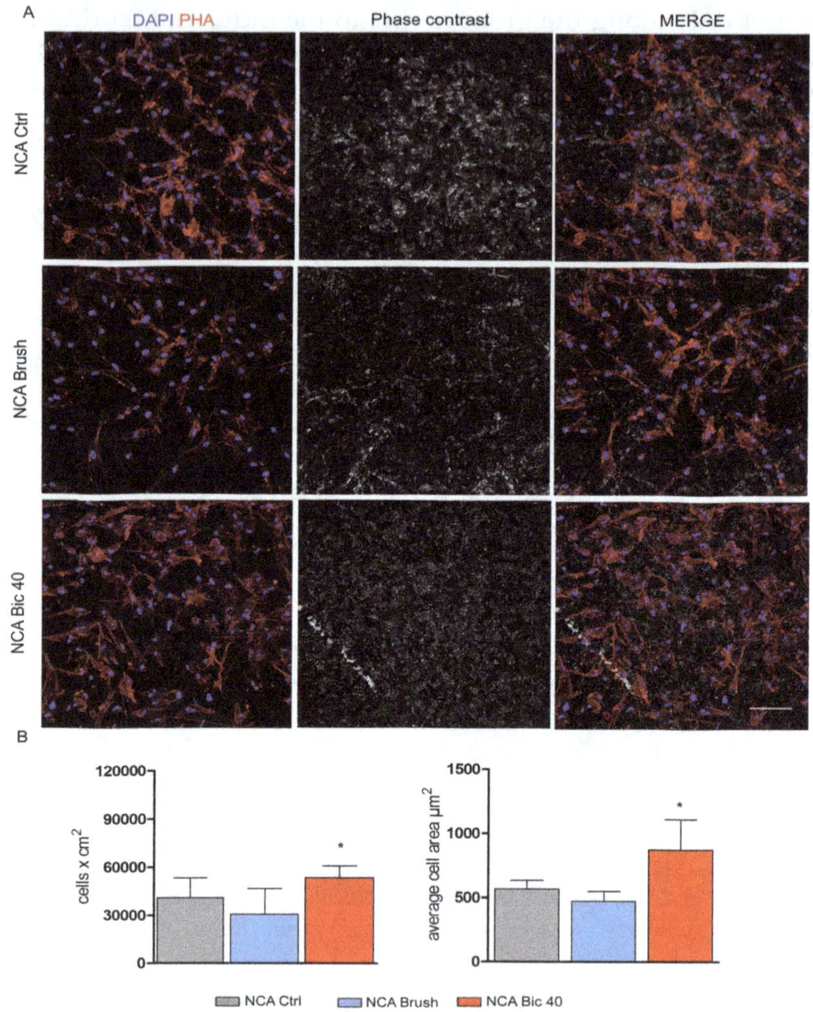

Figure 4. Evaluation of hDPSCs morphology and proliferation on NCA titanium surfaces. (**A**) hDPSCs morphology was assessed by confocal microscopy with phalloidin staining after 7 days of culture on NCA Ctrl, NCA Brush and NCA Bic40 surfaces. (**B**) Cell proliferation on titanium disks was measured by counting cell nuclei after DAPI staining. Histograms show cell numbers and average cell area after 7 days of culture on titanium surfaces from the three experimental groups. Values represent mean ± SD. * $p < 0.05$ NCA Bic 40 vs. NCA Brush, NCA Bic40 vs. NCA Ctrl; one-way ANOVA followed by the Newman-Keuls post-hoc test. Scale bar: 100 µm.

2.3. Expression of Stemness Markers

Human DPSCs were immune-selected against STRO-1 and c-Kit. After 7 days of culture on MCH and NCA surfaces, immunofluorescence analysis was performed in order to evaluate the maintenance of their biological properties. The expression of STRO-1 and c-Kit, two typical mesenchymal stem cells markers, were investigated in MCH and NCA after cleaning treatments.

As reported in Figure 5, hDPSCs cultured on MCH Ctrl showed the expression of both mesenchymal markers. These markers were still observed in hDPSCs cultured either on MCH Brush and MCH Bic40.

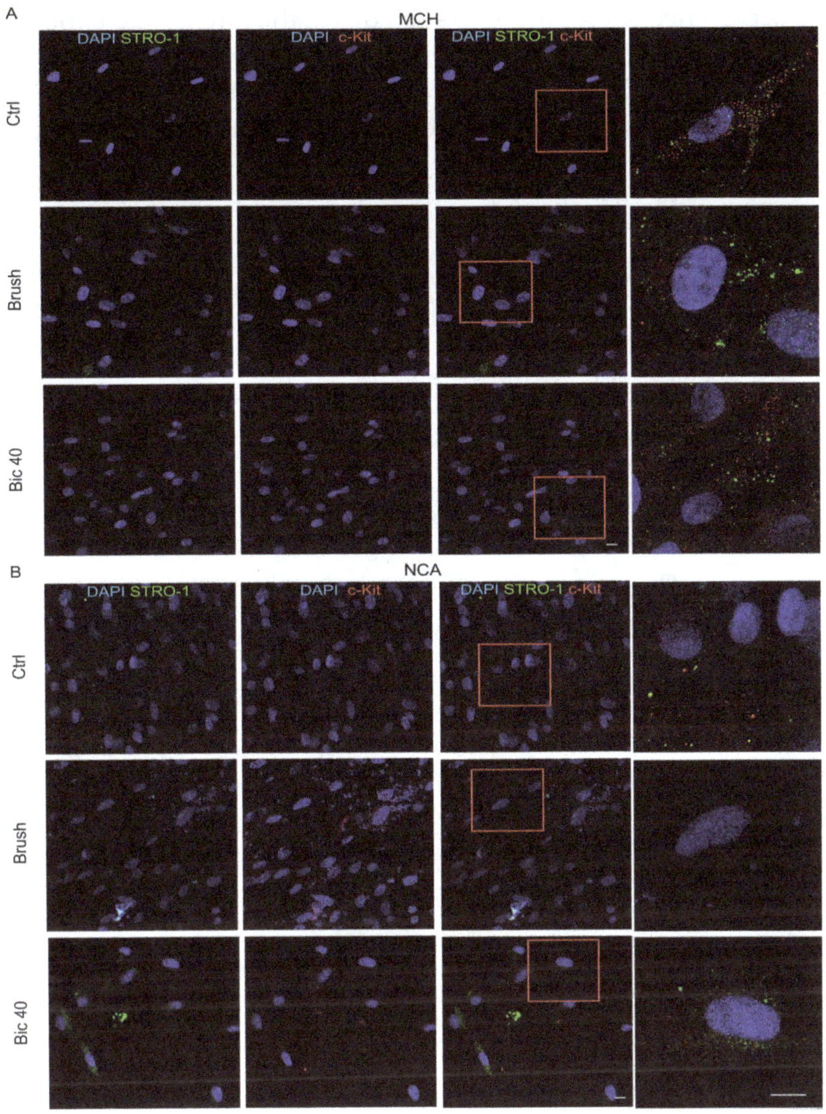

Figure 5. Evaluation of stemness markers of hDPSCs on titanium surfaces after cleaning treatments. Immunofluorescence analysis of STRO-1 and c-Kit in hDPSCs cultured for 7 days on MCH (**A**) and NCA (**B**) surfaces from the three experimental groups. Red squares indicate details reported at higher magnifications on the right. Nuclei were stained with DAPI. Scale bar: 10 μm.

On the contrary, we noticed a reduction in STRO-1 and c-Kit expression in hDPSCs grown on NCA Ctrl and NCA Brush after 7 days of culture. Conversely, the expression of these markers was evident in hDPSCs cultured on NCA Bic40. The morphology data in association with stemness evaluation indicate that after cleansing with Bic40, the NCA surface appeared more favourable/suitable to the growth of hDPSCs in their physiological microenvironment.

2.4. Microbial Biofilm Formation onto Titanium Disks

Based on the biological results concerning morphology, proliferation and stemness markers, it was then evaluated whether the polishing treatment with Bic40 on NCA surface may affect the microbial growth. Thus, *Pseudomonas aeruginosa* (10^6/mL) was seeded at time 0, in two sets of wells, containing or not the titanium disks; then, the plate was incubated at 35 °C for 24 h and microbial growth was assessed by bioluminescent analysis. As shown in Figure 6A, a superimposable trend was observed in the two groups of wells (control: no disks; sample: with disks); moreover, at 24 h, comparably high levels of total microbial load were achieved, being 2.6×10^8/mL and 3.4×10^8/mL the CFU/mL detected in control and sample groups, respectively. These data indicated that the presence of titanium disks did not affect microbial growth. To assess the occurrence of biofilm onto such disks, the latter were exposed to bacteria for 24 h, washed twice with PBS to eliminate the non-adherent microbial cells and then the residual bioluminescent signal was evaluated, as measure of formed biofilm. The obtained bioluminescent signal was converted in CFU and indicated that biofilm was produced at amounts as high as 1.95×10^8 CFU/mL (data not shown).

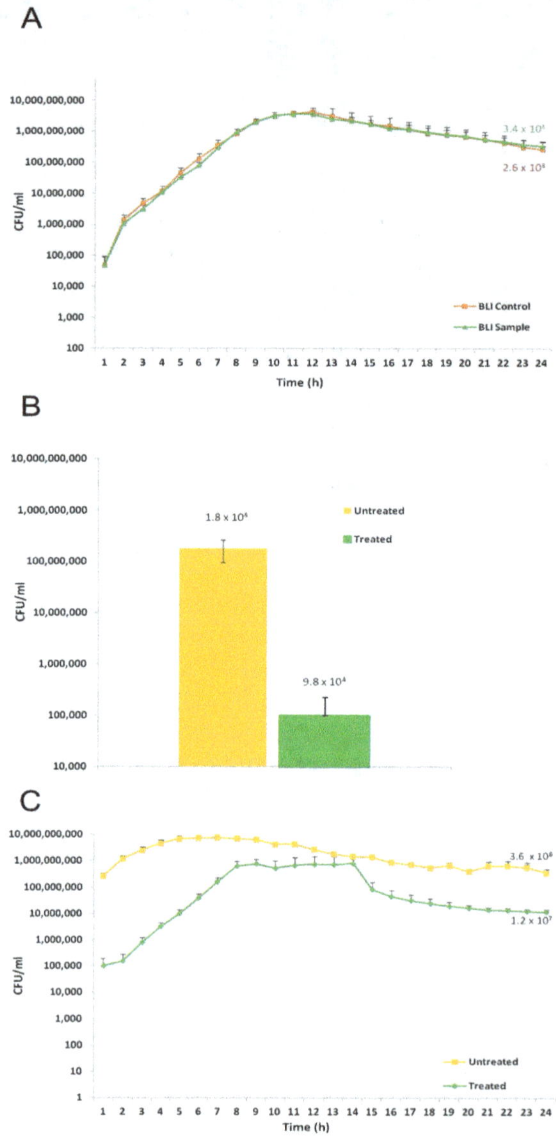

Figure 6. *P. aeruginosa* growth and biofilm formation on titanium disks, treated or not with Bic40 procedure, as assessed by a bioluminescent (BLI) bacterial strain. (**A**) *P. aeruginosa* growth was not affected by the presence of titanium disks. BLI-*Pseudomonas* (10^6/mL) in TSB plus 2% sucrose was seeded in 96 black well-plate and incubated at 35 °C in the presence (orange) or absence (green) of titanium disks (1/well). The plates were then incubated by Fluoroskan and the bioluminescent signal was recorded in real time (h), up to 24 h. By the calibration curve, the RLUs were converted in CFU/mL + SEM (Standard Error Mean), as indicated in the Y axis. (**B**) Effects of the cleaning procedure on titanium disks-associated biofilm. Microbial biofilm produced onto titanium disks (by 24 h incubation, as above) was exposed or not to the Bic40 cleaning procedure (treated vs. untreated group); the residual bioluminescent signal was measured and converted, by the calibration curve, in CFU/mL ± SEM, as indicated in the Y axis. (**C**) Real time monitoring of *P. aeruginosa* re-growth on treated and untreated titanium disks. The microbial re-growth, occurring in Bic40-treated and untreated disks, was evaluated in real time, for additional 24 h. Then, the bioluminescent signal was measured and converted in CFU, returning values of 3.6×10^8/mL and 1.2×10^7/mL, in untreated and treated groups, respectively.

2.5. Microbial Biofilm Removal from Titanium Disks

To assess the efficacy of the Bic40 cleaning procedure against a preformed biofilm, 4 disks containing a 24 h-old biofilm were treated with Bic40 procedure, as detailed above (treated group), while 3 disks, used as controls were not treated (untreated group); then, each disk was transferred in a new well with fresh medium and incubated for additional 24 h. As shown in Figure 6B, when compared to the untreated groups, the Bic40-treated disks displayed an about 3 logs drop in terms of CFU/mL.

2.6. Microbial Re-Growth on Treated and Untreated Titanium Disks

As detailed in Figure 6C, the microbial load in the untreated group remained almost constant during the subsequent 24 h range. In contrast, treated disks showed a delayed and time-related increase in CFU. In particular, the major differences between treated and untreated disks occurred within the first 5–6 h; then, microbial load on treated disks reached a plateau level, that consistently remained about 1 log below the values observed in the untreated disks until at 24 h.

3. Discussion

The peri-implant disease is due to the colonization of the implant surfaces by pathogens which constitute a biofilm [25]. Bacterial adhesion and biofilm formation play a fundamental role not only into the pathogenesis of peri-implantitis but also into the implant survival [12,13,26]. In a previous study [27] we observed that the biofilm occurred regardless of the degree of surface roughness. Therefore, the removal of the biofilm from the implant surface, indistinctly smooth or rough, is the primary objective. It is well known that the response of cells and tissues to a biomaterial depends on the properties of the material itself such as surface topography, chemical composition and capability to interact with body fluids [15,28]. Following bacterial contamination, the procedures used to decontaminate the implant surface can cause alterations of its topography and its chemical composition. To this regard and to the best of our knowledge the optimal cleansing approach is expected to effectively remove the bacteria biofilm without altering the chemical and physical properties of the implant and consequently the biological properties of cells involved in the osseointegration process. In this study we analysed two different titanium surfaces, before and after the treatment with two cleansing approaches, mimicking what physiologically occurs in terms of cells/implant interactions after decontamination procedures.

Qualitative analysis of surface morphology revealed how in both MCH and NCA groups the surfaces treated with Ni-Ti brushes are morphologically different from the untreated surfaces, in agreement with Park et al. [18]. In fact, SEM analysis showed the presence of deep grooves heterogeneously distributed over the MCH surface and flattened area over the NCA surface. Slight although not statistically significant differences were revealed by Ra, Rpv and Rsm physical parameters. Conversely, the treatment with Air-polishing system with Bic40 produced not significant alterations of both the MCH and NCA surfaces in terms of physical parameters. Subsequently, the aim of the study was to evaluate the biological features of stem cells that embryologically participate to the osseointegration process. The use of dental pulp stem cells represents a suitable choice in terms of stemness properties and ease of isolation. Although hDPSCs are a heterogeneous population, we used a stem cell population enriched for the expression of the stemness markers STRO-1 and c-Kit, which represent a strictly mesenchymal origin able to differentiate in bone, adipose and myogenic lineages. To the best of our knowledge, we noticed that on MCH titanium surface before and after both the cleansing treatments, hDPSCs maintained their fibroblast-like morphology without any alteration of cell proliferation. The only difference observed concerned the hDPSCs distribution pattern through the MCH Brush surface, in fact cells were spread along the grooves produced by Ni-Ti brush. On the contrary, hDPSCs grown on MCH Bic40 and MCH ctrl surfaces did not show any difference.

Regarding NCA surface, a change in cell morphology was observed in NCA ctrl and NCA brush, in accordance with our previous findings [15]. After the treatment with Bic40 hDPSCs showed their typical cell morphology and also demonstrated a statistically significant higher proliferation rate, when compared to NCA ctrl and NCA Brush surfaces: this phenomenon might be attributed to the interaction of calcium ions incorporated on the NCA surface with bicarbonate ions from the cleansing treatment with Bic40. These observations were confirmed by the evaluation of stemness markers on MCH and NCA surfaces before and after the cleansing treatments. In particular, whereas no differences were detected in any MCH group, we noticed that STRO-1 and c-Kit expression were maintained in NCA Bic40 group. As a matter of fact, the maintenance of stemness is a primary requirement to preserve the biological properties including self-renewal and differentiation capabilities and immunomodulatory properties and consequently to avoid cell senescence. Based on these results, Bic40 might represent the most suitable cleansing treatment. To further confirm the efficacy of Bic40, we also performed microbiology assays. Using a recently established model precious in assessing microbial biofilm formation onto medical devices [29], here we showed that BLI-*Pseudomonas* has the ability to adhere to the titanium disks and to form a consistent biofilm on their surface. Moreover, the cleaning treatment with BIC 40 μm is capable of reducing the biofilm of about 99% with respect to untreated control group (100% vs. 0.05%, respectively). In particular, the microbial load, evaluated as RLU and converted in CFU/mL, has been reduced of more than 3 logs in the treated groups as compared to their controls. Furthermore, microbial re-growth in treated disks remains consistently below the control values (difference of about 1 log). We may hypothesize that the combination of the physical treatment (dry spray) and the hypertonic condition (sodium bicarbonate accumulation onto titanium disks) negatively impact on microbial cell-viability. Furthermore, the enrichment of air-polishing powders with antimicrobial fillers such as Ciprofloxacin and/or mucosal defensive agents such as Zinc L-carnosine might improve the antibacterial action of the cleaning tool and its biocompatibility towards soft tissues [30]. In conclusion, we demonstrated that Bic40 provides a suitable cleansing approach either on smooth and rough surfaces.

4. Materials and Methods

4.1. Human DPSCs Isolation and Immune Selection

This study was carried out in compliance with the recommendations of Comitato Etico Provinciale—Azienda Ospedaliero-Universitaria di Modena (Modena, Italy), which provided the approval of the protocol (ref. number 3299/CE; 5 September 2017). Human DPSCs were isolated from third molars of adult subjects ($n = 3$; 30–35 years) undergoing routine dental extraction. All subjects gave written informed consent in accordance with the Declaration of Helsinki.

Cells were isolated from dental pulp as previously described [23]. Briefly, dental pulp was harvested from the teeth and underwent enzymatic digestion by using a digestive solution, (3 mg/mL type I collagenase plus 4 mg/mL dispase in α-MEM). Pulp was then filtered onto 100 μm Falcon Cell Strainers, in order to obtain a cell suspension. Cell suspension was then plated in 25 cm^2 culture flasks and expanded in standard culture medium [α-MEM supplemented with 10% heat inactivated foetal bovine serum (FBS), 2 mM L-glutamine, 100 U/mL penicillin, 100 μg/mL streptomycin] at 37 °C and 5% CO2. Following cell expansion, human DPSCs were immune-selected by using MACS® separation kit according to manufacturers' instructions. The immune-selections were performed by using primary antibodies: mouse IgM anti-STRO-1 and rabbit IgG anti-c-Kit (Santa Cruz, Dallas, TX, USA). The following magnetically labelled secondary antibodies were used: anti-mouse IgM and anti-rabbit IgG (Miltenyi Biotec, Bergisch Gladbach, Germany). The immune-selection resulted in the isolation of a homogeneous hDPSCs population expressing STRO-1 and c-Kit. All the experiments were performed using STRO-1^+/c-Kit^+ hDPSCs.

4.2. Titanium Surfaces Characterization

A total of 50 titanium disks (MegaGen Co. Ltd., Daegu, South Korea) measuring 13 mm in diameter and 3 mm in thickness were used in this study. Particularly, two different titanium surfaces were used: machined (MCH) and Ca2$^+$ incorporated (NCA). The treatment processes are hold by the manufacturer. For this study, titanium surfaces were divided into 3 different experimental groups: (1) control surfaces (Ctrl), (2) surfaces cleaned with Ni-Ti brushes (Brush) and (3) surfaces cleaned by air-polishing with $NaHCO_3$ 40 μm (Bic40).

The cleansing of the disks was carried out using two mechanical methods: (1) Nickel-Titanium Brushes (I.C.T. Brush micro, Hans Korea Co. Ltd., Gyeonggi-do, Korea/ De Ore, Verona, Italy) and (2) Air-Polishing System (Combi-Touch, Mectron spa, Carasco, Genova, Italy) with 40 μm bicarbonate powder.

Briefly, the "I.C.T." (Implant Cleaning Technique) nickel-titanium brushes, made up of about 40 super elastic filaments with a diameter of 0.07–0.13 mm, were used at 400 rpm and 600 rpm, respectively, for two sequential rounds of 45 s each. The total duration of each surface treatment was 90 s and a 25 g pressure calibrated on an electronic scale was used, with 100 N of torque. All the treatments were performed by the same operator under irrigation with buffer saline solution (0.9% NaCl).

The "Combi-Touch" air polishing system with sodium bicarbonate particles (ø 40 μm) was used for 30 s at a distance of 5 mm. In particular, the operating principle of "Combi Touch" air-polishing system consists in the mechanical action of compressed air spreading an accelerated flow of particles onto the titanium surface. When the particles hit the surface, their kinetic energy is dissipated almost completely, thus producing a gentle although effectively cleansing action. The cleaning treatment is completed by a water jet that is arranged in the form of a bell around the main flow and that uses the pressure drop originated around the nozzle to prevent the powder cloud from bouncing and being dispelled and, at the same time, to dissolve the powder by washing the surface.

After the cleansing treatments, surface morphology for each experimental group was qualitatively evaluated through Scanning Electron Microscopy (EVO MA 10—Carl Zeiss, Oberkochen, Germany) working at 25 keV. Moreover, surface roughness was determined by Atomic Force Microscopy (Nanoscope IIIa, Veeco, Santa Barbara, CA, USA) and Ra, Rpv and Rms parameters were obtained. Ra (Roughness average) measures the average surface roughness considering the peaks and the valley means. The Rpv (peak to valley distance) describes the maximum observed range in a sample area and it is given by the distance between the highest peak and the lowest valley on a measured surface. Rms parameter describes the density of micropores on the surface.

4.3. Cell Morphology and Proliferation

Undifferentiated STRO-1$^+$/c-Kit$^+$ hDPSCs at passage 1 were seeded at a density of 2.5×10^3 cell/cm^2 on titanium disks in 12-multiwell units and expanded under standard culture conditions. After 7 days of culture, cells were fixed in ice-cold paraformaldehyde 4% for 15 min without dissociating them from the titanium disks. The cells were subsequently permeabilized with 0.1% Triton X-100 in PBS for 5 min, stained with AlexaFluor546 Phalloidin (Thermo Fisher Scientific) and rinsed with PBS 1%. Nuclei were stained with 1 μg/mL 4′,6-diamidino-2-phenylindole (DAPI) in PBS 1%. Titanium disks were mounted with DABCO anti-fading medium on cover glasses. Cell proliferation and morphology were assessed using confocal microscopy (Nikon A1), as formerly described by Bianchi et al. [24].

Cell proliferation was measured by counting the DAPI-positive nuclei on 10 randomly selected fields measuring 2.85×10^5 μm^2 for each disk by a blind operator. At the same time, average cell area was measured on hDPSCs from 10 randomly selected fields, measuring 2.85×10^5 μm^2, on 3 disks for each experimental group.

4.4. Evaluation of Stemness Markers in hDPSCs Cultured on Titanium Disks

After 1 week of culture on each disk, cells were fixed in 4% ice-cold paraformaldehyde in PBS for 15 min and then processed as previously described [31]. The following primary Abs diluted 1:100 were used: mouse IgM anti-STRO-1 and rabbit IgG anti-c-Kit (Santa Cruz, Dallas, TX, USA). Secondary Abs (goat anti-mouse IgM Alexa488, goat anti-rabbit Alexa546) were diluted 1:200 (Thermo Fisher Scientific, Waltham, MA, USA). Nuclei were stained with 1 μg/mL 4′,6-diamidino-2-phenylindole

(DAPI) in PBS 1%. The multi-labelling immunofluorescence experiments were carried out avoiding cross-reactions between primary and secondary Abs.

Confocal imaging was performed using a Nikon A1 confocal laser scanning microscope, as previously described [32]. The confocal serial sections were processed with ImageJ software to obtain 3-dimensional projections and image rendering was performed by Adobe Photoshop Software.

4.5. Microbial Strain

We used the bioluminescent *Pseudomonas aeruginosa* strain (P1242) (BLI-*Pseudomonas*) previously engineered in order to express the luciferase gene and substrate under the control of a constitutive P1 integron promoter 2 [33]; thus, live cells constitutively produce a detectable bioluminescent signal. To quantify the bioluminescence emission by BLI-Pseudomonas in the experimental groups, a calibration curve was created allowing to express such values in terms of colony forming units (CFU)/mL; in particular, serial dilutions (starting from 1×10^8/mL) of a bacterial suspension in Tryptic Soy Broth (TSB) (OXOID, Milan, Italy) with 2% sucrose were prepared and a volume of 100 μL of each dilution was seeded in a black-well microtiter plate. The plate was immediately read by using a Fluoroskan Luminescence reader (Thermo Fisher Scientific, Waltham, MA, USA).

4.6. Biofilm Formation onto Titanium Disks

In order to allow biofilm formation onto Ca-structured titanium disks, 180 μL of overnight cultures of BLI-Pseudomonas (10^6/mL) in TSB plus 2% sucrose were seeded in 96 black well-plate, containing 1 disc/well. In parallel, BLI-Pseudomonas was seeded in wells without the titanium disks. The plates were then incubated at 35 °C for 24 h, into the Fluoroskan reader and the bioluminescence was detected at every hour to evaluate in real time, the total microbial load. After incubation, the disks were washed twice with phosphate buffered saline (PBS) (EuroClone, Wetherby, UK) at room temperature (RT), transferred into new wells and the bioluminescence signal was again measured; the obtained values were referred to the amounts of biofilm formed onto disk surfaces. Through the calibration curve, the relative luminescent units (RLU) obtained in each experiment were converted in CFU/mL.

4.7. Biofilm Re-Growth onto Treated and Untreated Titanium Disks

Following biofilm formation, the disks were split in two groups and the cleaning treatment was performed, as detailed above; then, controls (untreated) and cleaned (exposed to Bic40 μm for 30 s/surface) were transferred into new wells containing fresh medium and further assessed for microbial residual load and time-related re-growth. Briefly, treated and untreated disks were analysed by Fluoroskan reader, immediately (residual biofilm) and at any hour during a further 24 h incubation at 35 °C. Through the calibration curve, the RLU were converted in CFU/mL.

4.8. Statistical Analysis

All experiments were performed in triplicate. Data were expressed as mean ± standard deviation (SD). Differences between two experimental conditions were analysed by paired, Student's *t*-test. Differences among three or more experimental samples were analysed by ANOVA followed by Newman–Keuls post hoc test (GraphPad Prism Software version 5 Inc., San Diego, CA, USA). In any case, p value < 0.05 was considered statistically significant.

Author Contributions: Conceptualization, E.C., A.P., U.C. and G.C.; Methodology, E.C., A.P., G.C. and E.B.; Validation, A.P., G.C., A.M., B.C. and E.B.; Formal Analysis, A.P., E.B., A.d.P., P.B., U.C. and G.C.; Investigation, E.C., A.P., G.B., A.M., B.C. and E.B.; Data Curation, E.C., A.P., G.B., L.B. and E.B.; Writing—Original Draft Preparation, E.C., A.P., E.B. and G.C.; Writing—Review & Editing, E.C., A.P., L.B., G.B., A.M., B.C., E.B., A.d.P., P.B., U.C. and G.C.; Supervision, A.d.P., U.C. and G.C.; Funding Acquisition, U.C.

References

1. Albrektsson, T.; Donos, N. Implant survival and complications. The Third EAO consensus conference 2012. *Clin. Oral Implant. Res.* **2012**, *23*, 63–65. [CrossRef] [PubMed]
2. Lindhe, J.; Meyle, J.; on behalf of Group D of the European Workshop on Periodontology. Peri-implant diseases: Consensus Report of the Sixth European Workshop on Periodontology. *J. Clin. Periodontol.* **2008**, *35*, 282–285. [CrossRef]
3. Kumar, P.S. Systemic Risk Factors for the Development of Periimplant Diseases. *Implant. Dent.* **2019**, *28*, 115–119. [CrossRef] [PubMed]
4. Derks, J.; Tomasi, C. Peri-implant health and disease. A systematic review of current epidemiology. *J. Clin. Periodontol.* **2015**, *42*, 158. [CrossRef] [PubMed]
5. Dennison, D.K.; Huerzeler, M.B.; Quinones, C.; Caffesse, R.G. Contaminated Implant Surfaces: An In Vitro Comparison of Implant Surface Coating and Treatment Modalities for Decontamination. *J. Periodontol.* **1994**, *65*, 942–948. [CrossRef]
6. Toma, S.; Lasserre, J.F.; Taïeb, J.; Brecx, M.C. Evaluation of an air-abrasive device with amino acid glycine-powder during surgical treatment of peri-implantitis. *Quintessence Int* **2014**, *45*, 209–219.
7. Sahrmann, P.; Ronay, V.; Hofer, D.; Attin, T.; Jung, R.E.; Schmidlin, P.R. In vitro cleaning potential of three different implant debridement methods. *Clin. Oral Implant. Res.* **2015**, *26*, 314–319. [CrossRef] [PubMed]
8. Schwarz, F.; Ferrari, D.; Popovski, K.; Hartig, B.; Becker, J. Influence of different air-abrasive powders on cell viability at biologically contaminated titanium dental implants surfaces. *J. Biomed. Mater. Res. B Appl. Biomater.* **2009**, *88*, 83–91. [CrossRef] [PubMed]
9. Tastepe, C.S.; Liu, Y.; Visscher, C.M.; Wismeijer, D. Cleaning and modification of intraorally contaminated titanium disks with calcium phosphate powder abrasive treatment. *Clin. Oral Implant. Res.* **2013**, *24*, 1238–1246.
10. Wei, M.C.; Tran, C.; Meredith, N.; Walsh, L.J. Effectiveness of implant surface debridement using particle beams at differing air pressures. *Clin. Exp. Dent. Res.* **2017**, *3*, 148–153. [CrossRef]
11. Louropoulou, A.; Slot, D.E.; Van der Weijden, F. Influence of mechanical instruments on the biocompatibility of titanium dental implants surfaces: A systematic review. *Clin. Oral Implant. Res.* **2015**, *26*, 841–850. [CrossRef]
12. Mavrogenis, A.F.; Dimitriou, R.; Parvizi, J.; Babis, G.C. Biology of implant osseointegration. *J. Musculoskelet. Neuronal Interact.* **2009**, *9*, 61–71.
13. Wennerberg, A.; Albrektsson, T. Effects of titanium surface topography on bone integration: A systematic review. *Clin. Oral Implant. Res.* **2009**, *20*, 172–184. [CrossRef]
14. Feller, L.; Jadwat, Y.; Khammissa, R.A.G.; Meyerov, R.; Schechter, I.; Lemmer, J. Cellular Responses Evoked by Different Surface Characteristics of Intraosseous Titanium Implants. *Biomed Res. Int.* **2015**, *2015*, 1–8. [CrossRef]
15. Conserva, E.; Pisciotta, A.; Borghi, F.; Nasi, M.; Pecorini, S.; Bertoni, L.; de Pol, A.; Consolo, U.; Carnevale, G. Titanium Surface Properties Influence the Biological Activity and FasL Expression of Craniofacial Stromal Cells. *Stem Cells Int.* **2019**, *2019*, 4670560. [CrossRef]
16. John, G.; Becker, J.; Schwarz, F. Rotating titanium brush for plaque removal from rough titanium surfaces—An in vitro study. *Clin. Oral Implant. Res.* **2014**, *25*, 838–842. [CrossRef] [PubMed]
17. Duddeck, D.; Karapetian, V.; Grandoch, A. Time-saving debridment of implants with rotating titanium brushes. *Implants* **2012**, *3*, 20–22.
18. Park, J.-B.; Jeon, Y.; Ko, Y. Effects of titanium brush on machined and sand-blasted/acid-etched titanium disc using confocal microscopy and contact profilometry. *Clin. Oral Implant. Res.* **2015**, *26*, 130–136. [CrossRef] [PubMed]
19. Louropoulou, A.; Slot, D.E.; Van der Weijden, F. The effects of mechanical instruments on contaminated titanium dental implant surfaces: A systematic review. *Clin. Oral Implant. Res.* **2014**, *25*, 1149–1160. [CrossRef]
20. Tastepe, C.S.; Van Waas, R.; Liu, Y.; Wismeijer, D. Air powder abrasive treatment as an implant surface cleaning method: A literature review. *Int. J. Oral Maxillofac. Implant.* **2012**, *27*, 1461–1473.
21. Nemer Vieira, L.F.; Lopes de Chaves e Mello Dias, E.C.; Cardoso, E.S.; Machado, S.J.; Pereira da Silva, C.; Vidigal, G.M. Effectiveness of implant surface decontamination using a high-pressure sodium bicarbonate protocol: An in vitro study. *Implant Dent.* **2012**, *21*, 390–393. [CrossRef]

22. Pisciotta, A.; Bertoni, L.; Riccio, M.; Mapelli, J.; Bigiani, A.; La Noce, M.; Orciani, M.; De Pol, A.; Carnevale, G. Use of a 3D Floating Sphere Culture System to Maintain the Neural Crest-Related Properties of Human Dental Pulp Stem Cells. *Front. Physiol.* **2018**, *9*, 547. [CrossRef]
23. Pisciotta, A.; Carnevale, G.; Meloni, S.; Riccio, M.; De Biasi, S.; Gibellini, L.; Ferrari, A.; Bruzzesi, G.; De Pol, A. Human Dental pulp stem cells (hDPSCs): Isolation, enrichment and comparative differentiation of two sub-populations. *Bmc Dev. Boil.* **2015**, *15*, 14. [CrossRef]
24. Bianchi, M.; Pisciotta, A.; Bertoni, L.; Berni, M.; Gambardella, A.; Visani, A.; Russo, A.; De Pol, A.; Carnevale, G. Osteogenic Differentiation of hDPSCs on Biogenic Bone Apatite Thin Films. *Stem Cells Int.* **2017**, *2017*, 1–10.
25. Heitz-Mayfield, L.J.A.; Lang, N.P. Comparative biology of chronic and aggressive periodontitis vs. peri-implantitis. *Periodontology* **2010**, *53*, 167–181. [CrossRef]
26. Veerachamy, S.; Yarlagadda, T.; Manivasagam, G.; Yarlagadda, P.K. Bacterial adherence and biofilm formation on medical implants: A review. *Proc. Inst. Mech. Eng. H J. Eng. Med.* **2014**, *228*, 1083–1099. [CrossRef]
27. Conserva, E.; Generali, L.; Bandieri, A.; Cavani, F.; Borghi, F.; Consolo, U. Plaque accumulation on titanium disks with different surface treatments: An in vivo investigation. *Odontology* **2018**, *106*, 145–153. [CrossRef]
28. Anselme, K.; Ponche, A.; Bigerelle, M. Relative influence of surface topography and surface chemistry on cell response to bone implant materials. Part 2: Biological aspects. *Proc. Inst. Mech. Eng. H* **2010**, *224*, 1487–1507. [CrossRef]
29. Pericolini, E.; Colombari, B.; Ferretti, G.; Iseppi, R.; Ardizzoni, A.; Girardis, M.; Sala, A.; Peppoloni, S.; Blasi, E. Real-time monitoring of Pseudomonas aeruginosa biofilm formation on endotracheal tubes in vitro. *Bmc Microbiol.* **2018**, *18*, 84. [CrossRef]
30. Pagano, S.; Chieruzzi, M.; Balloni, S.; Lombardo, G.; Torre, L.; Bodo, M.; Cianetti, S.; Marinucci, L. Biological, thermal and mechanical characterization of modified glass ionomer cements: The role of nanohydroxyapatite, ciprofloxacin and zinc l-carnosine. *Mater. Sci. Eng. C Mater. Biol. Appl.* **2019**, *94*, 76–8516. [CrossRef]
31. Carnevale, G.; Riccio, M.; Pisciotta, A.; Beretti, F.; Maraldi, T.; Zavatti, M.; Cavallini, G.M.; La Sala, G.B.; Ferrari, A.; De Pol, A. In vitro differentiation into insulin-producing β-cells of stem cells isolated from human amniotic fluid and dental pulp. *Dig. Liver Dis.* **2013**, *45*, 669–676.
32. Carnevale, G.; Pisciotta, A.; Riccio, M.; Bertoni, L.; De Biasi, S.; Gibellini, L.; Zordani, A.; Cavallini, GM.; La Sala, GB.; Bruzzesi, G.; et al. Human dental pulp stem cells expressing STRO-1, c-kit and CD34 markers in peripheral nerve regeneration. *J. Tissue Eng. Regen. Med.* **2018**, *12*, e774–e785. [CrossRef]
33. Choi, K.-H.; Schweizer, H.P. mini-Tn7 insertion in bacteria with single attTn7 sites: Example Pseudomonas aeruginosa. *Nat. Protoc.* **2006**, *1*, 153–161. [CrossRef]

14

Human Dental Pulp Stem Cells Exhibit Different Biological Behaviours in Response to Commercial Bleaching Products

Carmen Llena [1], Mar Collado-González [2], Christopher Joseph Tomás-Catalá [2], David García-Bernal [2], Ricardo Elías Oñate-Sánchez [2], Francisco Javier Rodríguez-Lozano [2,3,*] and Leopoldo Forner [1]

1 Department of Stomatology, University de Valencia, 46010 Valencia, Spain; llena@uv.es (C.L.); forner@uv.es (L.F.)

2 School of Dentistry/Cellular Therapy and Hematopoietic Transplant Unit, Hematology Department, Virgen de la Arrixaca Clinical University Hospital, IMIB-Arrixaca, University of Murcia, 30120 Murcia, Spain; mdmcg1@um.es (M.C.-G.); ctc20203@um.es (C.J.T.-C.); redond@gmail.com (D.G.-B.); reosan@um.es (R.E.O.-S.)

3 School of Dentistry, Hospital Morales Meseguer 2pl. Av. Marqués de los Vélez s/n, University of Murcia, 30008 Murcia, Spain

* Correspondence: fcojavier@um.es

Abstract: The purpose of this study was to evaluate the diffusion capacity and the biological effects of different bleaching products on human dental pulp stem cells (*h*DPSCs). The bleaching gel was applied for 90, 30 or 15 min to enamel/dentine discs that adapted in an artificial chamber. The diffusion of hydrogen peroxide (HP) was analysed by fluorometry and the diffusion products were applied to *h*DPSCs. Cell viability, cell migration and cell morphology assays were performed using the eluates of diffusion products. Finally, cell apoptosis and the expression of mesenchymal stem cell markers were analysed by flow cytometry. Statistical analysis was performed using analysis of variance and Kruskal–Wallis or Mann–Whitney tests ($\alpha < 0.05$). Significant reductions of approximately 95% in cell viability were observed for the 3×15 min groups ($p < 0.001$), while 1×30 min of PerfectBleach and 1×90 min of PolaNight resulted in reductions of 50% and 60% in cell viability, respectively ($p < 0.001$). Similar results were obtained in the migration assay. Moreover, the 3×15 min group was associated with cell morphology alterations and reductions of >70% in cell live. Finally, *h*DPSCs maintained their mesenchymal phenotype in all conditions. Similar concentrations of carbamide peroxide (CP) and HP in different commercial products exhibited different biological effects on hDPSCs.

Keywords: bleaching products; diffusion; cytotoxicity; dental pulp; stem cells

1. Introduction

The first study examining the chemical mechanism of hydrogen peroxide (HP) when coming into contact with enamel was published in 1970, which demonstrated that HP reached the dentin structure to produce a whitening effect [1]. The permeability of hard dental tissues and the low molecular weight of HP explain HP diffusion [2,3]. The bleaching process occurs when the low molecular weight of HP diffuses through enamel and dentin as it releases reactive oxygen species (ROS) that react with other free or weakly bound substances before regaining molecular stability. This oxidant phenomenon may explain the complex mechanism of dental bleaching [4]. The presence of oxidising agents and the penetration capacity of HP are closely correlated with each other [5].

HP reaches the pulp chamber via the dentinal tubules, decreases cell metabolism and viability [6,7] and induces vascular permeability changes [8], DNA modifications and pulpal necrosis [9–12].

Dental pulp is a loose connective tissue that occupies the pulp chamber of the tooth, which originates from the embryonic dental papilla (ectomesenchymal tissue) [13]. It has a high capacity for repair since it exhibits a significant regenerative response in reaction to injury or trauma, which causes the secretion of tertiary dentine and promotion of the differentiation of dental pulp stem cells (*h*DPSCs) into odontoblast-like cells. In addition, *h*DPSCs are able to differentiate toward osteogenic, myogenic and adipogenic lineages, melanocytes, Schwann cells and neurons [14].

Previous studies have analysed the biocompatibility of several bleaching agents, although there are fewer investigations studying specific commercial products and the effect of different times of applications [15–19]. Furthermore, the different compositions of commercial bleaching products are often unknown and commercial bleaching products have provided differing results for their biocompatibility in vitro and in vivo.

Cell cultures are suitable for evaluating the effects of different dental products and materials on pulp tissues [20] and the biological response of human pulp cells to these products and materials. The results of these in vitro studies are not directly comparable to those in humans, but these studies provide a good model with which to analyse different products and techniques and their potential risks [21].

The literature has questioned whether the use of bleaching products with a high concentration of HP is necessary or even safe. However, these products have been applied and reapplied multiple times in the same clinical session in order to increase the speed of changing the colour of the teeth. Although the whitening effect is known to be related to the diffusion of peroxide through the dental tissues, studies suggest that the bleaching effect is not related to the constant reapplication of the gel because good results have been obtained with the technique of a single clinical application [22]. Thus, this finding might support the adoption of a new dosage that is based on a single application of the bleaching product. Thus, given that high concentrations of peroxide are potentially harmful to the pulp cells [7,23], a focus on the posology that is guided by the adoption of milder protocols is both appealing and justifiable in an effort to find safe alternatives to bleaching.

In addition to the discrepancy in the clinical application protocols, the diffusion of and pulp damage caused by different commercial products with similar HP concentrations is still not clear.

The present study evaluated the diffusion capacity and cytotoxicity of different high-concentration commercial bleaching products and different application protocols in vitro. The null hypothesis was that different commercial bleaching products with equal or similar concentrations of HP would not promote different responses in dental pulp stem cells. This study was conducted in order to determine if other substances contained in the product are responsible for the cytotoxicity of the commercial bleaching product.

There are no studies that have determined the toxicity of the excipients contained in different commercial bleaching products with equal or similar HP concentrations.

2. Materials and Methods

2.1. Specimen Selection and Preparation

We selected freshly impacted mandibular third molars ($n = 25$) from patients aged 18 to 35 years to obtain a homogeneous sample. Selected teeth were not subjected to the oral environment, occlusal loads or other functional aggressions. The study was approved by the Ethics Committee of the University of València (registration number H1443515306255).

Organic remains were removed from the teeth and the integrity of the dental structure was confirmed. Selected teeth were immersed in a 0.1% thymol solution and preserved at 4 °C for 48 h. Teeth were removed from the thymol solution and immersed in deionized water at 4 °C until use.

Twenty-five samples that contained 2 mm of enamel and 2 mm of dentin were prepared as follows. Each tooth was cut mesio-distally with a diamond disk mounted on a hand piece with water-cooling. Roots were discarded. The dentin surface was reduced with 400- and 600-grit silicon carbide paper Sof-lex™ discs (3M Dental Products, St. Paul, MN, USA) until the dentin thickness was 2 mm. The sample dimensions were in the range of 0.5–0.7 cm × 0.4–0.6 cm. The dentin surface was treated with 0.5 M ethylene diamine tetra-acetic acid (EDTA) at a pH of 7.4 for 30 s, which was subsequently rinsed with deionized water to remove the smear layer and stored in deionized water at 4 °C until use.

An artificial pulp chamber was prepared with heavy silicone (Panasil R Putty, Kettenbach, Huntington Beach, CA, USA) with a capacity of 100 µL. To stabilize the sample, a heavy silicone ring was fabricated to anchor the sample, which allowed the dentin to be in contact with the buffer and had an upper window for placing the study gel (Scheme 1). This ring fit perfectly in the artificial pulp chamber, which maintained the fixation of the sample, while additional sealing was performed between the sample and the ring by using wax.

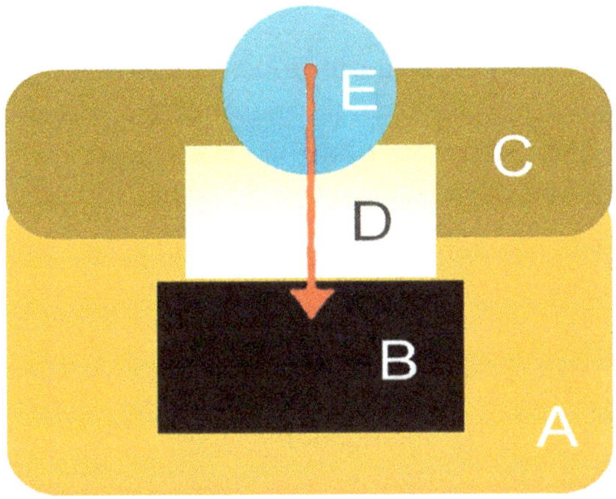

Scheme 1. Schematic representation of the artificial pulp chamber. Heavy silicone (A,C) was utilized to stabilize the sample (D), maintain the buffer (B) and prepare the artificial pulp chamber.

2.2. *Diffusion Evaluation*

The experimental specimens were randomized into five different groups ($n = 5$ each): group 1 was exposed to a neutral pH gel of 37.5% HP -Pola Office + (PO)- (SDI, Bayswater, VIC, Australia) for 30 min (PO30); group 2 was exposed to the same product as group 1 but with 3 applications of 15 min (PO3x15); group 3 was exposed to neutral pH gel of 35% HP -PerfectBleach (PB)- (Voco, Cuxhaven, Germany) for 30 min (PB30); group 4 was exposed to the same product as group 3 but with 3 applications of 15 min (PB3x15); and the group 5 was exposed to 16% carbamide peroxide (CP) -PolaNight (PN)- (SDI) for 90 min (PN90).

The diffusion of HP from different bleaching products was analysed using fluorimetry. The production of a homovanillic acid dimer from a reaction catalysed by peroxidase using HP as a substrate was measured as described by Barja [24]. Samples that had reacted with the peroxidase were measured using a fluorimeter (model F-4500 fluorescence spectrophotometer, Hitachi, Japan). A standard fluorimetry signal curve of HP (H1009-100ML, Sigma-Aldrich, St. Louis, MO, USA) was generated. The same dilutions were measured in a Helios Alpha UV−vis spectrophotometer (Thermo Fisher Scientific Inc., Waltman, MA, USA). Therefore, the fluorimetry signal was related to the concentration of the fluorescent dimer.

Phosphate-buffered saline (PBS; 400 µL) was placed in the buffer in the reservoir. Gel (0.5 µL) was applied to the external enamel surface and the film was coated (Parafilm M, Sigma-Aldrich, St. Louis, MO, USA). The HP in the PO15 and PB15 groups was replaced every 15 min without removal of the PBS from the reservoir. The HP remained for 30 min in the PO30 and PB30 groups and 90 min in the

PN90 group. The PBS containing the diffused HP from the reservoir was removed. The bleaching agent application process was performed at 37 °C.

A volume of 100 μL of the sample containing the diffused HP was removed and added to 1400 μL of the reaction buffer. Glycine—EDTA buffer (500 μL) was added after 15 min. Fluorescence intensity was measured, before the concentration value was extrapolated from the standard curve from the controls.

2.3. *Biological Assays*

2.3.1. Isolation and Culture of hDPSCs

hDPSCs were isolated and characterised as described previously [25]. Human DPSCs (hDPSCs) were obtained from impacted third molars collected from healthy subjects ($n = 15$). Donors provided written informed consent according to the guidelines of the Ethics Committee of our Institution. Briefly, the pulp chamber was exposed after removal of the tooth and the pulp tissue was retrieved, thoroughly minced and digested by means of a collagenase I (3 mg/mL) and dispase II (4 mg/mL) buffer (Invitrogen, Karlsruhe, Germany) for 45 min at 37 °C. The cells were cultured with a-MEM (Minimum Essential Media) medium (Invitrogen), supplemented with 15% fetal bovine serum (FBS, Invitrogen), 100 mM L-ascorbic acid phosphate (Sigma-Aldrich, Steinheim, Germany) and antibiotics/antimycotics (Complete Culture Medium, CCM) before incubating at 37 °C in 5% CO_2. This study was performed using hDPSCs from 4th passage of the culture.

2.3.2. Characterisation Assay

The mesenchymal immunophenotype of cultured human DPSCs was analyzed by flow cytometry. Single cell suspensions obtained by culture trypsinization were labelled or surface markers with fluorochrome-conjugated antibodies: CD73 (clone AD2), CD90 (clone DG3), CD105 (clone 43A4E1), CD14 (clone TÜK4), CD20 (clone LT20.B4), CD34 (clone AC136) and CD45 (clone 5B1) (Human Mesenchymal (MSC) Stem Cell Phenotyping Cocktail, Miltenyi Biotec, Bergisch-Gladbach, Germany), following the recommendations of the International Society of Cellular Therapy (ISCT) [26]. Flow cytometry analyses were performed using a FACSCanto II flow cytometer (BD Biosciences, San José, CA, USA).

2.3.3. Conditioned Medium

Culture medium conditioned with the bleaching products (BPs) was obtained as described by Cavalcanti et al. [27] in compliance with the ISO 10993-12 [28] proceedings. Briefly, 100 μL of the sample containing the diffused HP was removed and was collected into aliquots, before dilutions of 1%, 0.5% and 0.25% were created using cell culture medium. The conditioned medium was filtered in a sterile environment immediately and was used for cell culture exposure.

2.3.4. Cell Viability Assay

The metabolic activity of hDPSCs growing in the presence of different bleaching extracts was evaluated using the MTT assay (MTT Cell Growth Kit, Chemicon, Rosemont, IL, USA). hDPSCs were initially loaded with 1×10^3 cells per well and a volume of 180 μL in 96-well plates. Cells were starved for 24 h in serum-free medium at 37 °C in a humidified 5% CO_2 atmosphere prior to testing. The serum-free medium was replaced with different material elutes. Cells cultured in α-MEM medium containing 10% FBS were the negative control. After 24, 48 and 72 h, MTT (1 mg/mL in CCM) was added after cell seeding and incubated for 4 h at 37 °C and 5% CO_2. The MTT insoluble formazan was then dissolved by means of dimethyl sulfoxide DMSO that was applied for 2–4 h at 37 °C. The optical density (OD) was measured against blank (DMSO) at a wavelength of 570 nm (Abs570) and a reference filter of 690 nm by an automatic microplate reader (ELx800; Bio-Tek Instruments, Winooski, VT, USA)

2.3.5. Cell Migration

To study the chemotactic effect of bleaching extracts, *h*DPSCs were seeded on 12-well plastic dishes and incubated in culture medium for 24 h until until a monolayer formed. A pipette tip was used to generate a cross-shaped scratch or "wound" and the cell debris was removed with PBS. Plated cells were incubated with various dilutions of the eluates up to 48 h to allow cell migration back into the wounded area. Images of the scratched areas were captured at 0, 24 and 48 h using a phase-contrast microscope (Nikon, Tokyo, Japan). Two images photomicrographs per well were takenat each indicated time. ImageJ software (NIH, Bethesda, MD, USA) was used to evaluate the wound closure area.

2.3.6. Cell Morphology in Presence of Extracts

hDPSCs were plated on the glass coverslips at a low density and cultured in culture medium containing different material extracts to investigate morphological changes. The cells were fixed with 4% paraformaldehyde in phosphate-buffered saline (PBS) for 20 min at 2537 °C, permeabilized with 0.25% Triton X-100 (Sigma-Aldrich, St. Louis, MO, USA) for 3 min, and washed 3 times with PBS. For staining filamentous actin (F-actin), cells were incubated with CruzFluor594-conjugated phalloidin (Santa Cruz Biotechnology, Dallas, TX, USA). Nuclei were counterstained with 4,6-diamidino-2-phenylindole dihydrochloride (DAPI; Sigma-Aldrich). Fluorescent images were obtained using a confocal microscopy (Zeiss, Oberkochen, Germany).

2.3.7. Analysis of the Expression of Mesenchymal Stem Cell Surface Markers on hDPSCs Exposed to Bleaching Products Using Flow Cytometry

The expression of mesenchymal stem cell surface molecules was analysed in cultures of *h*DPSCs in 2nd–4th passages using flow cytometry. Briefly, cells were seeded at a density of 3×10^4 cells/cm^2 in 48-well plates and treated with the different eluates for 72 h at 37 °C. Cells were detached using a 0.25% *w*/*v* trypsin-EDTA solution. This was then rinsed twice with PBS and incubated in the dark at 4 °C for 30 min with fluorescence-conjugated specific monoclonal antibodies for human CD73, CD90 and CD105 (MiltenyiBiotec, BergischGladbach, Germany), as recommended by the International Society of Cellular Therapy (ISCT), to confirm the mesenchymal phenotype of the cells (Dominici et al., 2006). The lack of expression of the hematopoietic markers CD14, CD20, CD34 and CD45 was also analysed. Non-specific fluorescence was measured using specific-isotype monoclonal antibodies. Cells were acquired using a BD FACS Canto flow cytometer (BD Biosciences) and analysed using Kaluza analysis software (Beckman Coulter, Inc., Brea, CA, USA).

2.3.8. Detection of Apoptosis and Necrosis Using Flow Cytometry (Annexin-V/7-AAD Staining)

*h*DPSCs were cultured in different bleaching extracts for 72 h, which was followed by double staining with PE-conjugated Annexin-V and 7-AAD (BD Biosciences, Pharmingen). Percentages of live (Annexin-V$^-$/7-AAD$^-$), early apoptotic (Annexin-V$^+$/7-AAD$^-$) or late apoptotic and necrotic cells (Annexin-V$^+$/7-AAD$^+$ and Annexin-V$^-$/7-AAD$^+$) were determined using flow cytometry, before the percentages of each population were calculated.

2.4. Statistical Analysis

Two independent experiments were performed for all protocols in this study. Data were compiled and subjected to Levene's test to verify the homogeneity of variance. Data data were compiled and subjected to one-way ANOVA and Tukey's test (* $p < 0.05$, ** $p < 0.01$ and *** $p < 0.001$.)

3. Results

3.1. HP/CP Diffusion

All bleached groups differed in HP diffusion. We created a 1:2 dilution of the productions of one application, while we created 1:4 dilutions of the products of 3 applications to obtain unsaturated measures of fluorometry. Our results demonstrated variation in the quantification of homovanillic dimer (HD) between bleaching products (Figure 1). Table 1 shows that HD concentrations with PN were lower than those with the other products despite the longer exposure time (90 min). Pola Office exhibited no differences with different numbers of applications. Perfect Bleach exhibited great diffusion with three applications.

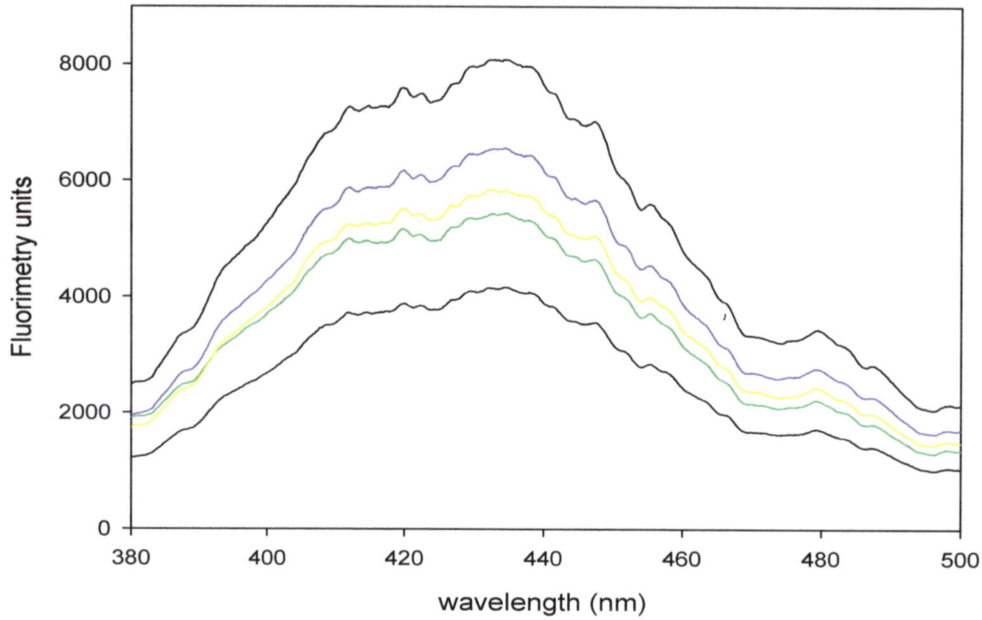

Figure 1. Fluorometric spectrum of samples of PO30 diluted 1:2 (black), PO3x15 diluted 1:4 (red), PB30 diluted 1:2 (green), PB3x15 diluted 1:4 (yellow) and PN90 diluted 1:2 (blue).

Table 1. Bleaching products diffusion.

Bleaching Products	Applications	Diffusion (mM)
Pola Office	1×30	38.4 ± 8.2
Pola Office	3×15	39.3 ± 1.2
Perfect Bleach	1×30	28.2 ± 6.5
Perfect Bleach	3×15	48.6 ± 1.7
Polanight	1×90	27.7 ± 0.4

3.2. Isolation and Characterisation of hDPSCs

Positive cell surface marker expression of the mesenchymal markers CD73, CD90 and CD105 and negative expression of the hematopoietic markers CD14, CD20, CD34 and CD45 were evaluated on *h*DPSCs using flow cytometry. More than 95% of viable *h*DPSCs were positive for the mesenchymal markers CD73, CD90 and CD105 and negative for the hematopoietic markers CD14, CD20, CD34 and CD45 (Figure 2).

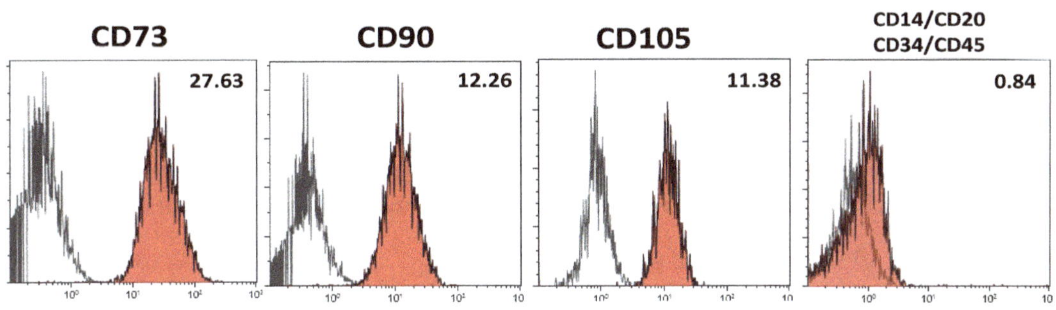

Figure 2. Immunophenotypic characterization of *h*DPSCs by flow cytometry for the expression of mesenchymal (CD73, CD90 and CD105) and hematopoietic (CD14, CD20, CD34 and CD45) stem cell (SC) markers (grey histogram: unstained control, red histogram: marker of interest). Results are means of triplicates of three independent experiments.

3.3. MTT Assays

MTT assays were performed to evaluate the effects of the eluates of different bleaching agents on *h*DPSC viability (Figure 3). The incubation of *h*DPSCs with 1% of each bleaching product yielded a significant reduction in cell viability rates compared with the control group at the indicated times (*** $p < 0.001$). In contrast, the 1%, 0.5% and 0.25% PB30 or PN allowed a slight but significant recovery of cell viability compared to PO30, PO3x15 or PB3x15 ($^{\Delta\Delta\Delta}$ $p < 0.001$). There was not difference in cell viability between 1 and 3 applications of the bleaching agents, except PO as there were significant differences in cell viability between 0.25% PO30 and PO3x15 (** $p < 0.01$). Our results revealed differences between bleaching agents with one application and PB30 produced better viability rates than PO30 and PN (*** $p < 0.001$).

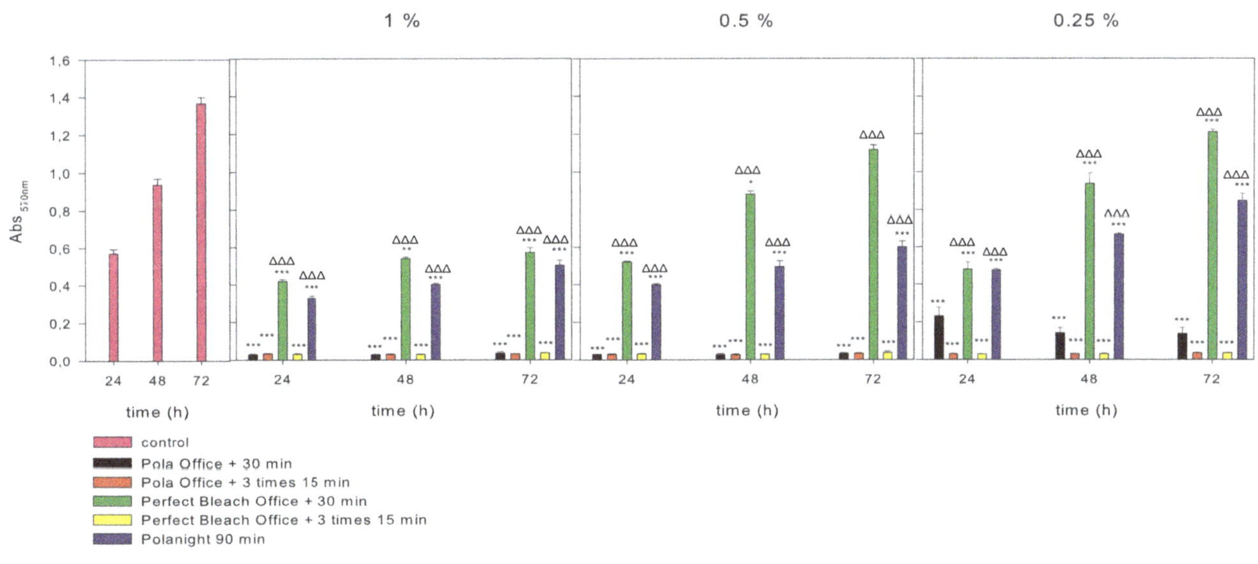

Figure 3. Cell viability was determined using the 3-(4,5-dimethyl-thiazol)-2,5-diphenyl-tetrazolium bromide (MTT) assay. The incubation of hDPSCs with 1% of each bleaching product revealed a significant reduction in cell viability rates compared with those in the control group at the indicated times of culture (*** $p < 0.001$). In contrast, a slight but significant recovery of cell viability was observed with 1%, 0.5% and 0.25% PB30 or PN compared to the others ($^{\Delta\Delta\Delta}$ $p < 0.001$).

3.4. Cell Migration

Compared to treatment with the complete medium (control), treatment with the different dilutions of PB3x15, PB30 and PO3x15 (except 0.25%) for 24 h induced a significantly lower cell migration rate

(** $p < 0.01$ and *** $p < 0.001$; Figure 4). Cell migration with PN and PO30 was still impaired but slightly higher at 24 h. Extracts of PO30 significantly promoted wound closure after 48 h of treatment and achieved comparable levels to control extracts. The PN group exhibited a slightly faster cell migration than the PB30 group, but both groups exhibited larger wound openings than the control group. Taken together, our results demonstrated that PO30 exerted a stronger effect on the migration ability of *h*DPSCs, while PN and PB30 produced values that were similar to those of the controls.

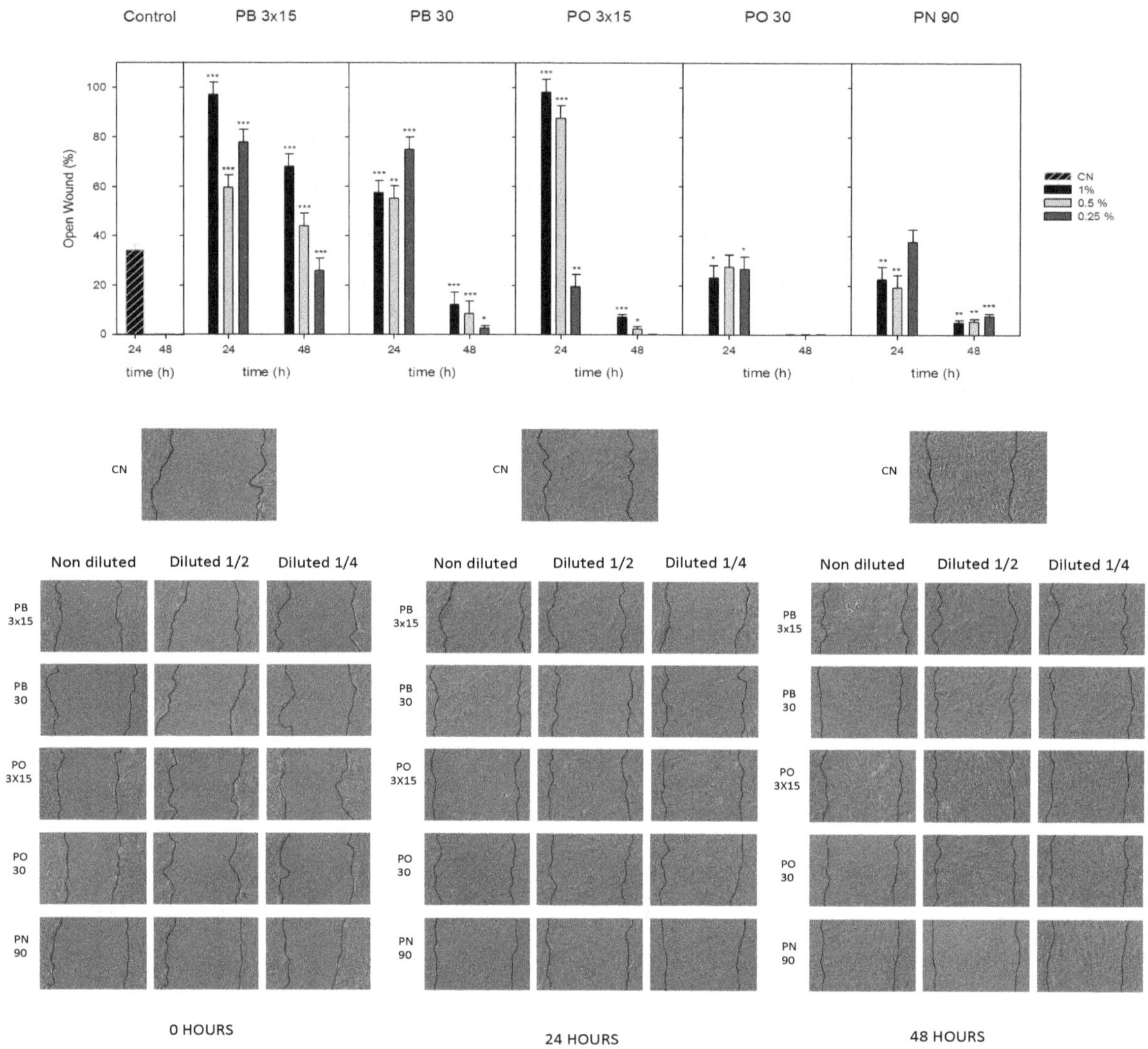

Figure 4. Wound-healing assay. Observation of wound closure change. Confluent hDPSCs were wounded and stimulated with bleaching extracts for up to 48 h. Cell migration is represented as the percentage of the open wound area under each condition compared with the control (* $p < 0.05$; ** $p < 0.01$; *** $p < 0.001$), which was analysed using one-way ANOVA.

3.5. Cell Morphology

The immunofluorescence assay was performed to detect changes in cellular morphology and cytoskeletal organisation of hDPSCs by phalloidin (red fluorescence) and DAPI (blue fluorescence). hDPSCs without bleaching extracts (control) showed a gradual increase in cell proliferation with fibroblastic morphology, a high expression of F-actin and confluency after 72 h of culture (Figure 5). Notably, treatment with extracts of PB3x15, PB30, PO3x15 and PO30 resulted in a small proportion of cells in both groups that lacked F-actin cytoskeleton staining and exhibited condensed or fragmented nuclei, which is typical of apoptotic cells. PN, especially at 0.25% and 0.5% concentrations, exhibited a similarly organised and stretched stress assembly of fibers compared with controls, which provides evidence for the optimal status of *h*DPSCs.

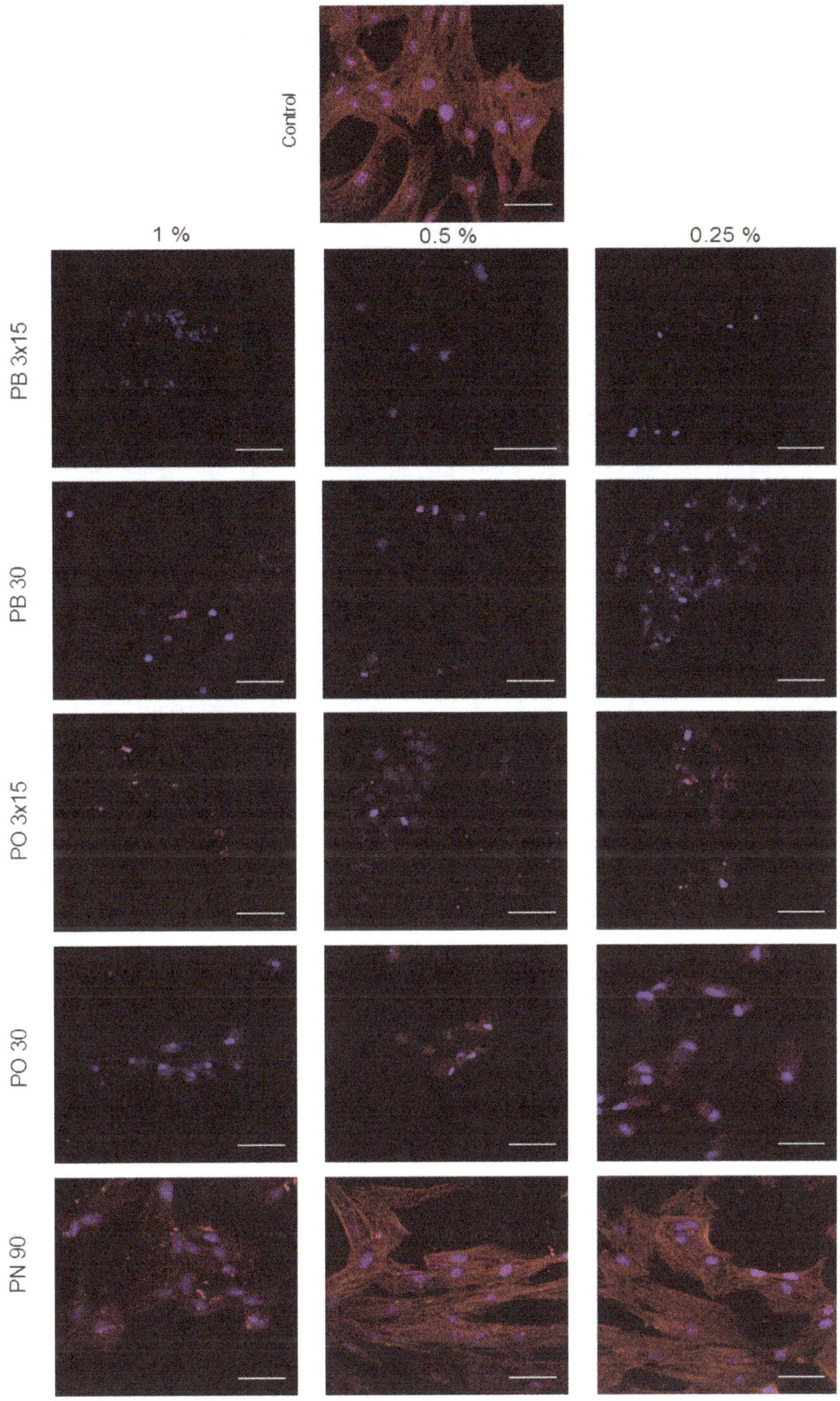

Figure 5. Representative immunofluorescence micrographs revealing the cytoskeletal organisation of *h*DPSCs exposed to control and bleaching products. Cultured *h*DPSCs were treated with undiluted extracts of bleaching products for 24 h. For staining filamentous actin (F-actin), cells were incubated with CruzFluor594-conjugated phalloidin (Santa Cruz Biotechnology, Dallas, TX, USA). Nuclei were counterstained with 4,6-diamidino-2-phenylindole dihydrochloride (DAPI) (blue). Scale bar = 150 μm.

3.6. Analysis of the Expression of Mesenchymal Stem Cell Surface Markers on hDPSCs Exposed to Bleaching Extracts Using Flow Cytometry

Flow cytometry studies were performed to determine possible phenotypic changes in viable *h*DPSCs after culture with the eluates of the different bleaching agents. MSC surface molecules CD73, CD90 and CD105 were expressed at levels greater than 95%, while the expression level of the hematopoietic markers CD14, CD20, CD34 and CD45 was lower than 5% (Figure 6). Notably, the incubation of *h*DPSCs with different dilutions of the extracts (1%, 0.5%, or 0.25%) did not significantly alter the percentage of positive expression of these mesenchymal markers compared to that in untreated *h*DPSCs (controls).

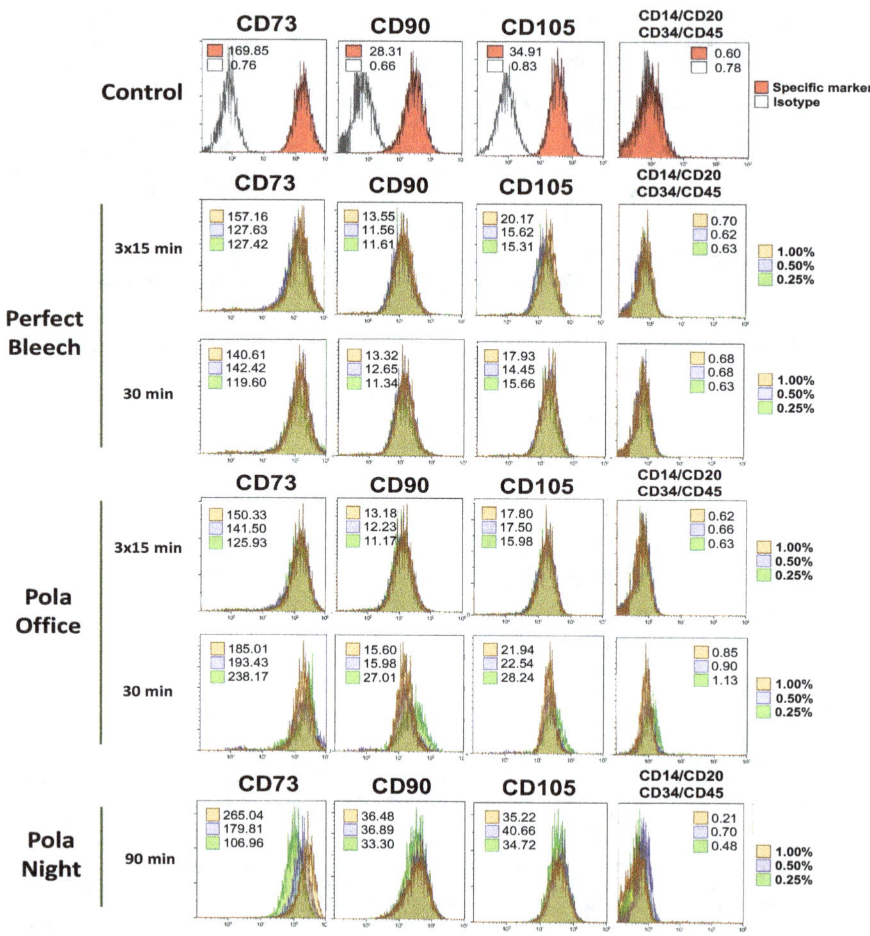

Figure 6. Mesenchymal phenotype analysis of *h*DPSCs after culture with bleaching products using flow cytometry. Cells were cultured for 72 h, detached and labelled with fluorescence-conjugated specific antibodies for the mesenchymal surface markers CD73, CD90 and CD105 and the hematopoietic markers CD14, CD20, CD34 and CD45. Inset numbers represent the mean fluorescence intensity values of viable cells. Histograms show representative flow cytometry results from three independent experiments.

3.7. Apoptosis/Necrosis of hDPSCs in the Presence of Bleaching Extracts

Figure 7 shows the representative 2D dot plots of the distribution of viable (Annexin-V^-/7-AAD^-), early apoptotic (Annexin-V^+/7-AAD^-) or late apoptotic/necrotic (Annexin-V^+/7-AAD^+ and Annexin-V^-/7-AAD^+) cells among the untreated *h*DPSCs (controls) or cells exposed to different dilutions of the bleaching extracts. The PN extract was associated with more than 90% of the cells remaining viable after 72 h. In contrast, the more concentrated eluates (1% and

0.5%) of the other bleaching agents decreased cell viability. This cytotoxic effect was minor in the most diluted extracts (0.25%).

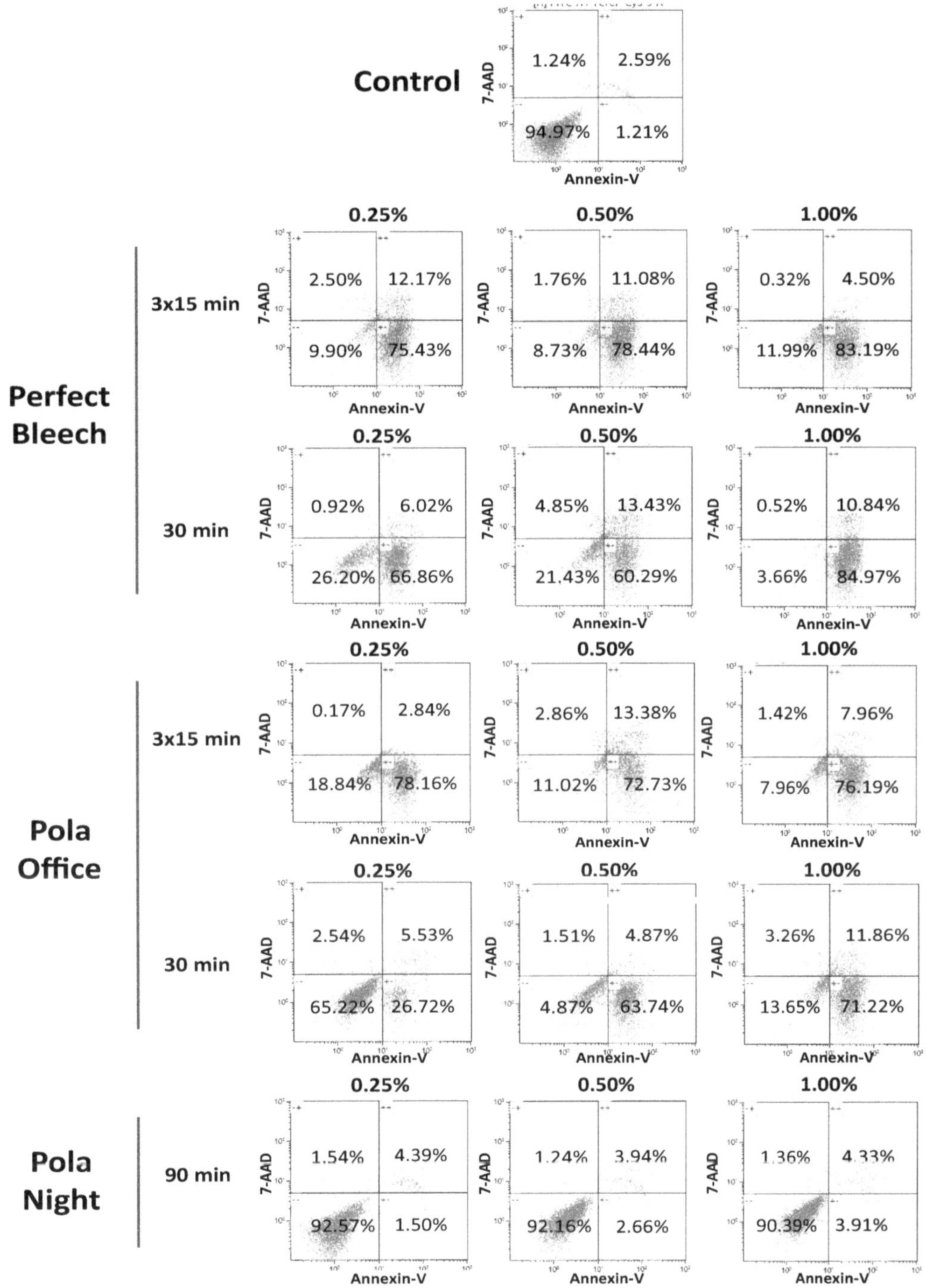

Figure 7. *h*DPSCs were cultured with bleaching extracts and plastic (control) for 72 h, before being labelled with Annexin-V and 7-AAD and analysed using flow cytometry. Numbers within the different quadrants represent the percentages of live (Annexin-V^-/7-AAD^-), early apoptotic (Annexin-V^+/7-AAD^-) or late apoptotic and necrotic (Annexin-V^+/7-AAD^+ and Annexin-V^-/7-AAD^+) cells. Dot-plots display representative flow cytometry results from three independent experiments. comma in the figure should be decimal point.

4. Discussion

To our knowledge, this is the first study to compare commercial bleaching products and their biological effects on stem cells from dental pulp. Little information on the diffusion capacity of commercial bleaching products and their effects on dental pulp tissue is available. Therefore, the present study quantified the diffusion of commercial bleaching products and their influence on the biological responses of hDPSCs.

The trans-enamel and trans-dentinal diffusion of bleaching products was based on a previously reported method [24], which is more sensitive than spectrophotometry. Our results demonstrated a higher diffusion of bleaching products after 3 applications. These results corroborate previous studies, which revealed that three applications of gels with greater HP concentrations produced greater diffusion of HP to the pulp chamber and increased damage to the dental pulp [11,12]. Therefore, the exposure time was less important than the number of applications. Our results demonstrated that PN (90 min) exhibited lower rates of diffusion than the other bleaching products. This is the less concentrated product as 16% CP is equivalent to 5–6% HP, but its diffusion was similar to that obtained with PB30.

Pulpal inflammation associated with local tissue necrosis was demonstrated in vivo by the application of high-concentration HP bleaching gels (35–38%) to human teeth [7,29]. hDPSCs are used as the cell line model to simulate clinical conditions because these cells play a major role in dental pulp inflammation and tooth hypersensitivity [25,30].

We analysed the biological cell responses of hDPSCs with respect to cell viability, cell migration, phenotype, apoptosis and morphology in the presence of three commercial bleaching products. The present investigation demonstrated that the PB3x15 and PO3x15 bleaching gel applications were cytotoxic to *h*DPSCs because cell viability was reduced. These results are clinically interesting because the number of applications may be involved with the occurrence of tooth sensitivity. In fact, Benetti et al. [31] demonstrated that major damage to rat dental pulp occurred after three applications of an HP gel, while de Oliveira et al. [6] also observed a significant reduction in cell viability following three applications of 10% HP gel for 15 min.

Previous studies demonstrated the healing of damaged pulp via the formation of a hard-tissue barrier or reparative dentine. The migration of pulp stem cells to substitute for irreversibly damaged odontoblasts after differentiation is an important step in this process [25]. In general, three applications of the bleaching gel produced lower cell migration than PN or PO30. However, we observed better cell migration in Pola Office groups than in Perfect bleach groups. Notably, Vaz et al. [32] reported that pulp inflammation was related to increased macrophage migration. These authors observed higher macrophage migration with in-office bleaching compared to at-home bleaching.

Optimising the state of dental pulp stem cells contributes to cell migration and dental pulp repair [21]. Immunofluorescence staining showed that undiluted extracts of cells treated with PN produced no morphological alterations and no changes in cytoskeletal organisation patterns compared to cells treated with the other bleaching products. Again, we observed better cell morphology in PO30 than PB30.

Analysis of the expression of mesenchymal stem cell markers is important in regenerative dentistry [33], which was performed in this study. The ISCT states that multipotent mesenchymal stromal cells must express CD105, CD73 and CD90 and should be devoid of the expression of hematopoietic markers, such as CD45, CD34, CD14 and CD11b [26]. We characterised the surface expression pattern of these markers using flow cytometry to evaluate possible changes in the expression. With commercial bleaching products, the MSC surface molecules CD73, CD90 and CD105 were expressed at levels greater than 95% following commercial bleaching, while the expression level of the hematopoietic markers CD34 and CD45 was less than 5%. Therefore, the bleaching products used in this study maintained the mesenchymal phenotype of hDPSCs.

Apoptosis plays an important role in the formation of reparative dentin by providing room for new dentin and preventing inflammation. Apoptosis also leads to the formation of mature dental pulp when exposed to extraneous stimuli [34]. Our results revealed that PN did not induce apoptosis, which is consistent with the results from Benneti et al. [31] as they demonstrated that the effects on pulp tissue varied with the HP concentration. These authors observed that higher HP concentrations produced pulp necrosis and had a prolonged effect on the apoptotic process, while lower HP concentrations induced moderate inflammation, cell proliferation and apoptosis. Nevertheless, in the present study, also in the apoptosis experiment, bleaching products with 35% HP concentration were more cytotoxic than 37% HP and caused membrane permeability-related apoptosis and necrosis. Thus, this effect is more dependent on the commercial product than on the composition.

5. Conclusions

In general, a low concentration of bleaching products, such as PN applied for 90 min, was less cytotoxic than other commercial bleaching products with 35–37.5% HP concentration. This effect occurred independently of the application protocol. For high concentration products, bleaching products with 35% HP concentration were more cytotoxic than 37% HP, which suggests that unknown agents in bleaching products could play an important role in determining their level of toxicity.

Author Contributions: C.L., M.C.-G., C.J.T.-C., D.G.-B., R.O.-S., F.J.R.-L., and L.F. conceived of and designed the experiments; M.C.-G., C.J.T.-C., and D.G.-B. performed the experiments; C.L. and F.J.R.-L. analysed the data; R.O.-S., F.J.R.-L., D.G.-B., and L.F. contributed materials/analysis tools; C.L., F.J.R.-L., and L.F. wrote the manuscript.

References

1. Cohen, S.C. Human pulpal response to bleaching procedures on vital teeth. *J. Endod.* **1979**, *5*, 134–138. [CrossRef]
2. Pugh, G., Jr.; Zaidel, L.; Lin, N.; Stranick, M.; Bagley, D. High levels of hydrogen peroxide in overnight tooth-whitening formulas: Effects on enamel and pulp. *J. Esthet. Restor. Dent.* **2005**, *17*, 40–45, discussion 46–47. [PubMed]
3. Kwon, S.R.; Li, Y.; Oyoyo, U.; Aprecio, R.M. Dynamic model of hydrogen peroxide diffusion kinetics into the pulp cavity. *J. Contemp. Dent. Pract.* **2012**, *13*, 440–445. [PubMed]
4. Azer, S.S.; Machado, C.; Sanchez, E.; Rashid, R. Effect of home bleaching systems on enamel nanohardness and elastic modulus. *J. Dent.* **2009**, *37*, 185–190. [CrossRef] [PubMed]
5. Sulieman, M. An overview of bleaching techniques: I. History, chemistry, safety and legal aspects. *Dent. Update* **2004**, *31*, 608–610, 612–604, 616. [CrossRef] [PubMed]
6. De Oliveira Duque, C.C.; Soares, D.G.; Basso, F.G.; Hebling, J.; de Souza Costa, C.A. Influence of enamel/dentin thickness on the toxic and esthetic effects of experimental in-office bleaching protocols. *Clin. Oral Investig.* **2017**, *21*, 2509–2520. [CrossRef] [PubMed]
7. Soares, D.G.; Basso, F.G.; Hebling, J.; de Souza Costa, C.A. Immediate and late analysis of dental pulp stem cells viability after indirect exposition to alternative in-office bleaching strategies. *Clin. Oral Investig.* **2015**, *19*, 1013–1020. [CrossRef] [PubMed]
8. Ferreira, V.G.; Nabeshima, C.K.; Marques, M.M.; Paris, A.F.; Gioso, M.A.; dos Reis, R.S.; Machado, M.E. Tooth bleaching induces changes in the vascular permeability of rat incisor pulps. *Am. J. Dent.* **2013**, *26*, 298–300. [PubMed]
9. Lima, A.F.; Marques, M.R.; Soares, D.G.; Hebling, J.; Marchi, G.M.; de Souza Costa, C.A. Antioxidant therapy enhances pulpal healing in bleached teeth. *Restor. Dent. Endod.* **2016**, *41*, 44–54. [CrossRef] [PubMed]
10. Costa, C.A.; Riehl, H.; Kina, J.F.; Sacono, N.T.; Hebling, J. Human pulp responses to in-office tooth bleaching. *Oral Surg. Oral Med. Oral Pathol. Oral Radiol. Endod.* **2010**, *109*, e59–e64. [CrossRef] [PubMed]

11. Cintra, L.T.A.; Ferreira, L.L.; Benetti, F.; Gastelum, A.A.; Gomes-Filho, J.E.; Ervolino, E.; Briso, A.L.F. The effect of dental bleaching on pulpal tissue response in a diabetic animal model. *Int. Endod. J.* **2017**, *50*, 790–798. [CrossRef] [PubMed]
12. Ferreira, L.L.; Gomes-Filho, J.E.; Benetti, F.; Carminatti, M.; Ervolino, E.; Briso, A.L.F.; Cintra, L.T.A. The effect of dental bleaching on pulpal tissue response in a diabetic animal model: A study of immunoregulatory cytokines. *Int. Endod. J.* **2018**, *51*, 347–356. [CrossRef] [PubMed]
13. Rodríguez-Lozano, F.J.; Insausti, C.L.; Iniesta, F.; Blanquer, M.; Ramírez, M.D.; Meseguer, L.; Meseguer-Henarejos, A.B.; Marín, N.; Martínez, S.; Moraleda, J.M. Mesenchymal dental stem cells in regenerative dentistry. *Med. Oral Patol. Oral Cir. Bucal* **2012**, *17*, e1062–e1067. [CrossRef] [PubMed]
14. Pisciotta, A.; Bertoni, L.; Riccio, M.; Mapelli, J.; Bigiani, A.; La Noce, M.; Orciani, M.; de Pol, A.; Carnevale, G. Use of a 3D Floating Sphere Culture System to Maintain the Neural Crest-Related Properties of Human Dental Pulp Stem Cells. *Front. Physiol.* **2018**, *9*, 547. [CrossRef] [PubMed]
15. Cintra, L.T.; Benetti, F.; Ferreira, L.L.; Rahal, V.; Ervolino, E.; Jacinto Rde, C.; Gomes Filho, J.E.; Briso, A.L. Evaluation of an experimental rat model for comparative studies of bleaching agents. *J. Appl. Oral Sci.* **2016**, *24*, 171–180. [CrossRef] [PubMed]
16. De Almeida, L.C.; Soares, D.G.; Gallinari, M.O.; de Souza Costa, C.A.; Dos Santos, P.H.; Briso, A.L. Color alteration, hydrogen peroxide diffusion, and cytotoxicity caused by in-office bleaching protocols. *Clin. Oral Investig.* **2015**, *19*, 673–680. [CrossRef] [PubMed]
17. Dias Ribeiro, A.P.; Sacono, N.T.; Lessa, F.C.; Nogueira, I.; Coldebella, C.R.; Hebling, J.; de Souza Costa, C.A. Cytotoxic effect of a 35% hydrogen peroxide bleaching gel on odontoblast-like mdpc-23 cells. *Oral Surg. Oral Med. Oral Pathol. Oral Radiol. Endod.* **2009**, *108*, 458–464. [CrossRef] [PubMed]
18. Hanks, C.T.; Fat, J.C.; Wataha, J.C.; Corcoran, J.F. Cytotoxicity and dentin permeability of carbamide peroxide and hydrogen peroxide vital bleaching materials, in vitro. *J. Dent. Res.* **1993**, *72*, 931–938. [CrossRef] [PubMed]
19. Kinomoto, Y.; Carnes, D.L., Jr.; Ebisu, S. Cytotoxicity of intracanal bleaching agents on periodontal ligament cells in vitro. *J. Endod.* **2001**, *27*, 574–577. [CrossRef] [PubMed]
20. Peters, O.A. Research that matters—Biocompatibility and cytotoxicity screening. *Int. Endod. J.* **2013**, *46*, 195–197. [CrossRef] [PubMed]
21. Tomas-Catala, C.J.; Collado-Gonzalez, M.; Garcia-Bernal, D.; Onate-Sanchez, R.E.; Forner, L.; Llena, C.; Lozano, A.; Moraleda, J.M.; Rodriguez-Lozano, F.J. Biocompatibility of new pulp-capping materials neomta plus, mta repair hp, and biodentine on human dental pulp stem cells. *J. Endod.* **2018**, *44*, 126–132. [CrossRef] [PubMed]
22. Marson, F.C.; Sensi, L.G.; Vieira, L.C.; Araujo, E. Clinical evaluation of in-office dental bleaching treatments with and without the use of light-activation sources. *Oper. Dent.* **2008**, *33*, 15–22. [CrossRef] [PubMed]
23. Soares, D.G.; Ribeiro, A.P.; Lima, A.F.; Sacono, N.T.; Hebling, J.; de Souza Costa, C.A. Effect of fluoride-treated enamel on indirect cytotoxicity of a 16% carbamide peroxide bleaching gel to pulp cells. *Braz. Dent. J.* **2013**, *24*, 121–127. [CrossRef] [PubMed]
24. Barja, G. The quantitative measurement of H_2O_2 generation in isolated mitochondria. *J. Bioenerg. Biomembr.* **2002**, *34*, 227–233. [CrossRef] [PubMed]
25. Collado-Gonzalez, M.; Pecci-Lloret, M.R.; Tomas-Catala, C.J.; Garcia-Bernal, D.; Onate-Sanchez, R.E.; Llena, C.; Forner, L.; Rosa, V.; Rodriguez-Lozano, F.J. Thermo-setting glass ionomer cements promote variable biological responses of human dental pulp stem cells. *Dent. Mater.* **2018**, *34*, 932–943. [CrossRef] [PubMed]
26. Dominici, M.; Le Blanc, K.; Mueller, I.; Slaper-Cortenbach, I.; Marini, F.; Krause, D.; Deans, R.; Keating, A.; Prockop, D.; Horwitz, E. Minimal criteria for defining multipotent mesenchymal stromal cells. The international society for cellular therapy position statement. *Cytotherapy* **2006**, *8*, 315–317. [CrossRef] [PubMed]
27. Cavalcanti, B.N.; Rode, S.M.; Marques, M.M. Cytotoxicity of substances leached or dissolved from pulp capping materials. *Int. Endod. J.* **2005**, *38*, 505–509. [CrossRef] [PubMed]
28. International Organization for Standardization. *10993-12. Biological evaluation of Medical Devices—Part 12: Sample Preparation and Reference Materials*; International Organization for Standardization: Geneva, Switzerland, 2007.

29. De Almeida, L.C.; Soares, D.G.; Azevedo, F.A.; Gallinari Mde, O.; Costa, C.A.; dos Santos, P.H.; Briso, A.L. At-home bleaching: Color alteration, hydrogen peroxide diffusion and cytotoxicity. *Braz. Dent. J.* **2015**, *26*, 378–383. [CrossRef] [PubMed]
30. Jha, N.; Ryu, J.J.; Choi, E.H.; Kaushik, N.K. Generation and role of reactive oxygen and nitrogen species induced by plasma, lasers, chemical agents, and other systems in dentistry. *Oxid. Med. Cell. Longev.* **2017**, *2017*, 7542540. [CrossRef] [PubMed]
31. Benetti, F.; Gomes-Filho, J.E.; Ferreira, L.L.; Ervolino, E.; Briso, A.L.F.; Sivieri-Araujo, G.; Dezan-Junior, E.; Cintra, L.T.A. Hydrogen peroxide induces cell proliferation and apoptosis in pulp of rats after dental bleaching in vivo: Effects of the dental bleaching in pulp. *Arch. Oral Biol.* **2017**, *81*, 103–109. [CrossRef] [PubMed]
32. Vaz, M.M.; Lopes, L.G.; Cardoso, P.C.; Souza, J.B.; Batista, A.C.; Costa, N.L.; Torres, E.M.; Estrela, C. Inflammatory response of human dental pulp to at-home and in-office tooth bleaching. *J. Appl. Oral Sci.* **2016**, *24*, 509–517. [CrossRef] [PubMed]
33. Rodríguez-Lozano, F.J.; Bueno, C.; Insausti, C.L.; Meseguer, L.; Ramírez, M.C.; Blanquer, M.; Marín, N.; Martínez, S.; Moraleda, J.M. Mesenchymal stem cells derived from dental tissues. *Int. Endod. J.* **2011**, *44*, 800–806. [CrossRef] [PubMed]
34. Wu, T.T.; Li, L.F.; Du, R.; Jiang, L.; Zhu, Y.Q. Hydrogen peroxide induces apoptosis in human dental pulp cells via caspase-9 dependent pathway. *J. Endod.* **2013**, *39*, 1151–1155. [CrossRef] [PubMed]

15

Effects of Ions-Releasing Restorative Materials on the Dentine Bonding Longevity of Modern Universal Adhesives after Load-Cycle and Prolonged Artificial Saliva Aging

Salvatore Sauro [1,2,*], Irina Makeeva [2], Vicente Faus-Matoses [3], Federico Foschi [2,4], Massimo Giovarruscio [2,4], Paula Maciel Pires [1,5], Maria Elisa Martins Moura [1,6], Aline Almeida Neves [5] and Vicente Faus-Llácer [3]

1 Departamento de Odontologia, Facultad de Ciencias de la Salud, Universidad CEU Cardenal Herrera, 46115 Valencia, SPAIN
2 Institute of Dentistry, I. M. Sechenov First Moscow State Medical University, 119146 Moscow, Russia; irina_makeeva@inbox.ru
3 Departamento de Estomatología, Facultad de Medicina y Odontología, Universitat de Valencia, 46010 Valencia, SPAIN; fausvj@uv.es (V.F.-M.); Vicente.J.Faus@uv.es (V.F.-L.)
4 Department of Restorative Dentistry, Faculty of Dentistry, Oral & Craniofacial Sciences at King's College London, Tower Wing, Guy's Hospital, Great Maze Pond, London SE1 9RT, UK; federico.foschi@kcl.ac.uk (F.F.); giovarruscio@me.com (M.G.)
5 Department of Pediatric Dentistry, Federal University of Rio de Janeiro, 21941-617 Rio de Janeiro, Brazil; paulinha_pmp@hotmail.com (P.M.P.); aline.neves@odonto.ufrj.br (A.A.N.)
6 Materiais Dentários, Universidade Federal do Ceará, Fortaleza, 60430-355 Ceará, Brazil; mariaelisa_martins@hotmail.com
* Correspondence: salvatore.sauro@uchceu.es

Abstract: This study aimed at evaluating the microtensile bond strength (MTBS) and fractographic features of dentine-bonded specimens created using universal adhesives applied in etch-and-rinse (ER) or self-etching (SE) mode in combination with modern ion-releasing resin-modified glass-ionomer cement (RMGIC)-based materials after load cycling and artificial saliva aging. Two universal adhesives (FTB: Futurabond M+, VOCO, Germany; SCU: Scotchbond Universal, 3M Oral Care, USA) were used. Composite build-ups were made with conventional nano-filled composite (AURA, SDI, Australia), conventional resin-modified glass ionomer cement (Ionolux VOCO, Germany), or a (RMGIC)-based composite (ACTIVA, Pulpdent, USA). The specimens were divided in three groups and immersed in deionized water for 24 h, load-cycled (350,000 cycles; 3 Hz; 70 N), or load-cycled and cut into matchsticks and finally immersed for 8 months in artificial saliva (AS). The specimens were cut into matchsticks and tested for microtensile bond strength. The results were analyzed statistically using three-way ANOVA and Fisher's LSD post hoc test ($p < 0.05$). Fractographic analysis was performed through stereomicroscope and FE-SEM. FTB showed no significant drop in bond strength after aging. Unlike the conventional composite, the two RMGIC-based materials caused no bond strength reduction in SCU after load-cycle aging and after prolonged aging (8 months). The SEM fractographic analysis showed severe degradation, especially with composite applied on dentine bonded with SCU in ER mode; such degradation was less evident with the two GIC-based materials. The dentine-bond longevity may be influenced by the composition rather than the mode of application (ER vs. SE) of the universal adhesives. Moreover, the choice of the restorative material may play an important role on the longevity of the finalrestoration. Indeed, bioactive GIC-based materials may contribute to maintain the bonding performance of simplified universal adhesives over time, especially when these bonding systems are applied in ER mode.

Keywords: adhesion; cycling mechanical stress; dentine; longevity; glass-ionomer cements; universal adhesives

1. Introduction

Direct restorations in modern operative dentistry are frequently accomplished using conventional resin composites due to their excellent mechanical and aesthetic properties [1,2]. Nevertheless, such restorative materials are still characterized by important downsides associated to polymerization shrinkage; a phenomenon that may induce stress at resin–dentine interfaces during the light-curing procedures and jeopardize their longevity [3–5]. Indeed, it has been widely demonstrated that the volumetric contraction of conventional resin composites can transfer polymerization stress directly to the adhesive-bonded interface, causing its innermost deformation due to a lack of proper bonding performance of some adhesive systems [3,6,7]. Consequently, the sealing between composite and dental hard tissues (i.e., dentine and enamel) can be seriously compromised. This will result in gaps and marginal leakage formation, which are pathways for microleakage of oral fluids, bacteria, and enzymes penetration [3,8–10]. Such issues may translate into important clinical problems such as post-operative sensitivity, marginal discoloration, recurrent caries, and advanced pulp pathology in all those cases that are seriously compromised by the caries process [11,12].

The recently introduced universal adhesive systems are currently very popular in general dental practices, as well as in dental hospitals, due to the fact that they can be applied both in self-etching (SE) and etch-and-rinse (ER) modes. Considering their compositions, universal adhesives can be also classified as simplified systems because all ingredients, including acidic functional monomers and solvents, are incorporated into one bottle. They are similar to one-step self-etching systems, so that they might still present issues related to bonding performance, degradation, and longevity [9,13]. However, application in self-etching mode minimizes recontamination of the dentine by blood and saliva during etch washing and drying. This makes SE a less technique-sensitive procedure compared to ER application mode. Moreover, SE systems present further benefits such as less post-operative sensitivity due to residual smear plugs, which are usually only partially removed from inside the dentinal tubules because of the mild acidic nature of SE systems. Indeed, the tubules remain occluded and the dentinal fluid movement is less evident compared to that usually experienced with ER systems [9,11].

On the other hand, great attention has been given to improve the effectiveness and longevity of resin–dentine bonds through several clinical strategies that may abate stress concentration at the resin–dentine interface during polymerization [14]. For instance, the use of flowable composites or resin-modified glass-ionomer cements (RMGIC) as liners or as dentine substitute materials may represent a suitable method to provide a sort of "stress-absorption" effect at the bonding interface [15,16]. This has been advocated to prevent stress development at the dentine-bonded interface and reduce gap formation, microleakage, and degradation over time [14,17,18]. Although RMGIC are self-adhesive materials, they are also often applied in dentine after etching and adhesive application, especially in those situations where the structure of the dental crown is highly compromised and a lack of mechanical retention is encountered [19–21].

It is also important to consider that occlusal stress during mastication, swallowing, as well as in cases of parafunctional habits, can affect the integrity of the bonding interface, making such a structure more susceptible to "quicker" degradation in the oral environment [22]. This seems to be of particular interest in modern, minimally invasive therapeutic restorative dentistry since it has been demonstrated that cyclic mechanical stress can promote gap formation at the margins along the composite restorations; bacteria penetration into narrow marginal gaps might ultimately promote secondary caries formation [23]. Recently, it has been advocated that ion-releasing resin-based restorative materials can reduce such biofilm penetration into marginal gaps of simulated tooth restorations; the risk for development and propagation of secondary caries is also reduced [24].

It is widely accepted that glass-ionomer cement (GIC)-based materials have a bioactive ability to release therapeutic ions such as fluoride. The presence of such ions has been associated with long-term caries inhibition when GIC-based materials are applied as a dentine substitute [25–27]. Moreover, GIC-based materials are an ideal dentine substitute as their physical properties, such as the coefficient of thermal expansion, dimensional stability, optical properties (i.e., opacity), and microhardness, are very close to that of dentine [28]. ACTIVA BioActive Restorative is a new type of restorative, bioactive, flowable, resin-based composite comparable to RMGICs. It contains fluoro-aluminum silicate particles and polyacid components of glass ionomer that undergo the acid-base setting reaction. Moreover, a bioactive ionic resin matrix is also contained in ACTIVA, which confers both light and chemical polymerization. According to the manufacturer, ACTIVA release calcium, phosphate, and fluoride when in contact with saliva. It has been advocated that restorative materials able to release specific "therapeutic" ions (e.g., calcium, phosphates, fluoride, strontium, and other minerals) into the dental hard tissues may buffer the constant assault of day-to-day ingestion of acidic food and beverages and encourage remineralization along the margins of the restoration with the tooth [29]. However, it is of great relevance that the use of ion-releasing materials in restorative dentistry may contribute to the reduced activity of proteases such as metalloproteinases (MMPs) and cathepsins involved in collagen degradation. Such enzymes are considered one of the main causes for reduction of bonding longevity when simplified bonding systems are applied in dentine with self-etching or etch-and-rinse protocols [30,31]. Moreover, there is a lack of knowledge about the effects of modern ion-releasing materials based on glass ionomer cements on resin–dentine interfaces created using current universal adhesives after mechanical load cycling and prolonged storage in artificial saliva.

Thus, the aim of this study was to evaluate, after short-term load-cycle aging or after load-cycle stress followed by prolonged aging (8 months) in artificial saliva (AS), the microtensile bond strength (MTBS) of resin–dentine bonded specimens created using universal adhesives applied in an etch-and-rinse or self-etching mode in combination with modern ion-releasing RMGIC-based materials. Fractographic analysis was also performed using field-emission scanning electron microscopy (FE-SEM).

The hypothesis tested was that compared to conventional resin composite, the use of modern ion-releasing materials would preserve the bonding performance of modern universal adhesives, applied in etch-and-rinse or self-etching, after mechanical load cycling and/or prolonged storage in artificial saliva (8 months).

2. Materials and Methods

2.1. Preparation of Dentine Specimens and Experimental Design

Sound human molars were extracted for periodontal or orthodontic reasons (ethical approval number: LEC № 11.18, 05/12/2018) and stored in distilled water at 5 °C for no longer than 3 months. The roots were removed 1 mm beneath the cemento–enamel junction using a diamond blade (XL 12205; Benetec, London, UK) mounted on a low-speed microtome (Remet evolution, REMET, Bologna, Italy). A second parallel cut was made to remove the occlusal enamel and expose mid-coronal dentine.

Three main groups (n = 72 specimens/group) were created based on the restorative materials used in this study: (i) RC: Resin composite (Aura SDI, Bayswater Victoria, Australia), applied in 2 mm increment layers up to 6 mm, and light-cured as per manufacturer's instructions; (ii) RMGIC: Resin-modified glass-ionomer cement (Ionolux; VOCO GmbH, Cuxhaven, Germany) mixed for 10 s in a trituration unit and applied in bulk. Two capsules of RMGIC were used and each one was light-cured as per manufacturer's instructions to obtain 6 mm build-ups; (iii) ACTIVA (ACTIVA BioActive Restorative, PULPDENT, Watertown, MA, USA) applied in 2 mm increment layers up to 6 mm and light-cured as per manufacturer's instructions. Light-curing was performed using an light-emitting diode (LED) light source (>1000 mW/cm^2) (Radii plus, SDI Ltd., Bayswater Victoria, Australia). The experimental design of this study required that the specimens in each main group were subsequently subdivided into four sub-groups (n = 18 specimens/group) based on the protocol employed for bonding procedures. Two modern universal adhesives were employed in this study: SCU (Scotchbond Universal, 3M Oral Care, St. Paul, MN, USA); FTB: (Futurabond M+, VOCO, Cuxhaven, Germany). These adhesives were applied as per manufacturer's instructions in self-etching (SE) or in etch-and-rinse (ER) mode (Table 1). In groups SCU–ER and FTB–ER, dentine was etched with 37% orthophosphoric acid for 15 s and subsequently rinsed with distilled water (15 s) and blotted, leaving the substrate moist. Adhesives were light-cured for 10 s. In groups SCU–SE and FTB–SE, the adhesives were applied with a microbrush for 20 s and air dried for 5 s to evaporate the solvent. These were finally light-cured for 10 s using am LED light source (>1000 mW/cm^2) (Radii plus, SID Ltd., Bayswater VIC, Australia). The specimens were finally restored with the selected restorative materials as aforementioned in the main groups. At this point, the specimens in each sub-group were furtherly divided into three groups (n = 6 specimens/group) based on the aging protocol: CTR: no aging (control, 24 h in deionized water); LC: Load cycling (350,000 cycles in artificial saliva); LC–AS: Load cycling (350,000 cycles in artificial saliva), followed by prolonged water storage (8 months in artificial saliva). A detailed description of the test groups can be found in Table 2 (Experimental design). The composition of the artificial saliva was AS: 0.103 g L^{-1} of $CaCl_2$, 0.019 g L^{-1} of $MgCl_2 \cdot 6H_2O$, 0.544 g L^{-1} of KH_2PO_4, 30 g L^{-1} of KCl, and 4.77 g L^{-1} HEPES (acid) buffer, pH 7.4] [32]. The specimens in the subgroup LC and LC–AS were mounted in plastic rings with acrylic resin for load cycle testing. A compressive load was applied to the flat surface (3 Hz; 70 N) using a 5 mm diameter spherical stainless-steel plunger attached to a cyclic-load machine (model S-MMT-250NB; Shimadzu, Tokyo, Japan) while immersed in AS [18,33].

Table 1. Adhesive system, composition, and application procedures.

Name	Composition	Application
Scotchbond Universal, 3M Oral Care, USA (lot: 627524)	10-MDP, HEMA, silane, dimethacrylate resins, Vitrebond™ copolymer, filler, ethanol, water, initiators, and catalysts (pH 2.7)	1. Apply the adhesive on the surface and rub it for 20 s. 2. Gently air-dry the adhesive for approximately 5 s for the solvent to evaporate. 3. Light cure for 10 s (>500 mW/cm^2).
FuturaBond M+, VOCO, Germany (lot: 1742551)	HEMA, BIS-GMA, ethanol, Acidic adhesive monomer (10-MDP), UDMA, catalyst ethanol, water, initiators, and catalysts (pH 2.8)	1. Apply the adhesive homogenously to the surface. 2. Rub for 20 s. 3. Dry off the adhesive layer with dry, oil-free air for at least 5 s. 4. Light cure for 10 s (>500 mW/cm^2).

Abbreviations: 10-MDP 10-methacryloxydecyl dihydrogen phosphate, Bis-GMA bisphenol A diglycidyl methacrylate, HEMA 2-hydroxyethyl methacrylate, UDMA urethane dimethacrylate.

2.2. *Micro-Tensile Bond Strength and Failure/Fractographic Analysis*

The specimens were cut after the aging period using a hard-tissue microtome (Remet evolution, REMET, Bologna, Italy) across the resin–dentine interface, obtaining approximately 15–18 matchstick-shaped specimens from each tooth (Ø 0.9 mm^2). These were submitted to microtensile bond strength tests using a device with a stroke length of 50 mm, peak force of 500 N, and a displacement resolution of 0.5 mm. Modes of failure were evaluated at 50× magnification using stereoscopic microscopy and conveyed in a percentage of adhesive (A), mixed (M), or cohesive (C) bonding fracture. Five representative fractured specimens from each sub-group were mounted on aluminum stubs with carbon glue after the critical-point drying process. The specimens were gold-sputter-coated and analyzed using field-emission scanning electron microscopy (FE-SEM S-4100; Hitachi, Wokingham, UK) at 10 kV and a working distance of 15 mm.

Bond strength values in MPa were initially assessed for normality distribution and variances homogeneity using Kolmogorov–Smirnov and Levene's tests, respectively. Data were then analyzed using a three-way Analysis of Variance (ANOVA Factors: restorative material, adhesive, and aging protocol) and Newman–Keuls multiple-comparison test ($\alpha = 0.05$). SPSS V16 for Windows (SPSS Inc., Chicago, IL, USA) was used.

Table 2. Experimental design. Distribution of specimens in groups and sub-groups for evaluation via microtensile bond strength (MTBS), interface confocal microscopy, and SEM fractographic analysis. CTR = control, no aging; LC = load-cycling; AS = artificial saliva.

Total Number of Specimens in Main Groups	**RESIN COMPOSITE (72 Specimens)**			**RMGIC (72 Specimens)**			**ACTIVA (72 Specimens)**		
Number of specimens in sub-groups (18/group)	Number of specimens in aging sub-groups (6/ group)								
SCU–ER: Scotchbond Etch and rinse	CTR 6 spec	LC 6 spec	LC+AS 6 spec	CTR 6 spec	LC 6 spec	LC+AS 6 spec	CTR 6 spec	LC 6 spec	LC+AS 6 spec
FTB–ER Futurabond M+ Etch and rinse	CTR 6 spec	LC 6 spec	LC+AS 6 spec	CTR 6 spec	LC 6 spec	LC+AS 6 spec	CTR 6 spec	LC 6 spec	LC+AS 6 spec
SCU–SE: Scotchbond Self-etch	CTR 6 spec	LC 6 spec	LC+AS 6 spec	CTR 6 spec	LC 6 spec	LC+AS 6 spec	CTR 6 spec	LC 6 spec	LC+AS 6 spec
FTB–SE: Futurabond M+ Self-etch	CTR 6 spec	LC 6 spec	LC+AS 6 spec	CTR 6 spec	LC 6 spec	LC+AS 6 spec	CTR 6 spec	LC 6 spec	LC+AS 6 spec

3. Results

Micro-Tensile Bond Strength (MTBS) and Failure Mode Analysis

There were no pre-test failures before the microtensile bond strength assessment. Three-way ANOVA revealed a significant effect of adhesive ($F = 28.75$, $p < 0.001$) and restorative material ($F = 6.68$, $p < 0.001$) on the bond strength, whereas the aging protocol was not statistically significant ($F = 8.17$; $p = 0.125$). The interactions between the three variables were significant ($p < 0.001$).

The results of the microtensile bond strength test (mean and $\pm$ SD) are depicted in Table 3. It was observed that there was no significant difference ($p > 0.05$) at 24 h testing between the two adhesives when applied in etch-and-rinse (ER) or self-etching (SE) mode and then restored using the conventional RC or the two RMGIC-based materials (IONOLUX and ACTIVA). Conversely, the specimens created with the conventional RMGIC presented no significant differences ($p > 0.05$) when bonded using the two adhesives applied in ER or SE mode. However, all the specimens created with the conventional RMGIC showed a significant lower bond strength compared to those created with RC or ACTIVA. The failure mode showed that all the specimens restored with the RMGIC failed mainly in the cohesive mode, leaving a clear presence of the material still bonded to the dentine. The specimens created with RC or ACTIVA failed mainly in the cohesive in composite and mixed mode, leaving part of the dentine still covered by the restorative material and the other part exposed.

The fractographic analysis showed that the restorative materials employed in this study had no influence on the outcomes in the control storage period (24 h), but all those specimens created with SCU in ER mode presented less resin infiltration within exposed acid-etched dentine collagen fibrils (Figure 1A,B), while the specimens bonded using the FTB applied in ER mode presented fractures mainly underneath the hybrid layer (Figure 1C). Moreover, in this latter case, there was mineralized peri-tubular dentine around the lumen of the dentine tubules and no demineralized and exposed collagen fibrils (Figure 1D). Conversely, all the specimens bonded with the two adhesives applied in SE or ER mode and then restored with RMGIC showed a surface still covered by the restorative material (cohesive mode within RMGIC) with no exposure of the dentine (Figure 1E,F) after microtensile bond strength testing. Furthermore, the fractographic analysis showed that the specimens created both with SCU (Figure 1F) and FTB (Figure 1G) applied in SE, and that failed in mixed or adhesive mode, presented a dentine surface still covered by a smear layer with no presence of collagen fibrils and/or exposed dentinal tubules (Figure 1I).

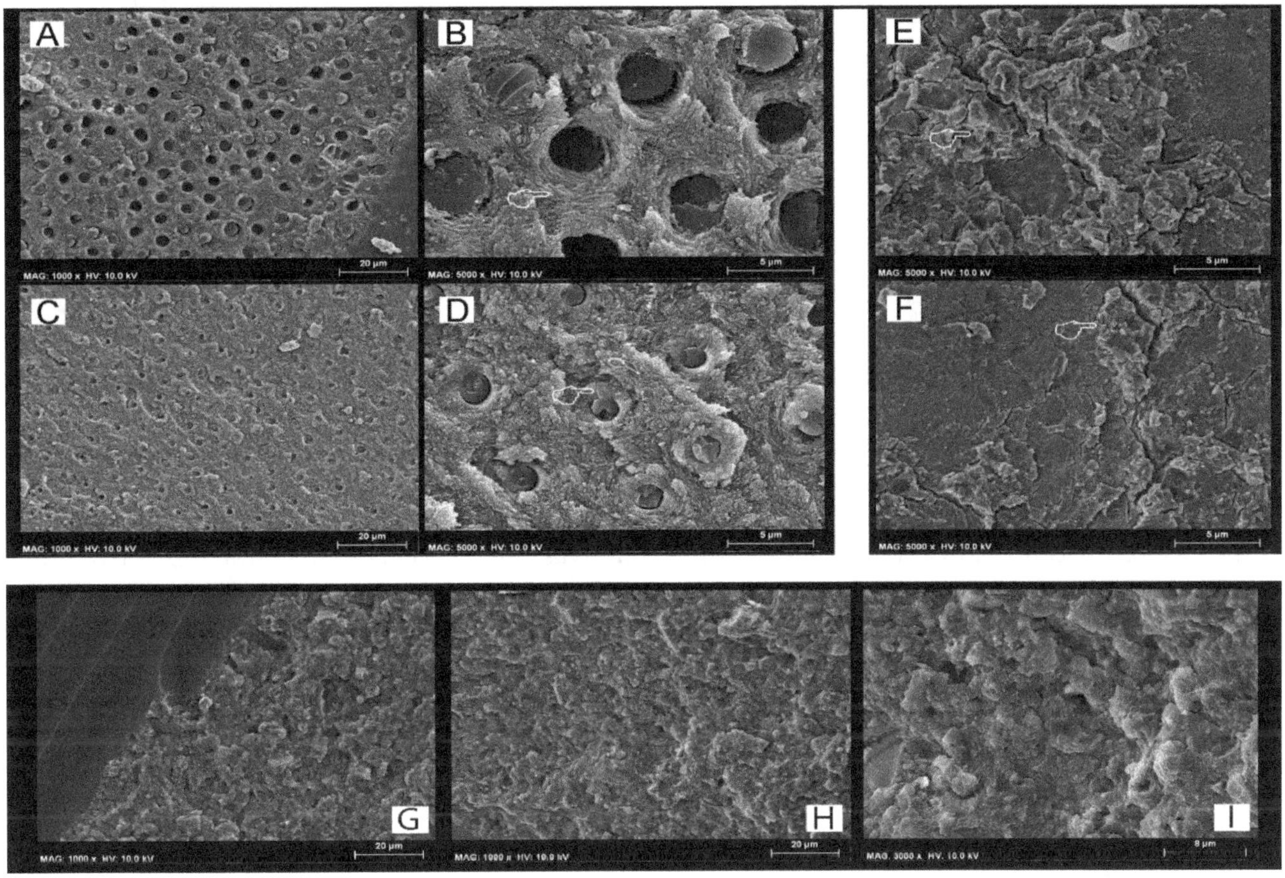

Figure 1. SEM fractographic analysis of the control specimens. (**A**) SEM fractography of a specimen created with SCU applied in ER mode and restored with resin composite (RC) showing the presence of exposed dentine and several resin tags still in the dentinal tubules. (**B**) At higher magnification, it is possible to note the presence of resin tags inside demineralized dentine tubules and collagen fibrils not well infiltrated by the SCU adhesive (pointer). This latter morphological characteristic may indicate that such resin–dentine interface would be affected by degradation over time and would drop in bond strength. (**C**) SEM fractography of a specimen created with FTB applied in ER mode and restored with ACTIVA showing the presence of exposed dentine and several resin tags still inside the small lumen of the dentinal tubules. (**D**) At higher magnification it is possible to observe a typical failure occurred at the bottom of the hybrid layer (HL) characterized by the presence of mineralized peritubular dentine (pointer), with tubules totally obliterated by resin tags and with no presence of demineralized exposed collagen fibrils. Conversely, the dentine specimens bonded with SCU (**E**) and FTB (**F**) applied in ER mode and restored with the RMGIC show the presence of the remaining RMGIC that totally covered the dentine surface. (**G**) SEM fractography of a specimen created with SCU applied in SE mode and restored with ACTIVA and (**H**) FTB applied in SE mode and restored with RC showing a characteristic failure in mixed mode. Note the presence of the remaining resin (**G**) and smear layer on the dentine surface; the latter was even more evident at higher magnification (**I**).

Table 3. The results show the mean (± SD) of the MTBS (MPa) to dentine and the percentage (%) of the failure mode analysis.

	RESIN COMPOSITE			RMGIC			ACTIVA		
	CTR	LC	LC+AS	CTR	LC	LC+AS	CTR	LC	LC+AS
SCU–ER: Scotchbond Etch and rinse	48.9 (7.6) A1 50/45/5	33.5 (5.6) B2 15/55/30	28.1 (5.7) B2 10/50/40	35.1 (7.1) B1 80/20/0	33.4 (7.8) B1 75/20/5	31.1 (8.8) B1 50/35/15	55.3 (6.1) A1 45/55/0	53.1 (7.1) A1 55/40/5	50.1 (6.8) A1 30/50/20
FTB–ER Futurabond M+ Etch and rinse	51.2 (5.9) A1 55/40/5	58.1 (7.3) A1 45/50/5	55.3 (6.5) A1 20/65/15	31.3 (6.7) B1 70/30/0	32.1 (6.6) B1 65/35/0	32.1 (7.1) B1 60/30/5	54.2 (5.7) A1 45/55/0	52.7 (6.2) A1 55/40/5	52.1 (5.6) A1 30/50/20
SCU–SE: Scotchbond Self-etch	45.1 (5.2) A1 45/50/5	44.4 (6.2) A1 40/50/10	34.1 (5.9) B1 10/55/35	32.3 (7.4) B1 70/30/0	34.4 (7.2) B1 65/30/5	29.6 (7.9) B1 50/45/5	46.1 (6.2) A1 40/55/5	49.8 (7.4) A1 30/65/5	49.5 (6.9) A1 45/50/5
FTB–SE: Futurabond M+ Self-etch	49.2 (4.9) A1 40/50/10	48.3 (9.3) A1 45/50/5	45.6 (7.5) A1 25/60/15	34.1 (6.2) B1 75/25/0	31.5 (7.7) B1 70/30/50	30.5 (7.5) B1 60/35/5	48.1 (6.2) A1 40/55/5	51.1 (7.4) A1 45/50/5	50.5 (7.4) A1 45/50/5

Failure mode [Cohesive/Mixed/Adhesive]. The same number indicates no significance in column, while the same letter indicates no significance in row ($p > 0.05$).

After submitting the specimens to load-cycle aging, the only group that showed a significant bond strength drop ($p < 0.05$) was that created with the SCU applied in ER mode and restored using the conventional RC. In this group, an important change in the failure mode was also observed; only 15% of the specimens failed in cohesive mode, while failure in mixed and adhesive modes were 55% and 30%, respectively (Table 3). This situation was not evident in the specimens bonded with the same adhesive but restored using IONOLUX (RMGIC) or ACTIVA; no significant bond strength drop ($p > 0.05$) and no radical change in failure mode was observed. The SEM fractography showed no important ultra-morphological changes in most of the fractured resin–dentine interfaces of these groups compared to the control group. Conversely, the specimens created with the SCU applied in ER mode (Figure 2A) and restored with the conventional RC, which failed prevalently in mixed and adhesive mode, showed that the fracture occurred underneath the hybrid layer with no sign of demineralized and/or poorly infiltrated collagen fibrils (Figure 2B,C).

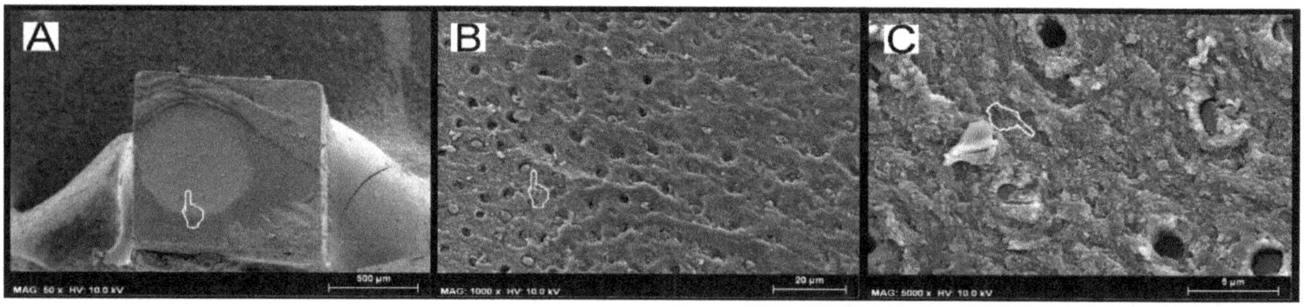

Figure 2. SEM Fractographic analysis after load-cycle aging. (**A**) SEM fractography of a specimen created with SCU applied in ER mode and restored with RC showing a characteristic failure in mixed mode. The finger pointer indicates a brighter area of greater and more evident aging (pointer), which was probably induced by the cycling load. However, when we observed that specific area at higher magnifications (**B**), it was possible to observe that the fracture occurred underneath the hybrid layer (pointer), which is characterized by the presence of mineralized dentine (pointer), with tubules totally obliterated by resin tags and with no presence of demineralized exposed collagen fibrils (**C**).

The prolonged aging in artificial saliva performed subsequent load-cycling stress induced important changes on microtensile bond strength as well as on the ultramorphology of the fracture of some specific groups. In particular, the specimens bonded with SCU applied both in ER and SE mode and then restored with the conventional composite had a significant drop in bond strength compared to the specimens in the groups CTR and LC ($p < 0.05$). Moreover, the number of failures in mixed and adhesive modes increased in the aforementioned groups compared to the control

(CTR) group. The SEM fractography showed evident signs of dentine degradation in the group of specimens created with SCU applied in ER mode and then restored with the conventional composite (Figure 3(A1,A2)). The SEM fractography showed that specimens created with SCU applied in SE mode and then restored with the RC presented degradation both of the adhesive (Figure 3B) and dentine hybrid layers (Figure 3C). Conversely, the same specimens restored with the RMGIC or ACTIVA presented a stable bond strength with no significant drop ($p < 0.05$), and the type of failure remained quite similar to the control group. The SEM fractography showed no drastic changes in all those groups for the ultramorphology of fractured resin–dentine interfaces compared to the control group (Figure 3D,E). In particular, the SEM fractography of a specimen created with SCU applied in ER mode and restored with ACTIVA and RMGIC showed the presence of dentine that was well mineralized with no sign of demineralized collagen fibrils, but with the presence of mineral debrides as a possible result of the bioactivity of such GIC-based materials (Figure 3D).

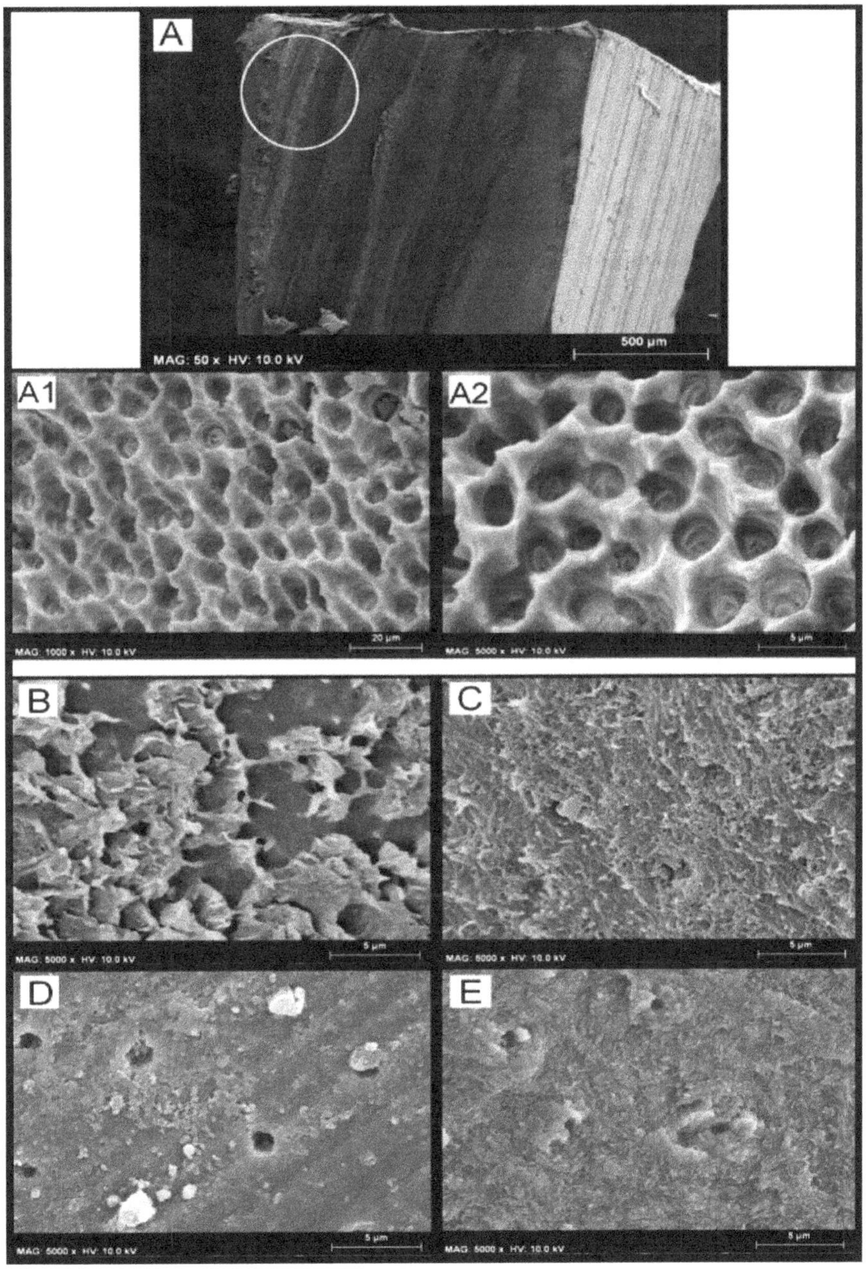

Figure 3. SEM Fractographic analysis after load cycling and aging in artificial saliva. (**A**) SEM fractography of a specimen created with SCU applied in ER mode and restored with RC showing

a characteristic failure in adhesive mode. Note that the white circle indicates no physical difference in the material; it was added to show the reader that images (**A1**,**A2**) were obtained by higher magnification in that zone. Indeed, in (**A1**,**A2**) it is possible to see severe collagen degradation without the presence of any resin residual. (**B**) SEM fractography of a specimen created with SCU applied in SE mode where it is possible to see a failure between composite and adhesive, probably due to degradation induced by excessive water sorption upon mechanical stress and prolonged AS storage. However, it was also possible to see, in those specimens that failed in mixed mode, signs of degradation of the collagen fibrils underneath the hybrid/interdiffusion layer (**C**). (**D**) SEM fractography of a specimen created with SCU applied in ER mode and restored with ACTIVA showing that the failure occurred underneath the hybrid layer, but the exposed dentine is well mineralized with no sign of exposed demineralized collagen fibrils. Note also the presence of mineral debrides that are a possible result of the bioactivity of ACTIVA, which released ions and diffused through the resin-bonded dentine. (**E**) SEM fractography of a specimen created with FTB applied in SE mode and restored with RMGIC. The specimens of this group failed mainly in cohesive and mixed mode; this latter zone is characterized by a fracture occurring underneath the hybrid layer, leaving behind a dentine surface completely mineralized with no sign of exposed, denatured, or demineralized collagen fibrils. Please note the presence of a well mineralized intratubular dentine inside the lumen of the dentine tubules.

4. Discussion

This study showed that the use of modern ion-releasing materials such as conventional RMGIC or RMGIC-based composite (ACTIVA) preserved the bonding performance of only one (SCU) of the two modern universal adhesives bonded to dentine in etch-and-rinse or self-etching mode, after the two aging protocols employed in the experimental design. Conversely, the dentine-bonded specimens created with the FTB universal bonding system applied in etch-and-rinse or self-etching showed no significant drop in bonding performance after aging, regardless the restorative material employed or the aging protocol. Hence, the hypothesis tested in this study needs to be partially accepted as the use of a specific new generation universal bonding systems may confer a stable dentine-bonded interface over time. Nevertheless, the use of modern ion-releasing restorative materials such as RMGIC or ACTIVA may preserve the bonding performance of those universal adhesives that are more prone to degradation after aging.

The effects of the load-cycle aging protocol on the bonding performance of the SCU system applied in ER mode and restored with the conventional RC were relevant; the bond strength of this group of specimens dropped significantly ($p < 0.05$). Moreover, only the specimens bonded using SCU applied both in ER and SE mode and then restored with the conventional composite showed a significant drop in bond strength compared to the specimens in the control (CTR, 24 h) group after prolonged aging in artificial saliva. The ultramorphology analysis performed in the specimens of the control group (24 h), created using the SCU system applied in ER mode and restored with RC showed the presence of demineralized-acid-etched dentine collagen that was not well resin-infiltrated (Figure 1A,B). While the same specimens submitted to LC aging showed no exposed collagen, but mineralized dentine with resin tags that obliterated the dentinal tubules (Figure 2). This was an interesting result, so we hypothesize that a possible explanation to the difference in bonding performance observed between these two latter situations (LC-only aging vs. CTR) may be attributed to the fact that the hybrid layer created using simplified adhesives applied in etch-and-rinse mode can represent the critical part of the resin–dentine interface, as it probably remains only partially polymerized [33–35]. Indeed, it has been advocated that during cycling loading such un-polymerized monomers within the hybrid layer, created with simplified, highly hydrophilic etch-and-rinse adhesives, may be mechanically "intruded" into the demineralized dentine causing a more compact and performant hybrid layer. However, such a morphological change within the resin–dentine interface may favor higher stress concentrations during the cycling load at the bottom of the hybrid layer, causing an accelerated mechanically-induced degradation phenomenon in this specific zone that often remains partially demineralized and poorly infiltrated by adhesive monomers [34,35]. Indeed, the absence of a proper, partially demineralized bottom of the hybrid layer may explain why the dentine bonded with SCU or FTB in SE mode showed no bond-strength drop after load-cycle aging, regardless of the restorative material and the protocol employed for aging [33,34]. Our results seem to be in accordance with those of Dorfer et al. [36] who demonstrated water diffusion within the resin–dentine interface and hybrid layer during flexure; this promoted chemical/mechanical degradation and washout of "poorly" polymerized water-soluble monomers.

Apparently, such type of degradation mentioned above was improbable in dentine etched with phosphoric acid and bonded using the same simplified adhesive (SCU), but restored with RMGIC or ACTIVA. Indeed, such restorative materials may have absorbed some of the stress generated by the load-cycle aging due to their lower modulus of elasticity, thereby reducing the risk for degradation at the bonding interface [14,15]. The fact that the two GIC-based materials with lower moduli of elasticity may have distributed stresses within their bulk structure lowering the tension concentration at the interface created with the SCU adhesive, applied both in ER and SE mode and subsequently submitted to a cycling load followed by prolonged storage in AS. This observation was supported by the absence of reduction in bonding performance compared to those specimens restored with the conventional composite; this latter group presented a significant bond strength drop ($p < 0.05$) after such a prolonged aging protocol. In addition to the significant bond strength reduction (Table 3), the results of this current study also showed the presence of funneled dentinal tubules, with no presence of collagen fibrils and no residual of restorative material on the dentine surface (Figure 1), which are all typical morphological signs that indicate collagen hydrolysis and proteolytic denaturation caused by the activity of proteases such as MMPs and cathepsins [34,35,37]. Conversely, the SCU adhesive applied in ER mode and restored with ACTIVA failed mainly in mixed mode or in cohesive/mixed mode when restored with the RMGIC. The SEM fractographic analysis highlighted in those specimens the presence of exposed dentine due to a fracture that occurred underneath the hybrid layer, which left behind a well mineralized dentine with no sign of collagen degradation. Indeed, in this latter case, mineralized peri-tubular dentine around the lumen of the dentine tubules and with no demineralized and exposed collagen fibrils was often observed; this is a typical ultramorphological aspect of failure occurring away from the hybrid layer in resin–dentine interface characterized by high bonding stability [37].

Furthermore, mineral debris were detected as a possible result of the bioactivity of ACTIVA and RMGIC (Figure 3D). Indeed, glass-ionomer materials are considered the main bioactive ion-releasing restorative materials currently available in clinics, since they may be able to induce mineral growth within the bonded-dentine interface [18]. We speculate that the results of this study may be somehow correlated to the those hypothesized by Toledano et al. [22,33], who showed that when bioactive materials are submitted to mechanical cycling load, they may promote diffusion of ions through the adhesive-bonded dentine due to the permeable nature of simplified all-in-one bonding systems [37], increasing the mineral–matrix ratio, and reduce nanoleakage and permeability at the resin–dentine interface. Moreover, it has been demonstrated that fluoride ions may inhibit both pro- and active metalloproteinases (MMP-2 and MMP-9) [38], thus reducing the enzymatic degradation at the bonding interface. It may be also possible that in the case of diffusion of calcium and phosphate ions through permeable hybrid layers, these may precipitate and crystallize in complex calcium-phosphates and inhibit MMPs through the formation of a Ca-PO/MMP complex [39].

On the other hand, a possible explanation for the differences in bonding performance attained in this study with the two simplified universal adhesives when restored with a conventional RC may be related to their different chemical compositions. Unlike FTB, the SCU system, which was the only adhesive that both when applied in ER and SE mode in combination with RC presented a significant bond strength drop after prolonged aging protocol, contains a polyalkenoic acid copolymer (PAC).

It has been shown that PAC contained in adhesives tends to accumulate primarily on the outer surface of the hybrid layer and creates "isles" between dentine and the adhesive layer [39]. It is also well known that PAC has multiple pendent carboxylic acids along a linear backbone that bind water, which causes important water sorption and solubility. Moreover, the high molecular weight of PAC [40] precludes its penetration into interfibrillar spaces within the acid-etched dentine.

Several reports indicated that simplified adhesives containing relatively high amount of bisphenol A diglycidyl methacrylate (Bis-GMA) in combination with PAC and 2-hydroxyethyl methacrylate (HEMA) do not infiltrate well into acid-etched dentine, so creating HEMA-rich/Bis-GMA-poor hybrid layers. It is also believed that HEMA, mixing with water within the hybrid layer, may produce hydrogels able to absorb water, which in turn enable hydrolytic and enzymatic degradation processes that jeopardize the longevity of resin–dentine interfaces [41–43]. Furthermore, it is generally well known that water-containing and acidic, single-bottle, pre-hydrolyzed silane coupling agents have a relatively short shelf life because both water and lower pH media can cause silane to degrade over time [44]. A modern, universal adhesive such as SCU contains both free silane and silaned nanofillers. Thus, we believe that water sorption at the adhesive layer may have accelerated polymer hydrolysis and filler debonding, reducing the durability of its bonding performance [44,45].

The information obtained in this study, along with all the observations discussed above, may also be relevant to the contemporary philosophy in atraumatic restorative dentistry. This is based on the preparation of minimally invasive cavities in order to preserve as much sound dental tissue as possible. However, such an ultraconservative intervention should always be followed by restorative treatments performed using therapeutic restorative approaches that protect the resin–dentine interface from degradation processes and prevent the reoccurrence of secondary carious lesions [46,47]. It is well known that the bonding performance of adhesive systems applied to caries-affected dentine (CAD) is not as strong as that attained when such materials are used in sound dentine; the bonding performance seems correlated to the low biomechanical properties of CAD (e.g., modulus of elasticity) [47].

Therefore, such a situation leads to failure of the restoration over time, so that improvements and suitable alternative restorative procedures are necessary in order to improve the durability of the bonding between adhesives and CAD. Wang et al [48] demonstrated distinct differences in the depth of dentine demineralization and degree of adhesive infiltration in non-carious and CAD. Because of the structural alteration and porosities in CAD, deeper, demineralized layers occurred. The deeper the demineralized collagen, the poorer the resin infiltration into the deepest part of the CAD. This resulted in phase separation of resin adhesives and "weak" bond strength. However, Tekçe et al. [49] showed that in such circumstances, the use of flowable resin-based composites, RMGICs, and compomers may provide stronger dentine-bond strength and better margin sealing than conventional glass-ionomer cement and resin composites due to the ability of such materials to dissipate the occlusal stress and the therapeutic effect of ions released over time.

In conclusion, within the limitations of this study, it is possible to affirm that the choice of appropriate materials from a chemical and mechanical point of view can make a difference on the bonding performance/durability of dentine-bonded interfaces. Indeed, the application of well-formulated modern adhesive systems in combination with ion-releasing dentine-replacement materials might offer to clinicians the possibility to perform more long-lasting adhesive restorations. However, these concepts must be corroborated by future in vivo and/or clinical trial studies in order to evaluate their true suitability in a clinical scenario.

Author Contributions: Conceptualization, S.S. and V.F.-L.; Data curation, F.F., M.E., and M.M.; Formal Analysis, A.A.N. and M.G.; Investigation, P.M.P. and I.M.; Methodology, M.G. and S.S.; Resources I.M.; Project Administration, V.F.-M.; Supervision, S.S.; Validation, M.G.; Writing–Original Draft Preparation, S.S. and F.F.; Writing–Review and Editing, S.S., F.F., and M.G.

References

1. Arhun, N.; Celik, C.; Yamanel, K. Clinical evaluation of resin-based composites in posterior restorations: Two-year results. *Oper. Dent.* **2010**, *35*, 397–404. [CrossRef] [PubMed]
2. Ferracane, J.L. Resin composite–state of the art. *Dent. Mater.* **2011**, *27*, 29–38. [CrossRef] [PubMed]
3. Kakaboura, A.; Rahiotis, C.; Watts, D.; Silikas, N.; Eliades, G. 3D-marginal adaptation versus setting shrinkage in light-cured microhybrid resin composites. *Dent. Mater.* **2007**, *23*, 272–278. [CrossRef] [PubMed]
4. Boaro, L.C.; Froes-Salgado, N.R.; Gajewski, V.E.; Bicalho, A.A.; Valdivia, A.D.; Soares, C.J.; Miranda Junior, W.G.; Braga, R.R. Correlation between polymerization stress and interfacial integrity of composites restorations assessed by different in vitro tests. *Dent. Mater.* **2014**, *30*, 984–992. [CrossRef] [PubMed]
5. Van Dijken, J.W.; Lindberg, A. A 15-year randomized controlled study of a reduced shrinkage stress resin composite. *Dent. Mater.* **2015**, *31*, 1150–1158. [CrossRef] [PubMed]
6. He, Z.; Shimada, Y.; Sadr, A.; Ikeda, M.; Tagami, J. The effects of cavity size and filling method on the bonding to Class I cavities. *J. Adhes. Dent.* **2008**, *10*, 447–453. [PubMed]
7. Sakaguchi, R.L.; Peters, M.C.; Nelson, S.R.; Douglas, W.H.; Poort, H.W. Effects of polymerization contraction in composite restorations. *J. Dent.* **1992**, *20*, 178–182. [CrossRef]
8. Davidson, C.L.; de Gee, A.J.; Feilzer, A. The competition between the composite-dentin bond strength and the polymerization contraction stress. *J. Dent. Res.* **1984**, *63*, 1396–1399. [CrossRef] [PubMed]
9. De Munck, J.; Van Landuyt, K.; Coutinho, E.; Poitevin, A.; Peumans, M.; Lambrechts, P.; Van Meerbeek, B. Micro-tensile bond strength of adhesives bonded to Class-I cavity-bottom dentin after thermo-cycling. *Dent. Mater.* **2005**, *21*, 999–1007. [CrossRef] [PubMed]
10. Fleming, G.J.; Cara, R.R.; Palin, W.M.; Burke, F.J. Cuspal movement and microleakage in premolar teeth restored with resin-based filling materials cured using a 'soft-start' polymerisation protocol. *Dent. Mater.* **2007**, *23*, 637–643. [CrossRef] [PubMed]
11. Bernardo, M.; Luis, H.; Martin, M.D.; Leroux, B.G.; Rue, T.; Leitao, J.; DeRouen, T.A. Survival and reasons for failure of amalgam versus composite posterior restorations placed in a randomized clinical trial. *J. Am. Dent. Assoc.* **2007**, *138*, 775–783. [CrossRef] [PubMed]
12. He, Z.; Shimada, Y.; Tagami, J. The effects of cavity size and incremental technique on micro-tensile bond strength of resin composite in Class I cavities. *Dent. Mater.* **2007**, *23*, 533–538. [CrossRef] [PubMed]
13. Chen, C.; Niu, L.N.; Xie, H.; Zhang, Z.Y.; Zhou, L.Q.; Jiao, K.; Chen, J.H.; Pashley, D.H.; Tay, F.R. Bonding of universal adhesives to dentine–Old wine in new bottles? *J. Dent.* **2015**, *43*, 525–536. [CrossRef] [PubMed]
14. Nikolaenko, S.A.; Lohbauer, U.; Roggendorf, M.; Petschelt, A.; Dasch, W.; Frankenberger, R. Influence of c-factor and layering technique on microtensile bond strength to dentin. *Dent. Mater.* **2004**, *20*, 579–585. [CrossRef] [PubMed]
15. Irie, M.; Suzuki, K.; Watts, D.C. Immediate performance of self-etching versus system adhesives with multiple light-activated restoratives. *Dent. Mater.* **2004**, *20*, 873–880. [CrossRef] [PubMed]
16. Irie, M.; Suzuki, K.; Watts, D.C. Marginal gap formation of light-activated restorative materials: Effects of immediate setting shrinkage and bond strength. *Dent. Mater.* **2002**, *18*, 203–210. [CrossRef]
17. Sampaio, P.C.; de Almeida Junior, A.A.; Francisconi, L.F.; Casas-Apayco, L.C.; Pereira, J.C.; Wang, L.; Atta, M.T. Effect of conventional and resin-modified glass-ionomer liner on dentin adhesive interface of Class I cavity walls after thermocycling. *Oper. Dent.* **2011**, *36*, 403–412. [CrossRef] [PubMed]
18. Sauro, S.; Faus-Matoses, V.; Makeeva, I.; Nunez Marti, J.M.; Gonzalez Martinez, R.; Garcia Bautista, J.A.; Faus-Llacer, V. Effects of Polyacrylic Acid Pre-Treatment on Bonded-Dentine Interfaces Created with a Modern Bioactive Resin-Modified Glass Ionomer Cement and Subjected to Cycling Mechanical Stress. *Materials* **2018**, *11*, 1884. [CrossRef] [PubMed]
19. Boksman, L.; Jordan, R.E.; Suzuki, M.; Charles, D.H. A visible light-cured posterior composite resin: Results of a 3-year clinical evaluation. *J. Am. Dent. Assoc.* **1986**, *112*, 627–631. [CrossRef] [PubMed]
20. Boksman, L.; Jordan, R.E.; Suzuki, M. Posterior composite restorations. *Compend. Contin. Educ. Dent.* **1984**, *367*, 372–373.
21. Jordan, R.E.; Suzuki, M.; Gwinnett, A.J. Conservative applications of acid etch-resin techniques. *Dent. Clin. N. Am.* **1981**, *25*, 307–336. [PubMed]
22. Toledano, M.; Cabello, I.; Aguilera, F.S.; Osorio, E.; Osorio, R. Effect of in vitro chewing and bruxism events on remineralization, at the resin-dentin interface. *J. Biomech.* **2015**, *48*, 14–21. [CrossRef] [PubMed]

23. Khvostenko, D.; Salehi, S.; Naleway, S.E.; Hilton, T.J.; Ferracane, J.L.; Mitchell, J.C.; Kruzic, J.J. Cyclic mechanical loading promotes bacterial penetration along composite restoration marginal gaps. *Dent. Mater.* **2015**, *31*, 702–710. [CrossRef] [PubMed]
24. Khvostenko, D.; Hilton, T.J.; Ferracane, J.L.; Mitchell, J.C.; Kruzic, J.J. Bioactive glass fillers reduce bacterial penetration into marginal gaps for composite restorations. *Dent. Mater.* **2016**, *32*, 73–81. [CrossRef] [PubMed]
25. Browning, W.D. The benefits of glass ionomer self-adhesive materials in restorative dentistry. *Compend. Contin. Educ. Dent.* **2006**, *27*, 308–314. [PubMed]
26. Forsten, L. Resin-modified glass ionomer cements: Fluoride release and uptake. *Acta Odontol. Scand.* **1995**, *53*, 222–225. [CrossRef] [PubMed]
27. Forss, H.; Jokinen, J.; Spets-Happonen, S.; Seppa, L.; Luoma, H. Fluoride and mutans streptococci in plaque grown on glass ionomer and composite. *Caries Res.* **1991**, *25*, 454–458. [CrossRef] [PubMed]
28. Cho, S.Y.; Cheng, A.C. A review of glass ionomer restorations in the primary dentition. *J. Can. Dent. Assoc.* **1999**, *65*, 491–495. [PubMed]
29. Fuss, M.; Wicht, M.J.; Attin, T.; Derman, S.H.M.; Noack, M.J. Protective Buffering Capacity of Restorative Dental Materials In Vitro. *J. Adhes. Dent.* **2017**, *19*, 177–183. [PubMed]
30. Tezvergil-Mutluay, A.; Agee, K.A.; Hoshika, T.; Tay, F.R.; Pashley, D.H. The inhibitory effect of polyvinylphosphonic acid on functional matrix metalloproteinase activities in human demineralized dentin. *Acta Biomater.* **2010**, *6*, 4136–4142. [CrossRef] [PubMed]
31. Osorio, R.; Yamauti, M.; Sauro, S.; Watson, T.F.; Toledano, M. Experimental resin cements containing bioactive fillers reduce matrix metalloproteinase-mediated dentin collagen degradation. *J. Endod.* **2012**, *38*, 1227–1232. [CrossRef] [PubMed]
32. Sauro, S.; Watson, T.; Moscardo, A.P.; Luzi, A.; Feitosa, V.P.; Banerjee, A. The effect of dentine pre-treatment using bioglass and/or polyacrylic acid on the interfacial characteristics of resin-modified glass ionomer cements. *J. Dent.* **2018**, *73*, 32–39. [CrossRef] [PubMed]
33. Toledano, M.; Aguilera, F.S.; Sauro, S.; Cabello, I.; Osorio, E.; Osorio, R. Load cycling enhances bioactivity at the resin-dentin interface. *Dent. Mater.* **2014**, *30*, e169–e188. [CrossRef] [PubMed]
34. Sauro, S.; Osorio, R.; Watson, T.F.; Toledano, M. Assessment of the quality of resin-dentin bonded interfaces: An AFM nano-indentation, muTBS and confocal ultramorphology study. *Dent. Mater.* **2012**, *28*, 622–631. [CrossRef] [PubMed]
35. Sauro, S.; Toledano, M.; Aguilera, F.S.; Mannocci, F.; Pashley, D.H.; Tay, F.R.; Watson, T.F.; Osorio, R. Resin-dentin bonds to EDTA-treated vs. acid-etched dentin using ethanol wet-bonding. Part II: Effects of mechanical cycling load on microtensile bond strengths. *Dent. Mater.* **2011**, *27*, 563–572. [CrossRef] [PubMed]
36. Dorfer, C.E.; Staehle, H.J.; Wurst, M.W.; Duschner, H.; Pioch, T. The nanoleakage phenomenon: Influence of different dentin bonding agents, thermocycling and etching time. *Eur. J. Oral Sci.* **2000**, *108*, 346–351. [CrossRef] [PubMed]
37. Sauro, S.; Pashley, D.H.; Mannocci, F.; Tay, F.R.; Pilecki, P.; Sherriff, M.; Watson, T.F. Micropermeability of current self-etching and etch-and-rinse adhesives bonded to deep dentine: A comparison study using a double-staining/confocal microscopy technique. *Eur. J. Oral Sci.* **2008**, *116*, 184–193. [CrossRef] [PubMed]
38. Tezvergil-Mutluay, A.; Seseogullari-Dirihan, R.; Feitosa, V.P.; Cama, G.; Brauer, D.S.; Sauro, S. Effects of Composites Containing Bioactive Glasses on Demineralized Dentin. *J. Dent. Res.* **2017**, *96*, 999–1005. [CrossRef] [PubMed]
39. Makowski, G.S.; Ramsby, M.L. Differential effect of calcium phosphate and calcium pyrophosphate on binding of matrix metalloproteinases to fibrin: Comparison to a fibrin-binding protease from inflammatory joint fluids. *Clin. Exp. Immunol.* **2004**, *136*, 176–187. [CrossRef] [PubMed]
40. Larraz, E.; Deb, S.; Elvira, C.; Roman, J.S. A novel amphiphilic acrylic copolymer based on Triton X-100 for a poly(alkenoate) glass-ionomer cement. *Dent. Mater.* **2006**, *22*, 506–514. [CrossRef] [PubMed]
41. Wang, Y.; Spencer, P. Quantifying adhesive penetration in adhesive/dentin interface using confocal Raman microspectroscopy. *J. Biomed. Mater. Res.* **2002**, *59*, 46–55. [CrossRef] [PubMed]
42. Wang, Y.; Spencer, P. Effect of acid etching time and technique on interfacial characteristics of the adhesive-dentin bond using differential staining. *Eur. J. Oral Sci.* **2004**, *112*, 293–299. [CrossRef] [PubMed]
43. Sattabanasuk, V.; Vachiramon, V.; Qian, F.; Armstrong, S.R. Resin-dentin bond strength as related to different surface preparation methods. *J. Dent.* **2007**, *35*, 467–475. [CrossRef] [PubMed]

44. Yoshihara, K.; Nagaoka, N.; Sonoda, A.; Maruo, Y.; Makita, Y.; Okihara, T.; Irie, M.; Yoshida, Y.; Van Meerbeek, B. Effectiveness and stability of silane coupling agent inc'orporated in universal adhesives. *Dent. Mater.* **2016**, *32*, 1218–1225. [CrossRef] [PubMed]
45. Van Landuyt, K.L.; De Munck, J.; Mine, A.; Cardoso, M.V.; Peumans, M.; Van Meerbeek, B. Filler debonding & subhybrid-layer failures in self-etch adhesives. *J. Dent. Res.* **2010**, *89*, 1045–1050. [PubMed]
46. Eick, J.D.; Robinson, S.J.; Chappell, R.P.; Cobb, C.M.; Spencer, P. The dentinal surface: Its influence on dentinal adhesion. Part III. *Quintessence Int.* **1993**, *24*, 571–582. [PubMed]
47. Erhardt, M.C.; Toledano, M.; Osorio, R.; Pimenta, L.A. Histomorphologic characterization and bond strength evaluation of caries-affected dentin/resin interfaces: Effects of long-term water exposure. *Dent. Mater.* **2008**, *24*, 786–798. [CrossRef] [PubMed]
48. Wang, Y.; Spencer, P.; Walker, M.P. Chemical profile of adhesive/caries-affected dentin interfaces using Raman microspectroscopy. *J. Biomed. Mater. Res. A* **2007**, *81*, 279–286. [CrossRef] [PubMed]
49. Tekçe, N.; Tuncer, S.; Demirci, M.; Pashaev, D. The bonding effect of adhesive systems and bulk-fill composites to sound and caries-affected dentine. *J. Adhes. Sci. Technol.* **2016**, *30*, 171–185. [CrossRef]

16

A Novel Dental Sealant Containing Dimethylaminohexadecyl Methacrylate Suppresses the Cariogenic Pathogenicity of *Streptococcus mutans* Biofilms

Maria Salem Ibrahim [1,2], Ahmed S. Ibrahim [3], Abdulrahman A. Balhaddad [1,4], Michael D. Weir [1,5], Nancy J. Lin [6], Franklin R. Tay [7], Thomas W. Oates [5], Hockin H. K. Xu [1,5,8,9] and Mary Anne S. Melo [1,10,*]

1 Ph.D Program in Dental Biomedical Sciences, University of Maryland School of Dentistry, Baltimore, MD 21201, USA
2 Department of Preventive Dental Sciences, College of Dentistry, Imam Abdulrahman Bin Faisal University, Dammam 34212, Saudi Arabia
3 Medical Microbiology Department, Health Monitoring Centers, Ministry of Health, Jeddah 21176, Saudi Arabia
4 Department of Restorative Dental Sciences, College of Dentistry, Imam Abdulrahman Bin Faisal University, Dammam 34212, Saudi Arabia
5 Department of Advanced Oral Sciences and Therapeutics, Division of Biomaterials and Tissue Engineering, University of Maryland School of Dentistry, Baltimore, MD 21201, USA
6 Biosystems and Biomaterials Division, National Institute of Standards and Technology, Gaithersburg, MD 20899, USA
7 Department of Endodontics, The Dental College of Georgia, Augusta University, Augusta, GA 30912, USA
8 Center for Stem Cell Biology and Regenerative Medicine, University of Maryland School of Medicine, Baltimore, MD 21201, USA
9 University of Maryland Marlene and Stewart Greenebaum Cancer Center, University of Maryland School of Medicine, Baltimore, MD 21201, USA
10 Division of Operative Dentistry, Department of General Dentistry, University of Maryland School of Dentistry, Baltimore, MD 21201, USA
* Correspondence: mmelo@umaryland.edu

Abstract: Cariogenic oral biofilms are strongly linked to dental caries around dental sealants. Quaternary ammonium monomers copolymerized with dental resin systems have been increasingly explored for modulation of biofilm growth. Here, we investigated the effect of dimethylaminohexadecyl methacrylate (DMAHDM) on the cariogenic pathogenicity of *Streptococcus mutans* (*S. mutans*) biofilms. DMAHDM at 5 mass% was incorporated into a parental formulation containing 20 mass% nanoparticles of amorphous calcium phosphate (NACP). *S. mutans* biofilms were grown on the formulations, and biofilm inhibition and virulence properties were assessed. The tolerances to acid stress and hydrogen peroxide stress were also evaluated. Our findings suggest that incorporating 5% DMAHDM into 20% NACP-containing sealants (1) imparts a detrimental biological effect on *S. mutans* by reducing colony-forming unit counts, metabolic activity and exopolysaccharide synthesis; and (2) reduces overall acid production and tolerance to oxygen stress, two major virulence factors of this microorganism. These results provide a perspective on the value of integrating bioactive restorative materials with traditional caries management approaches in clinical practice. Contact-killing strategies via dental materials aiming to prevent or at least reduce high numbers of cariogenic bacteria may be a promising approach to decrease caries in patients at high risk.

Keywords: antibacterial agents; biofilm; dental caries; sealant; quaternary ammonium compounds; *Streptococcus mutans*

1. Introduction

Dental caries is a biofilm-triggered oral disease with an international pandemic distribution, primarily affecting school-age children [1]. The World Health Organization reports that dental caries is the most common oral condition included in the Global Burden of Disease Study [2]. Carious lesions of permanent teeth (2.3 billion people) ranks as the most prevalent oral condition, while carious lesions on deciduous teeth (560 million children) ranks 12th [2]. The pits and fissures on children's teeth present a topography with deep and narrow features, making the mechanical removal of plaque bacteria by brushing very challenging [3].

In efforts toward pediatric caries prevention, dental sealants were introduced for application on the occlusal surface. The sealants act as a physical barrier for microorganisms at the pits and fissures of the teeth. Evidence-based clinical recommendations, stated by the American Dental Association and the American Academy of Pediatric Dentistry, support sealants as a practical approach in preventing and arresting pit-and-fissure occlusal caries lesions [4]. Although sealants are a widely used preventive approach against occlusal carious lesions, the failure rate is high. Longitudinal data [5,6] show reasons for failure related to bacterial colonization underneath the sealed fissures with the progressive demineralization and development of cavitation.

Exploring the potential opportunities for new biotechnologies and biomaterials to improve dental outcomes requires an enhanced understanding of caries etiology and bacteria-material interactions. A material that can detrimentally affect the oral bacteria on or near its surface is a promising area of dental material development. For instance, bioactive or bioinductive materials can help reduce cariogenic biofilm formation at the sealant-tooth interface [7]. Likewise, contact-active dental materials that inhibit the growth of acid-producing bacteria can potentially disturb and even correct the localized dysbiosis (imbalance) of the oral microflora that may lead to caries around dental sealants [8,9]. Quaternary ammonium compounds are highly antimicrobial when applied in solution and also demonstrate antimicrobial activity when immobilized on a surface [10]. In the last decade, quaternary ammonium-based methacrylate monomers have been investigated to impart antibacterial surfaces to dental materials.

Recent works have demonstrated the application of dimethylaminohexadecyl methacrylate (DMAHDM) and amorphous calcium phosphate (NACP) as an antibacterial strategy for resin-based materials [8,11,12]. DMAHDM, an antibacterial monomer, acts primarily through direct contact killing [13]. It has been previously hypothesized that a positively charged DMAHDM structure may interact with negatively charged bacteria to lead to cell membrane leakiness and rupture [14,15]. Our previous report [16] has tuned sealant formulations to reach acceptable values for physical and mechanical properties using DMAHDM at 5 mass% and NACP at 20 mass%, respectively. However, the antibacterial performance of these formulations was not investigated.

The targeted cariogenic biofilm is a densely packed community of oral microbial cells with predominantly acid-tolerant, acid-producing bacteria surrounded by an exopolysaccharide (EPS)-rich matrix [13,17,18]. Within cariogenic dental plaque, *Streptococcus mutans* (*S. mutans*) has been strongly linked to cariogenic biofilm formation and carious lesion progression [19]. The main observable characteristics associated with *S. mutans* cariogenic pathogenicity include adhesion to tooth surfaces, synthesis of EPS via glucosyltransferases, biofilm formation, efficient use of sucrose to create an acidic environment, and aciduricity via acid tolerance response [13,20]. These virulence factors under a sucrose-rich environment contribute to the structural integrity and pathogenicity of the biofilm produced by *S. mutans* [17,18]. The remarkable ability of *S. mutans* to cope with significant and constant environmental variations, including changes in pH and oxygen tension, further leads it to be one of the primary cariogenic pathogens in this context [20].

The ability to reduce or modulate the virulence and viability of *S. mutans* biofilms using bioactive dental sealants could reduce caries associated with sealants. In the present study, we hypothesized that the formation and cariogenicity of *S. mutans* biofilms (acidogenicity, EPS production, aciduricity and tolerance to oxygen stress) would be reduced when the biofilms are in contact with sealant formulations containing 5% DMAHDM. Accordingly, this study aimed to investigate the effect of sealant formulations with 5% DMAHDM and 20% NACP on the virulence properties and viability of *S. mutans* biofilms.

2. Results

2.1. DMAHDM Reduced Biofilm Formation

Multiple properties of *S. mutans* were strongly reduced when the biofilms were cultured on the surfaces of sealants containing DMAHDM, relative to sealants without DMAHDM. Figure 1 shows the CFU counts for the 48 h *S. mutans* biofilms formed on the various sealants. The CFU values for groups containing 5% DMAHDM were significantly lower than those for control groups (commercial and experimental) and for groups containing 20% NACP ($p < 0.05$). A two-way ANOVA found a significant effect for 5% DMAHDM (F (1,58) = 5.453; $p = 0.23$) but no significant effect for 20% NACP (F (1,58) = 0.884; $p = 0.351$) or for the interaction between these factors ($p = 0.88$) on CFU counts.

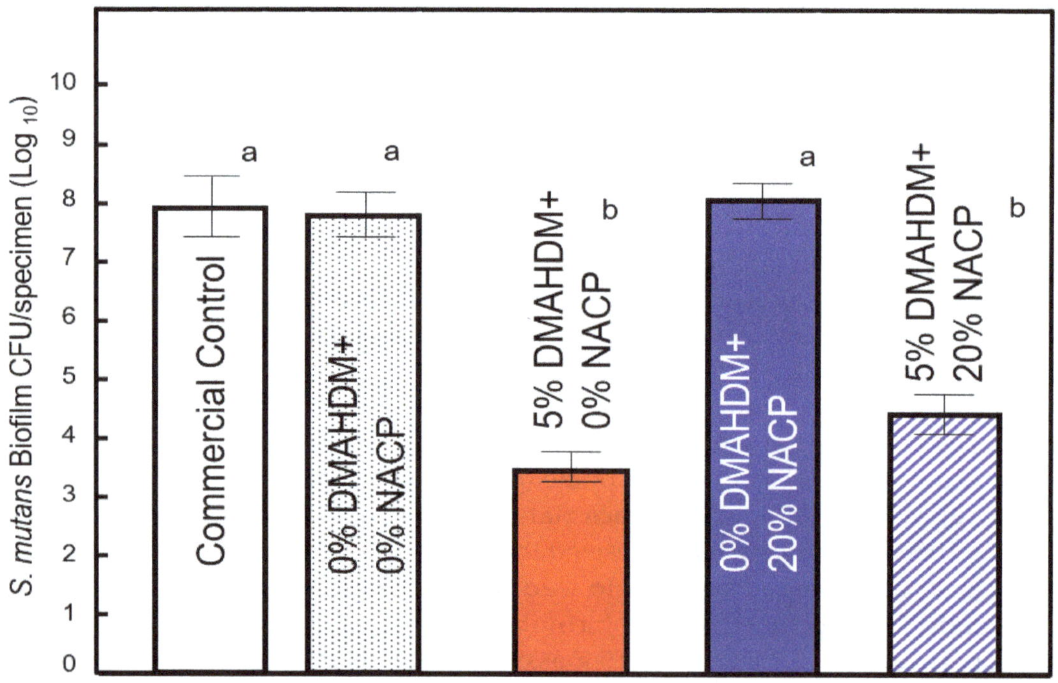

Figure 1. Colony-forming units per sealant specimen for *S. mutans* biofilms (mean ± SD of three independent experiments; $n = 6$ per group/experiment). Different lowercase letters denote a significant difference at a level of $\propto = 0.05$ among groups.

Figure 2 shows the results from the MTT assay reflecting active metabolizing (respiring) *S. mutans* cells in the biofilms adherent to the sealant specimens. For the two formulations containing 5% DMAHDM, the MTT values were lower in comparison to the control ($p < 0.05$), representing approximately 82% and 87% reduction in biofilm metabolic activity for 5% DMAHDM + 0% NACP and 5% DMAHDM + 20% NACP, respectively. There is no main effect for the presence of 20% NACP (F (1,64) = 0.784; $p = 0.467$).

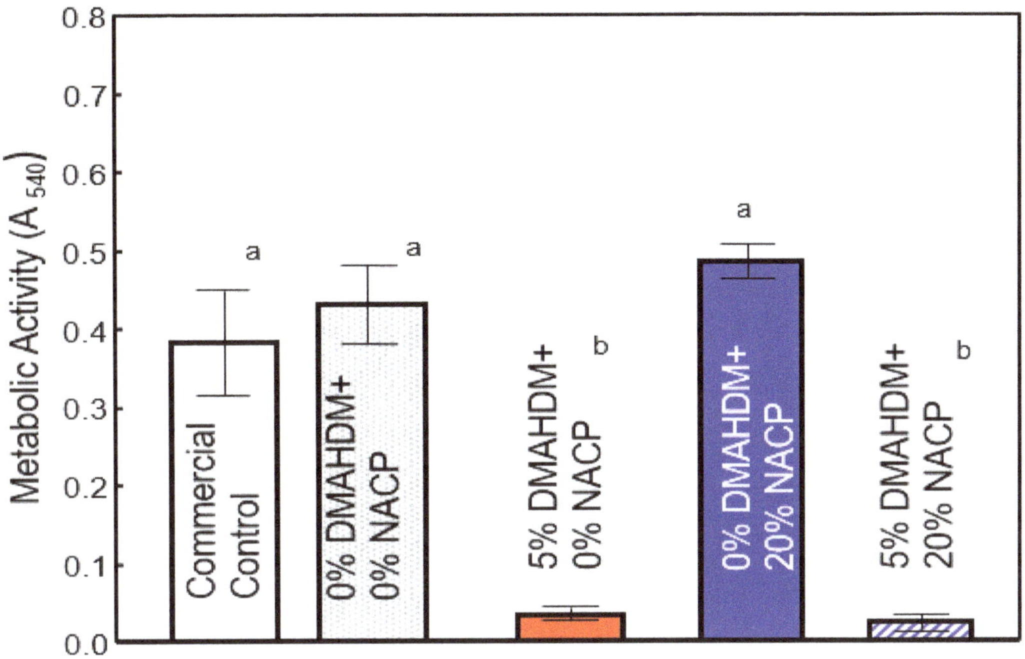

Figure 2. The metabolic activity of the 48 h *S. mutans* biofilms measured by MTT assay (mean ± SD of three independent experiments; $n = 6$ per group/experiment; non-normalized values). Different lowercase letters denote a significant difference at a level of $\propto = 0.05$ among groups.

2.2. DMAHDM Alone and in Combination with NACP Alters Acid and Oxygen Tolerance of *S. mutans*

Figure 3A uses the change in CFU (normalized to time zero) to represent the *S. mutans* biofilm survival rate after exposure to pH 2.8 for up to 45 min. *S. mutans* biofilms grown on sealant specimens containing 5% DMAHDM displayed lower survival at 10 min (38% and 44%, respectively) compared with the control and NACP only groups (60% and 65%, respectively). This difference was not as pronounced at later time points.

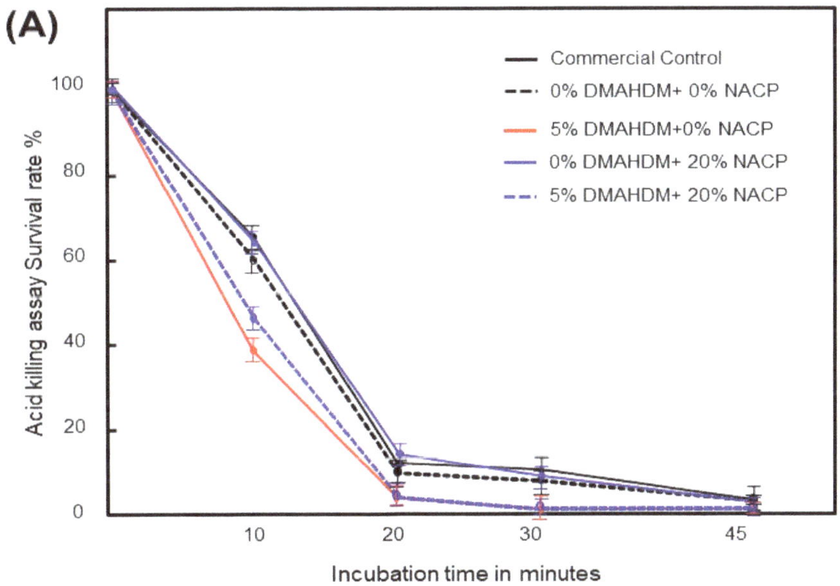

Figure 3. *Cont.*

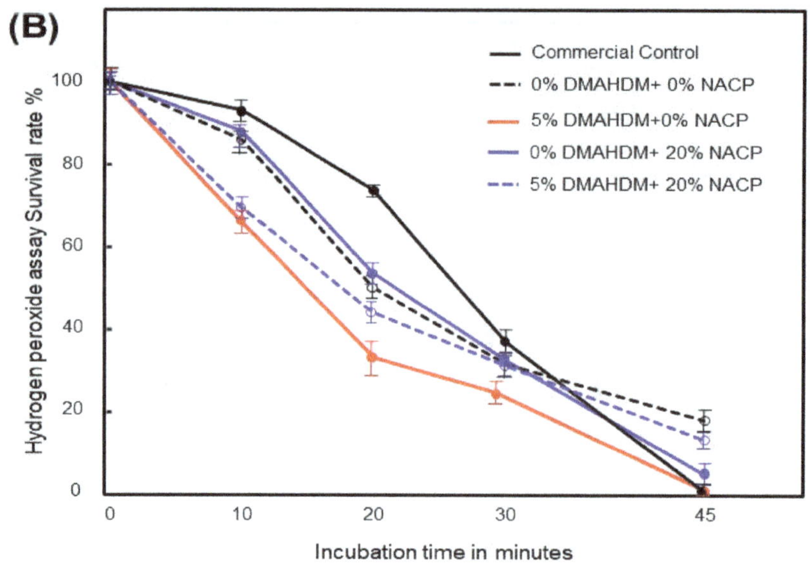

Figure 3. *S. mutans* biofilm survival expressed as the percent change in CFUs after exposure to (**A**) acid (pH 2.8) and (**B**) 0.2% H_2O_2 for up to 45 min (Mean ± SD of three independent experiments; $n = 8$ per group/experiment). Lines were drawn to improve readability.

For the hydrogen peroxide killing assay, Figure 3B depicts the survival rate of *S. mutans* biofilms exposed to an H_2O_2 concentration of 0.2% for 45 min. *S. mutans* biofilms formed on sealant specimens containing 5% DMAHDM exhibited lower survival than the control sealant specimens at all timepoints except at 30 min and 45 min.

2.3. Attenuation of Exopolysaccharide Produced by *S. mutans*

Measurements of EPS levels in the biofilms are plotted in Figure 4. Biofilms on the control sealant specimens had high exopolysaccharide production. Adding only 20% NACP to the formulation did not change the production of the polysaccharide ($F_{1,23} = 0.626$, $P = 0.436$) substantially from the controls. Incorporation of DMAHDM significantly decreased the water-insoluble polysaccharide synthesis from *S. mutans* ($p < 0.05$). There was no significant interaction between DMAHDM and NACP content for polysaccharide production.

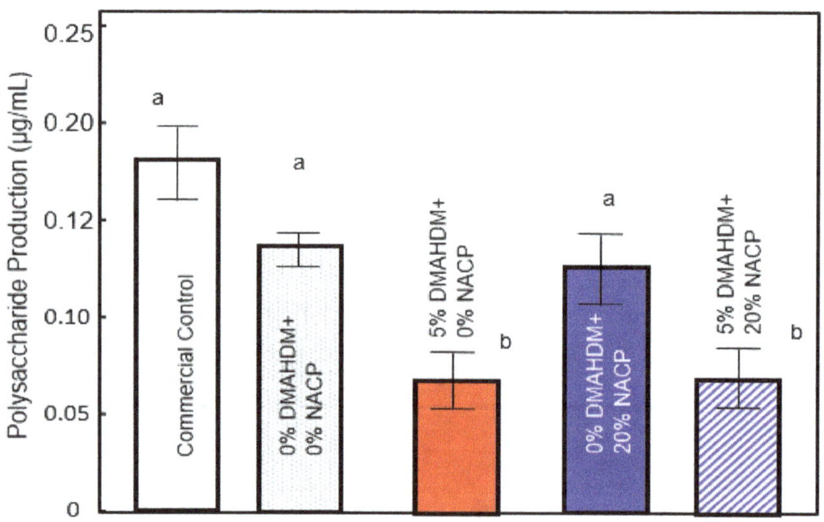

Figure 4. The polysaccharide production of 48 h *S. mutans* biofilms expressed as µg/mL (mean ± SD of three independent experiments; $n = 6$ per group/experimental). Different lowercase letters denote a significant difference at a level of ∝ = 0.05 among groups.

Figure 5 plots the pH of the culture medium during biofilm formation. Biofilms in commercial and experimental control groups had the highest acid production, leading to a drop in pH sustained over 48 h. The addition of 20% NACP supported a near neutral pH over the 48-hour time course ($p < 0.05$). The addition of 5% DMAHDM had a minimal effect when NACP was present, but without NACP the initial pH drop within the first 8 h matched that of the controls. At 24 h and 48 h, however, the pH in the 5% DMAHDM only-sealant specimens increased relative to the controls, with pH values above 5.5.

The lactic acid production of biofilms on the sealants is presented in Figure 6. Biofilms on the control groups and the group containing 20% NACP only produced the most acid ($p < 0.05$), and 20% NACP had no significant effect on lactic acid production. Analysis of the lactic acid concentration indicates a significant effect of DMAHDM incorporation ($F_{1,40} = 4.611$, $P = 0.027$) on the biofilm lactic acid production. Low lactic acid concentrations at levels approximately 10% of those on the control groups were observed. There was no interaction for lactic acid production between DMAHDM content and NACP content.

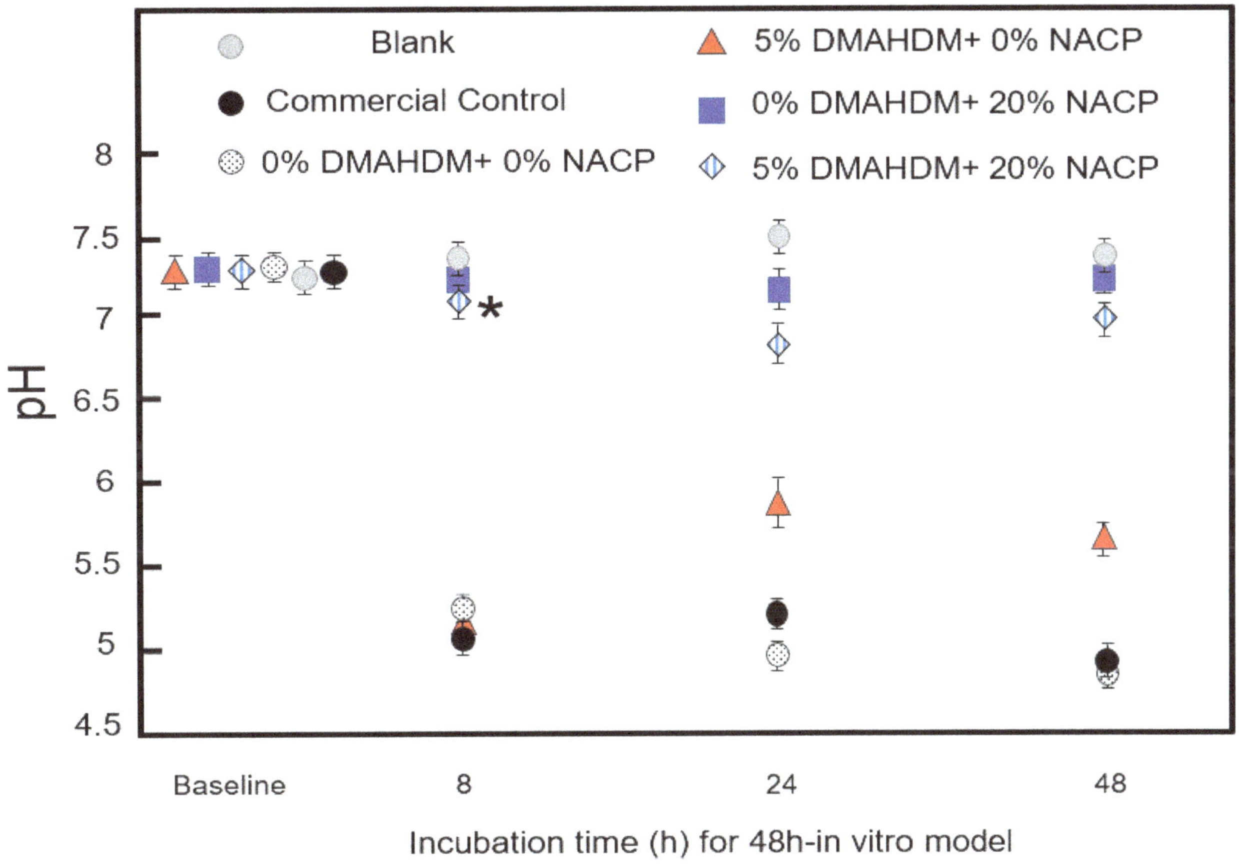

Figure 5. pH measurements (mean ± SD; $n = 3$) of growth medium from *S. mutans* biofilms grown on the various sealant specimens for 0 h, 8 h, 24 h, and 48 h. The blank represents growth medium incubated alongside tested groups. The asterisk represents a significant difference at a level of $\alpha = 0.05$ for 0% DMAHDM + 20% NACP and 5% DMAHDM + 20% NACP.

Imaging of green fluorescent protein (GFP)-expressing *S. mutans* was used to visualize the biofilm structures. The 48 h *S. mutans* biofilms formed on the 5% DMAHDM + 20% NACP sealant specimens (Figure 7A) were qualitatively reduced in visible biomass as compared to biofilms that grew on the control sealant specimens (Figure 7B). The biofilms on the control sealants (Figure 7C) appeared denser and thicker in comparison to biofilms on the DMAHDM + NACP sealant (Figure 7D).

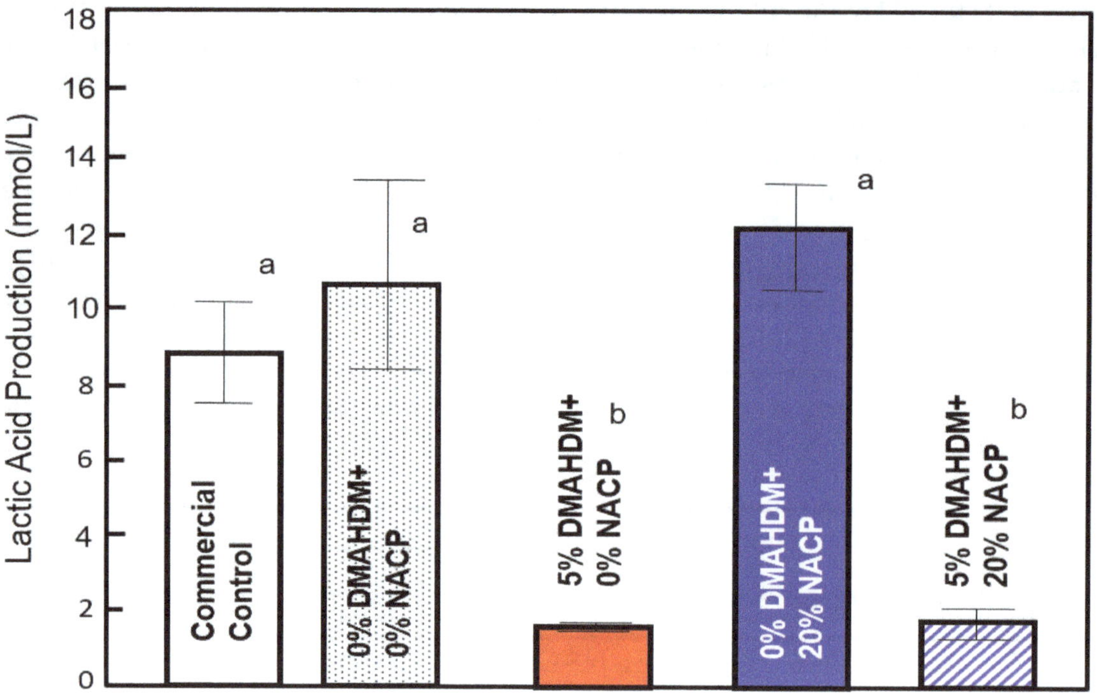

Figure 6. Lactic acid production of the 48 h *S. mutans* biofilms expressed as mmol/L (mean ± SD of three independent experiments; $n = 6$ per group/experimental). Different lowercase letters denote a significant difference at a level of $\propto = 0.05$ among groups.

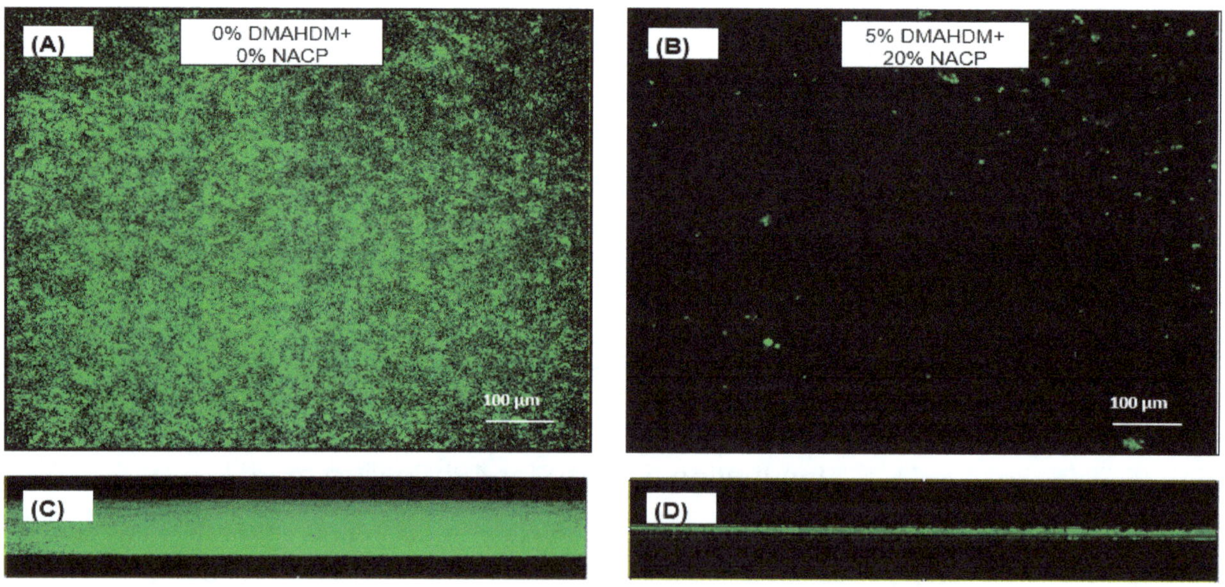

Figure 7. Scanning confocal laser microscope images of *S. mutans* biofilms formed on 0% DMAHDM + 0% NACP (control) and 5% DMAHDM + 20% NACP. (**A**,**B**) Random, representative images in the x-y plane (top view); (**C**,**D**) random, representative images in the x-z plane (side view).

3. Discussion

In this study, we explored the influence of an antibacterial contact killing approach for sealant formulations on virulence factors of *S. mutans*. The antibacterial strategy of incorporating 5% DMAHDM into a parental formulation containing 20% NACP resulted in an overall significant reduction of acid-producing biofilms. The data obtained from the CFU (Figure 1) and metabolic activity (Figure 2) assays showed that 5% DMAHDM, alone or combined with 20% NACP, can remarkably inhibit the activity of *S. mutans* biofilms, surpassing the clinically relevant greater-than-3-log (99.9%) reduction [21]. These results are consistent with previous reports for oral biofilms exposed to dental bonding formulations containing DMAHDM [22,23].

Subsequently, we examined whether the in vitro antibiofilm activity of DMAHDM would translate into changes in the ability of *S. mutans* to survive and resist high acid and oxygen stresses. *S. mutans* needs to present aciduricity to avoid falling victim to its own acidogenic metabolism. However, biofilms grown on DMAHDM-containing sealants were generally less tolerant of acidic and oxidative stresses (Figure 4). Upon exposure to acid, *S. mutans* promotes many changes at the transcriptional and physiological levels to respond to the threat of acid damage to sensitive and critical cytoplasmic molecules, such as metabolic organelles and DNA [24,25]. *S. mutans* protects itself from the damaging effects of acids through the maintenance of a cytoplasm that is more alkaline relative to the extracellular space [26]. This alkaline environment is mainly reached via plasma membrane mechanisms such as F1F0 ATPase for proton extrusion and changes in unsaturated fatty acid percentage [24]. The harmful interactions between DMAHDM and the *S. mutans* membrane can hypothetically damage a cell's ability to maintain the intracellular alkaline environment. Similarly, *S. mutans* makes changes to its membrane composition to limit the formation of hydrogen peroxide, promote its safe elimination, and repair damage [27]. If the membrane is dysfunctional, such as via perturbation by quaternary ammonium compounds like DMAHDM, the cell may have a reduced ability to survive in H_2O_2 environments, as seen here.

S. mutans relies on exopolysaccharide matrix synthesis to help it attach firmly to tooth surfaces. *S. mutans'* ability to synthesize exopolysaccharide is essential for a biofilm's structural stability and may limit antibacterial strategies [28]. According to the results of the EPS assay (Figure 5), the DMAHDM monomer lowers the level of extracellular polysaccharide production, which may make these biofilms less stable and may potentially be beneficial for the non-cariogenic microbial community. The representative confocal microscopy images (Figure 7) qualitatively support the results from the bioassays by showing reduced biofilm growth on the DMAHDM materials. The images suggest a reduced ability of *S. mutans* to form a dense biofilm architecture.

The presence of NACP alone (without DMAHDM) did not affect biofilm parameters including CFUs, metabolic activity, or polysaccharide production; however, an effect of NACP was observed on the pH values for the 48 h biofilm model where the pH stayed neutral for all time points tested when NACP was included in the formulation. NACP can affect pH through the release of supersaturating levels of calcium and phosphate ions. NACP is expected to enhance the remineralizing capacity relative to larger amorphous calcium phosphate particles due to the higher surface area-to-volume ratio of NACP. For instance, NACP has a relatively high specific surface area of 17.76 m^2/g, compared to about 0.5 m^2/g of traditional CaP particles [29]. The higher proportion of exposed surface area for NACP requires lower filler levels (by mass) to reach the same surface area and therefore expected outcome as compared to amorphous calcium phosphate on the micro scale. Previous studies showed that nanocomposites with NACP filler fraction of 20 mass% were able to reduce demineralization [30,31]. The importance of the calcium reservoir relies on the fact that Ca^{2+}, being one of the ions of hydroxyapatite, may reduce the driving force for tooth demineralization that occurs during a pH drop in dental biofilm. During demineralization, calcium release precedes phosphate release from enamel, dentin, and cementum, and calcium-deficient carbonated hydroxyapatite comprises the major substitution activity that takes place [32]. The presence of carbonates and other ionic substitutions significantly disrupts the crystal lattice in hydroxyapatite, weakening the hydroxyapatite and increasing its susceptibility to acid attack and solubility. Therefore, using high-calcium release materials to suppress the demineralization process could be beneficial.

Collectively, our data support the hypothesis that sealants with DMAHDM are able to disrupt *S. mutans* biofilm formation, thereby reducing their virulence potential. This outcome helps open the door for an important pathway to suppress dental caries via biofilm modulation and not only total biofilm eradication. A previous study conducted to investigate the antibacterial effect of DMAHDM on multispecies biofilms revealed that biofilms had a reduced relative amount of *S. mutans* when grown in contact with 3% DMAHDM as compared to the control, suggesting that DMAHDM may also be able to modulate the biofilm species composition toward a non-cariogenic tendency [33]. Shifting the biofilm composition from a cariogenic/acidogenic phenotype to a less virulent or even non-cariogenic biofilm is essential. However, the *S. mutans*/quaternary ammonium interactions involve various complex mechanisms where specific mechanisms and pathways are not clear and are still under debate [10,34]. While this study focused on the ability of sealant formulations with 5% DMAHDM and 20% NACP to alter the virulence-related traits of *S. mutans*, further research on the underlying mechanisms of bacterial/quaternary ammonium interactions is needed to optimize materials and achieve desired outcomes of improved oral health.

4. Materials and Methods

4.1. Development of Dental Resin Sealant Formulations

The parental resin matrix [16] consisted of (% by mass): 44.5% of pyromellitic glycerol dimethacrylate (PMGDM) (Hampford, Stratford, CT, USA); 39.5% of ethoxylated bisphenol a dimethacrylate (EBPADMA) (Sigma-Aldrich, St. Louis, MO, USA); 10% of 2-hydroxyethyl methacrylate (HEMA) (Esstech, Essington, PA, USA); 5% of bisphenol a glycidyl dimethacrylate (Esstech), and 1% of phenyl bis (2,4,6-trimethyl benzoyl)-phosphine oxide (BAPO) (Sigma-Aldrich) as a photo-initiator. For some formulations, DMAHDM at 5 mass% was added. The mass ratio of resin to filler was 1:1, where the filler fraction consisted of silanized barium boroaluminosilicate glass particles (average size of 1.4 μm (Caulk/Dentsply, Milford, DE, USA)) with or without the addition of NACP. DMAHDM and NACP were synthesized according to previous studies [16,22].

The tested dental sealant formulations were prepared as follows (% by mass):

1. Commercial High-viscosity Sealant/Flowable Composite control termed "Commercial Control" (Virtuoso, DenMat, Lompoc, CA, USA).
2. Experimental Control Sealant termed "0% DMAHDM + 0% NACP; Experimental Control" (50% PEHB + 0% DMAHDM + 50% Glass + 0% NACP).
3. Experimental Sealant termed "5% DMAHDM + 0% NACP" (45% PEHB + 5% DMAHDM + 50% Glass + 0% NACP).
4. Experimental Sealant termed "0% DMAHDM + 20% NACP" (50% PEHB + 0% DMAHDM + 30% Glass + 20% NACP).
5. Experimental Sealant termed "5% DMAHDM + 20% NACP" (45% PEHB + 5% DMAHDM + 30% Glass + 20% NACP).

4.2. Sample Preparation

Sealant specimens (diameter = 9 mm; thickness = 2 mm) were prepared using polytetrafluoroethylene molds covered with Mylar strips and glass slides [35]. Each sealant specimen was light-cured (1200 mW/cm^2; 60 s; Labolight DUO, GC America, Alsip, IL, USA) on each side. Specimens were sterilized using ethylene oxide (24-h cycle; Andersen Sterilizers, Inc., Haw River, NC, USA) and allowed to de-gas for at least seven days after sterilization.

4.3. *S. mutans* Biofilm Formation

An *S. mutans* biofilm model was used [36] with modifications. *S. mutans* UA159 from the American Type Culture Collection (ATCC, Manassas, VA, USA) was cultured overnight (≈18 h) in brain heart infusion (BHI) broth (Sigma-Aldrich) at 37 °C and 5% CO_2 (by volume). This *S. mutans* culture was adjusted to an optical density at 600 nm (OD_{600}) of 0.9 (≈1×10^8 CFU/mL according to growth curves monitored by spectrophotometry) and diluted in biofilm medium containing BHI broth supplemented with 2% (by mass) sucrose to prepare the inoculum.

The inoculum (1.5 mL) was added to wells of a 24-well culture plate containing the sterilized sealant specimens, and the well plates were incubated in an anaerobic chamber (37 °C; gas composition by volume: 10% H_2, 5% CO_2, 85% N_2; Whitley Workstation DG250; Microbiology International, Frederick, MD, USA) for 48 h without agitation to form a more established biofilm. The growth medium was changed at 8 h and 24 h. Control groups included wells with 1.5 mL of inoculum without sealants (Control inoculum) and wells with 1.5 mL of BHI + 2% sucrose without bacteria (Control BHI). Sealant specimens with the 48-hour biofilms were characterized as described in Sections 4.4–4.10.

4.4. Colony-Forming Unit Counts

After the sealant specimens (n = 6) had been incubated for 48 h, each sealant specimen with the attached biofilm was washed in 1 mL of phosphate-buffered saline (PBS), transported to a vial containing 2 mL of PBS, sonicated for 5 min (Branson 3510-DTH Ultrasonic Cleaner), and vortexed (5 s; maximum speed) to harvest the biofilm [37]. The resultant bacterial suspensions were serially diluted 10^1- through 10^6-fold, drop-plated onto BHI agar plates, and anaerobically incubated at 37 °C. After 48 h, the number of colony-forming units (CFU) was determined [37]. The results were calculated based on the number of CFU and the dilution factor; $\log_{10}$ transformed data are expressed as CFU/specimen.

4.5. Metabolic Activity

Metabolic activity was assessed via MTT (3-[4,5-dimethylthiazol-2-yl]-2,5-diphenyltetrazolium bromide) assay [37]. Briefly, each sealant specimen (n = 6) was washed in 1 mL of PBS and transported to a new 24-well plate containing 1 mL of tetrazolium dye (0.5 mg/mL) in PBS. Then, sealant specimens were incubated anaerobically for 1 h and transferred to a new 24-well plate. To solubilize the formazan crystals, 1 mL of dimethyl sulfoxide (DMSO) was added to each well, and the plate was incubated for 20 min at 37 °C. After that, 200 μL of the DMSO solution was collected from each specimen to measure the absorbance at 540 nm [37] (SpectraMax, Molecular Devices LLC, San Jose, CA, USA). The OD_{540} of DMSO defines the blanks for the spectrophotometric method. Values were not normalized prior to analysis.

4.6. Acid Stress and Oxygen Stress Tolerance

The differences in acid tolerance of *S. mutans* UA159 biofilms on the various formulations were evaluated using the method described by Kim et al. [38]. After 48 h of incubation, sealant specimens (n = 8) were washed once with 0.1 mol/L glycine (pH 7.0) and switched to 0.1 mol/L glycine at pH 2.8. Wells with biofilms but not treated with glycine served as controls. Specimens were incubated at room temperature, and 100 μL aliquots were collected at 0 min, 10 min, 20 min, 30 min, and 45 min. CFU was determined per Section 4.4.

The differences in oxidative stress tolerance of *S. mutans* UA159 biofilms were evaluated via hydrogen peroxide killing assay (n = 8) [38]. Sealant specimens were washed once with 0.1 mol/L glycine (pH 7.0) and placed in 5 mL of the same buffer. After that, hydrogen peroxide was added for a final concentration of 0.2%, and 100-μL aliquots were collected at 0 min, 10 min, 20 min, 30 min, and 45 min after the addition of hydrogen peroxide. Ten microliters of catalase (5 mg/mL) were added to each aliquot to inactivate the hydrogen peroxide immediately after aliquot collection. CFU was determined per Section 4.4.

4.7. Polysaccharide Production

The water-insoluble polysaccharide production in the 48 h *S. mutans* biofilms was measured using a phenol-sulfuric acid method [9] with modifications. Each sealant specimen (n = 6) was rinsed with 2 mL of PBS, transferred to a vial containing 1 mL of PBS, sonicated (Branson 3510-DTH Ultrasonic Cleaner) for 5 min, and vortexed (5 s; maximum speed) to harvest the biofilm. Centrifugation (10,000× g (~10,000 r.c.f.) at 4 °C for 5 min) yielded a precipitate that was rinsed with PBS and resuspended in 1 mL of de-ionized water. Then, 1 mL of 6% (by volume) phenol solution was added to the vial, followed by 5 mL of 95–97% (by volume) sulfuric acid. After 30 min of incubation at 23 °C, 100 μL were transferred to a 96-well plate, and absorbance was measured at OD_{490} using a spectrophotometer. Standard glucose concentrations were used to convert OD readings to polysaccharide concentrations.

4.8. Acid-Neutralizing Activity

The pH of the biofilm growth medium (n = 3) was measured at 0 h, 8 h, 24 h, and 48 h using a digital pH meter (accuracy ± 5%; Accumet XL25, Thermo Fisher Scientific, Waltham, MA, USA). During the experiments, the pH meter was calibrated at regular intervals using commercial standard buffer solutions of pH 4, pH 7, and pH 10 at room temperature.

4.9. Lactic Acid Production

Lactate concentrations were determined using an enzymatic (lactate dehydrogenase) method [33]. After the sealant specimens had incubated for 48 h, each specimen (n = 6) with the attached biofilm was washed in 1.5 mL of cysteine peptone water (by mass: yeast extract 0.5%, peptone 0.1%, sodium chloride 0.85%, cysteine 0.005%), transferred to a new plate containing 1.5 mL of buffered peptone water (BPW) with 0.2% (by mass) sucrose, and incubated for 3 h at 37 °C in 5% CO_2 [37]. The lactic acid concentrations in the BPW solution were then measured based on the absorbance at 340 nm using a spectrophotometer. A standard curve was prepared using lactic acid standard solution (46937; Sigma) [39].

4.10. Confocal Laser Scanning Microscopy

Confocal laser scanning microscopy (CLSM) was performed for qualitative visualization of fully-hydrated, living cultures for two groups of sealants: the experimental control and 5% DMAHDM + 20% NACP. The qualitative approach was chosen to support the microbiological assay results. Biofilms were grown as described apart from the bacterial strain. For imaging, a green fluorescent protein (*gfp*)-expressing strain of *S. mutans* UA159 (*gfp*-UA159) was used in the biofilm model. *Gfp*-UA159 cells continually exhibit green fluorescence throughout growth.

The fluorescence of *gfp*-UA159 48 h biofilms was captured with a Yokogawa Spinning Disk Field Scanning Confocal System (CSU-W1) (Nikon Instruments Inc. Melville, NY, USA) on a Nikon Ti2 inverted microscope (Nikon Instruments Inc. Melville, NY, USA) using a 20× (numerical aperture, 1.00) water immersion objective. Biofilms were imaged four times on two sealant specimens. Biofilm slices in the x-y and x-z planes were collected at random locations on the biofilms.

4.11. Statistical Analysis

All experiments were performed with six to eight repetitions (sealant specimens) in each of three independent experiments. The average of the three experiments per specimen was considered as a statistical unit. The data satisfied the assumption of the equality of variances and normal distribution of errors. Factors included DMAHDM incorporation at two levels (0% and 5%) and NACP incorporation at two levels (0% and 20% NACP). Interactions between these two factors were also considered. To assess the *S. mutans* biofilm biological response, the following dependent variables were analyzed: Log CFU/specimen, metabolic activity, lactic acid production, and exopolysaccharide synthesis. The means and standard deviations (which serve as an estimate of the measurement uncertainty) for the dependable variables were analyzed by two-way ANOVA. Statistical significance was pre-set at $\alpha = 5\%$. All the statistical analyses were performed by SPSS statistics software (IBM version 26, Armonk, NY, USA).

4.12. Disclaimer

Certain commercial equipment, instruments, and materials are identified in this paper in order to specify the experimental procedure. Such identification does not imply recommendation or endorsement by the National Institute of Standards and Technology (NIST), nor does it imply that the material or equipment identified is necessarily the best available for the purpose.

5. Conclusions

S. mutans relies on its virulence-related traits to change oral plaque biofilms and promote the development and increase the severity of carious lesions in children. This study investigated the antibacterial strategy of incorporating 5% DMAHDM into dental sealants containing 20% NACP to reduce virulence and viability of *S. mutans* biofilms. Our findings suggest that sealants with 5% DMAHDM were able to impart a detrimental biological effect on *S. mutans* biofilms by significantly reducing the biofilm formation, metabolic activity, and EPS production. The antibacterial sealants were also able to reduce the aciduricity and the tolerance to oxygen stress. This less virulent phenotype is expected to reflect on the clinical pathogenicity of *S. mutans* and to play a key role in improving the longevity and integrity of dental sealants. Contact-killing strategies via dental materials aiming to prevent or modulate pathogenic biofilms are a promising approach in patients at high risk of caries.

Author Contributions: Conceptualization, M.A.S.M. and H.H.K.X.; Methodology, M.A.S.M., H.H.K.X., M.D.W., A.S.I. and N.J.L.; Investigation, M.S.I.; Analysis and Graphs—M.S.I., A.A.B. and M.A.S.M.; Writing—M.S.I., M.A.S.M. and H.H.K.X.; Writing—Review & Editing, H.H.K.X., N.J.L. and M.A.S.M.; Funding Acquisition, H.H.K.X., and M.A.S.M.; Resources, F.R.T.; M.D.W. and T.W.O.; Supervision, M.D.W. and T.W.O.; Project Administration, H.H.K.X. and M.A.S.M.

Acknowledgments: The authors thank Mary Ann Jabra-Rizk for providing the *gfp*-expressing strain of *S. mutans* and Joseph Mauban for his assistance with the confocal microscopic images. M.S.I acknowledges the scholarship from the Imam AbdulRahman bin Faisal University, Dammam, Saudi Arabia, and the Saudi Arabia Cultural Mission (#428237).

References

1. Manton, D.J. Child dental caries—A global problem of inequality. *EClinicalMedicine* **2018**, *1*, 3–4. [CrossRef] [PubMed]
2. WHO. Sugars and Dental Caries. Available online: http://www.who.int/oral_health/publications/sugars-dental-caries-keyfacts/en/ (accessed on 21 February 2019).
3. Papageorgiou, S.N.; Dimitraki, D.; Kotsanos, N.; Bekes, K.; van Waes, H. Performance of pit and fissure sealants according to tooth characteristics: A systematic review and meta-analysis. *J. Dent.* **2017**, *66*, 8–17. [CrossRef] [PubMed]
4. Wright, J.T.; Crall, J.J.; Fontana, M.; Gillette, E.J.; Nový, B.B.; Dhar, V.; Donly, K.; Hewlett, E.R.; Quinonez, R.B.; Chaffin, J.; et al. Evidence-based clinical practice guideline for the use of pit-and-fissure sealants: A report of the American dental association and the American academy of pediatric dentistry. *J. Am. Dent. Assoc.* **2016**, *147*, 672–682. [CrossRef] [PubMed]
5. Alves, L.S.; Giongo, F.C.M.D.S.; Mua, B.; Martins, V.B.; Barbachan e Silva, B.; Qvist, V.; Maltz, M. A randomized clinical trial on the sealing of occlusal carious lesions: 3–4-year results. *Braz. Oral Res.* **2017**, *31*, e44. [CrossRef] [PubMed]
6. Fontana, M.; Platt, J.A.; Eckert, G.J.; González-Cabezas, C.; Yoder, K.; Zero, D.T.; Ando, M.; Soto-Rojas, A.E.; Peters, M.C. Monitoring of sound and carious surfaces under sealants over 44 months. *J. Dent. Res.* **2014**, *93*, 1070–1075. [CrossRef] [PubMed]
7. Cheng, Y.; Feng, G.; Moraru, C.I. Micro-and nanotopography sensitive bacterial attachment mechanisms: A review. *Front. Microbiol.* **2019**, *10*. [CrossRef] [PubMed]
8. Melo, M.A.S.; Weir, M.D.; Li, F.; Cheng, L.; Zhang, K.; Xu, H.H.K. Control of biofilm at the tooth-restoration bonding interface: A question for antibacterial monomers? A critical review. *Rev. Adhes. Adhes.* **2017**, *5*, 303–324. [CrossRef]

9. Wang, L.; Xie, X.; Imazato, S.; Weir, M.D.; Reynolds, M.A.; Xu, H.H.K. A protein-repellent and antibacterial nanocomposite for class-V restorations to inhibit periodontitis-related pathogens. *Mater. Sci. Eng. C* **2016**, *67*, 702–710. [CrossRef]
10. Inácio, Â.S.; Domingues, N.S.; Nunes, A.; Martins, P.T.; Moreno, M.J.; Estronca, L.M.; Fernandes, R.; Moreno, A.J.M.; Borrego, M.J.; Gomes, J.P.; et al. Quaternary ammonium surfactant structure determines selective toxicity towards bacteria: mechanisms of action and clinical implications in antibacterial prophylaxis. *J. Antimicrob. Chemother.* **2016**, *71*, 641–654. [CrossRef]
11. Melo, M.A.; Orrego, S.; Weir, M.D.; Xu, H.H.K.; Arola, D.D. Designing multiagent dental materials for enhanced resistance to biofilm damage at the bonded interface. *ACS Appl. Mater. Interfac.* **2016**, *8*, 11779–11787. [CrossRef]
12. Melo, M.A.S.; Guedes, S.F.F.; Xu, H.H.K.; Rodrigues, L.K.A. Nanotechnology-based restorative materials for dental caries management. *Trends Biotechnol.* **2013**, *31*, 459–467. [CrossRef] [PubMed]
13. Kuramitsu, H.K.; Wang, B.Y. The whole is greater than the sum of its parts: dental plaque bacterial interactions can affect the virulence properties of cariogenic Streptococcus mutans. *Am. J. Dent.* **2011**, *24*, 153–154. [PubMed]
14. Lin, W.; Yuan, D.; Deng, Z.; Niu, B.; Chen, Q. The cellular and molecular mechanism of glutaraldehyde-didecyldimethylammonium bromide as a disinfectant against Candida albicans. *J. Appl. Microbiol.* **2019**, *126*, 102–112. [CrossRef] [PubMed]
15. Li, J.; Zhao, L.; Wu, Y.; Rajoka, M.S.R. Insights on the ultra high antibacterial activity of positionally substituted 2′-O-hydroxypropyl trimethyl ammonium chloride chitosan: A joint interaction of -NH2 and -N + (CH3)3 with bacterial cell wall. *Colloids Surf. B Biointerf.* **2019**, *173*, 429–436. [CrossRef] [PubMed]
16. Ibrahim, M.S.; AlQarni, F.D.; Al-Dulaijan, Y.A.; Weir, M.D.; Oates, T.W.; Xu, H.H.K.; Melo, M.A.S. Tuning nano-amorphous calcium phosphate content in novel rechargeable Antibacterial dental sealant. *Materials* **2018**, *11*, 1544. [CrossRef] [PubMed]
17. Xiao, J.; Klein, M.I.; Falsetta, M.L.; Lu, B.; Delahunty, C.M.; Yates, J.R.; Heydorn, A.; Koo, H. The exopolysaccharide matrix modulates the interaction between 3D architecture and virulence of a mixed-species oral biofilm. *PLoS Pathog.* **2012**, *8*, e1002623. [CrossRef]
18. Klein, M.I.; Hwang, G.; Santos, P.H.S.; Campanella, O.H.; Koo, H. Streptococcus mutans-derived extracellular matrix in cariogenic oral biofilms. *Front. Cell. Infect. Microbiol.* **2015**, *5*, 10. [CrossRef]
19. Valdez, R.M.A.; Duque, C.; Caiaffa, K.S.; dos Santos, V.R.; de Aguiar Loesch, M.L.; Colombo, N.H.; Arthur, R.A.; de Negrini, T.C.; Boriollo, M.F.G.; Delbem, A.C.B. Genotypic diversity and phenotypic traits of *Streptococcus mutans* isolates and their relation to severity of early childhood caries. *BMC Oral Health* **2017**, *17*, 115. [CrossRef]
20. Krzyściak, W.; Jurczak, A.; Kościelniak, D.; Bystrowska, B.; Skalniak, A. The virulence of *Streptococcus mutans* and the ability to form biofilms. *Eur. J. Clin. Microbiol. Infect. Dis.* **2014**, *33*, 499–515. [CrossRef]
21. Michels, H.T.; Keevil, C.W.; Salgado, C.D.; Schmidt, M.G. From laboratory research to a clinical trial. *HERD* **2015**, *9*, 64–79. [CrossRef]
22. Wu, J.; Zhou, H.; Weir, M.D.; Melo, M.A.S.; Levine, E.D.; Xu, H.H.K. Effect of dimethylaminohexadecyl methacrylate mass fraction on fracture toughness and antibacterial properties of CaP nanocomposite. *J. Dent.* **2015**, *43*, 1539–1546. [CrossRef] [PubMed]
23. Zhou, H.; Li, F.; Weir, M.D.; Xu, H.H.K. Dental plaque microcosm response to bonding agents containing quaternary ammonium methacrylates with different chain lengths and charge densities. *J. Dent.* **2013**, *41*, 1122–1131. [CrossRef] [PubMed]
24. Baker, J.L.; Faustoferri, R.C.; Quivey, R.G. Acid-adaptive mechanisms of *Streptococcus mutans*-the more we know, the more we don't. *Mol. Oral Microbiol.* **2017**, *32*, 107–117. [CrossRef] [PubMed]
25. Len, A.C.L.; Harty, D.W.S.; Jacques, N.A. Stress-responsive proteins are upregulated in *Streptococcus mutans* during acid tolerance. *Microbiology* **2004**, *150*, 1339–1351. [CrossRef] [PubMed]
26. Kajfasz, J.K.; Rivera-Ramos, I.; Abranches, J.; Martinez, A.R.; Rosalen, P.L.; Derr, A.M.; Quivey, R.G.; Lemos, J.A. Two Spx proteins modulate stress tolerance, survival, and virulence in *Streptococcus mutans*. *J. Bacteriol.* **2010**, *192*, 2546–2556. [CrossRef] [PubMed]
27. Kajfasz, J.K.; Ganguly, T.; Hardin, E.L.; Abranches, J.; Lemos, J.A. Transcriptome responses of *Streptococcus mutans* to peroxide stress: Identification of novel antioxidant pathways regulated by Spx. *Sci. Rep.* **2017**, *7*, 16018. [CrossRef] [PubMed]

28. Hwang, G.; Klein, M.I.; Koo, H. Analysis of the mechanical stability and surface detachment of mature *Streptococcus mutans* biofilms by applying a range of external shear forces. *Biofouling* **2014**, *30*, 1079–1091. [CrossRef]
29. Sun, L.; Chow, L.C.; Frukhtbeyn, S.A.; Bonevich, J.E. Preparation and properties of nanoparticles of calcium phosphates with various Ca/P ratios. *J. Res. Natl. Inst. Stand. Technol.* **2010**, *115*, 243–255. [CrossRef]
30. Melo, M.A.S.; Weir, M.D.; Rodrigues, L.K.A.; Xu, H.H.K. Novel calcium phosphate nanocomposite with caries-inhibition in a human in situ model. *Dent. Mater.* **2013**, *29*, 231–240. [CrossRef]
31. Weir, M.D.; Chow, L.C.; Xu, H.H.K. Remineralization of demineralized enamel via calcium phosphate nanocomposite. *J. Dent. Res.* **2012**, *91*, 979–984. [CrossRef]
32. Abou Neel, E.A.; Aljabo, A.; Strange, A.; Ibrahim, S.; Coathup, M.; Young, A.M.; Bozec, L.; Mudera, V. Demineralization-remineralization dynamics in teeth and bone. *Int. J. Nanomed.* **2016**, *11*, 4743–4763. [CrossRef] [PubMed]
33. Wang, H.; Wang, S.; Cheng, L.; Jiang, Y.; Melo, M.A.S.; Weir, M.D.; Oates, T.W.; Zhou, X.; Xu, H.H.K. Novel dental composite with capability to suppress cariogenic species and promote non-cariogenic species in oral biofilms. *Mater. Sci. Eng. C* **2019**, *94*, 587–596. [CrossRef] [PubMed]
34. Wilkosz, N.; Jamróz, D.; Kopeć, W.; Nakai, K.; Yusa, S.I.; Wytrwal-Sarna, M.; Bednar, J.; Nowakowska, M.; Kepczynski, M. Effect of polycation structure on interaction with lipid membranes. *J. Phys. Chem. B* **2017**, *121*, 7318–7326. [CrossRef] [PubMed]
35. Al-Dulaijan, Y.A.; Cheng, L.; Weir, M.D.; Melo, M.A.S.; Liu, H.; Oates, T.W.; Wang, L.; Xu, H.H.K. Novel rechargeable calcium phosphate nanocomposite with antibacterial activity to suppress biofilm acids and dental caries. *J. Dent.* **2018**, *72*, 44–52. [CrossRef] [PubMed]
36. Wang, S.; Zhou, C.; Ren, B.; Li, X.; Weir, M.D.; Masri, R.M.; Oates, T.W.; Cheng, L.; Xu, H.K.H. Formation of persisters in *Streptococcus mutans* biofilms induced by antibacterial dental monomer. *J. Mater. Sci. Mater. Med.* **2017**, *28*, 178. [CrossRef] [PubMed]
37. Al-Qarni, F.D.; Tay, F.; Weir, M.D.; Melo, M.A.S.; Sun, J.; Oates, T.W.; Xie, X.; Xu, H.H.K. Protein-repelling adhesive resin containing calcium phosphate nanoparticles with repeated ion-recharge and re-releases. *J. Dent.* **2018**, *78*, 91–99. [CrossRef] [PubMed]
38. Kim, K.; An, J.S.; Lim, B.S.; Ahn, S.J. Effect of bisphenol a glycol methacrylate on virulent properties of *Streptococcus mutans* UA159. *Caries Res.* **2019**, *53*, 84–95. [CrossRef]
39. Melo, M.A.S.; Cheng, L.; Weir, M.D.; Hsia, R.C.; Rodrigues, L.K.A.; Xu, H.H.K. Novel dental adhesive containing antibacterial agents and calcium phosphate nanoparticles. *J. Biomed. Mater. Res. B Appl. Biomater.* **2013**, *101*, 620 629. [CrossRef]

Localized Delivery of Pilocarpine to Hypofunctional Salivary Glands through Electrospun Nanofiber Mats: An Ex Vivo and In Vivo Study

Sujatha Muthumariappan [1], Wei Cheng Ng [2], Christabella Adine [1], Kiaw Kiaw Ng [1], Pooya Davoodi [2], Chi-Hwa Wang [2] and Joao N. Ferreira [1,3,4,*]

[1] Department of Oral and Maxillofacial Surgery, Faculty of Dentistry, National University of Singapore, Singapore 119085, Singapore; email2sujatha227@gmail.com (S.M.); christabella.adine@u.nus.edu (C.A.); kiawkiaw.ng@gmail.com (K.K.N.)

[2] Department of Chemical and Biomolecular Engineering, National University of Singapore, Singapore 117585, Singapore; weicheng.ng@gmail.com (W.C.N.); davoodi.pooya@u.nus.edu (P.D.); chewch@nus.edu.sg (C.-H.W.)

[3] Faculty of Dentistry, Chulalongkorn University, Bangkok 10330, Thailand

[4] National Institute of Dental and Craniofacial Research, National Institutes of Health, Bethesda, MD 20892-4370, USA

* Correspondence: Joao.F@chula.ac.th

Abstract: Dry mouth or xerostomia is a frequent medical condition among the polymedicated elderly population. Systemic pilocarpine is included in the first line of pharmacological therapies for xerostomia. However, the efficacy of existing pilocarpine formulations is limited due to its adverse side effects and multiple daily dosages. To overcome these drawbacks, a localized formulation of pilocarpine targeting the salivary glands (SG) was developed in the current study. The proposed formulation consisted of pilocarpine-loaded Poly(lactic-*co*-glycolic acid) (PLGA)/poly(ethylene glycol) (PEG) nanofiber mats via an electrospinning technique. The nanofiber mats were fully characterized for their size, mesh porosity, drug encapsulation efficiency, and in vitro drug release. Mat biocompatibility and efficacy was evaluated in the SG organ ex vivo, and the expression of proliferation and pro-apoptotic markers at the cellular level was determined. In vivo short-term studies were performed to evaluate the saliva secretion after acute SG treatment with pilocarpine-loaded nanofiber mats, and after systemic pilocarpine for comparison purposes. The outcomes demonstrated that the pilocarpine-loaded mats were uniformly distributed (diameter: 384 ± 124 nm) in a highly porous mesh, and possessed a high encapsulation efficiency (~81%). Drug release studies showed an initial pilocarpine release of 26% (4.5 h), followed by a gradual increase (~46%) over 15 d. Pilocarpine-loaded nanofiber mats supported SG growth with negligible cytotoxicity and normal cellular proliferation and homeostasis. Salivary secretion was significantly increased 4.5 h after intradermal SG treatment with drug-loaded nanofibers in vivo. Overall, this study highlights the strengths of PLGA/PEG nanofiber mats for the localized daily delivery of pilocarpine and reveals its potential for future clinical translation in patients with xerostomia.

Keywords: electrospinning; nanomaterials; nanofibers; drug delivery; pilocarpine; salivary glands; hypofunction; dry mouth; xerostomia

1. Introduction

Dry mouth syndrome or xerostomia is a common global health problem that arises most commonly within an ageing population [1–3]. At the age of 70, 16% of men and 25% of women report xerostomia symptoms [2]. Xerostomia is mostly triggered by diuretic medication regimens, radiotherapy for head and neck cancers, auto-immune disorders, and uncontrolled diabetes, among other diseases [4,5]. Currently, muscarinic agonists like pilocarpine are the first line of pharmacological therapy for xerostomia [4]. Pilocarpine is only available in oral formulations, which upon ingestion produce significant systemic adverse effects, leading to low tolerability and reducing patient adherence to the drug [6,7]. Furthermore, pilocarpine tablets are contra-indicated in many medical conditions affecting the elderly, including cardiovascular disease, chronic obstructive pulmonary disease, and glaucoma [4,7]. Only half of the patients respond well to pilocarpine tablets, probably due to its short duration of action (3–5 h), requiring multiple daily administrations [8]. To this end, a localized pilocarpine formulation, specifically targeting the SG and bypassing systemic adsorption, is mandatory to make the saliva secretion more long-lasting. A recent double-blind randomized clinical trial showed that 0.1% pilocarpine mouthwash was not more effective than 0.9% saline after four weeks of treatment [9]. However, when pilocarpine dosing is increased to 1–2% in studies using mouthwash, there is a significant increase in salivation and high tolerability due to the absence of adverse side effects [10,11]. Several studies have tested the efficacy of topical pilocarpine administration via mouthwash or oral rinses, but they show contradicting outcomes [8,12], perhaps because pilocarpine mouthwashes only target the minor SG present in the oral mucosa, which are glands that in normal conditions do not significantly contribute to the whole saliva output (<1%) [13]. Major SG located underneath the facial skin should be targeted instead, potentially via an intradermal or transdermal route [14]. To meet this need, a new localized and SG-targeted pilocarpine drug delivery system is needed.

Poly(lactic-*co*-glycolic acid) (PLGA) and poly(ethylene glycol) (PEG) are advantageous materials for use as drug carriers due to their favorable biodegradability and biocompatibility, which ensure safe therapies [15,16]. Various carriers in the form of particles and fiber meshes fabricated in our previous works using electrohydrodynamic atomization (EHDA) techniques have been proven to work effectively for sustained and controlled drug release with hydrophilic drugs like pilocarpine [17,18]. In EHDA, the solution is subjected to high voltage, and the charged droplet disintegrates into fine jets or aerosols in a Taylor cone-like fashion, which upon immediate evaporation of the solvent leads to the formation of the desired solid carriers [19,20]. EHDA can be operated in the electrospraying or electrospinning mode to obtain different products (particles or fibers) of different sizes (microns, sub-microns, etc.) and morphologies, depending on the operating parameters (flow rates, voltage, etc.) and properties of material used (concentration, electrical conductivity, surface tension, viscosity, etc.) [21,22]. For instance, highly concentrated and viscous liquid favors the electrospinning regime to form fibers, as the liquid easily solidifies at the onset of jetting owing to a sufficiently strong elastic network that stabilizes the jet against breakup [22].

In this study, we present a new approach for the localized and controlled delivery of pilocarpine and successfully evaluated it ex vivo and in vivo. The proposed formulation was composed of homogenous pilocarpine-loaded PLGA/PEG nanofiber mats using electrohydrodynamic atomization techniques in electrospinning mode. Next, we aimed to (1) characterize the diameter distribution, porosity and in vitro drug release of this localized nanofiber mat formulation, to (2) evaluate its biocompatibility in ex vivo SG organs, and to (3) compare the in vivo saliva secretion rates of this localized formulation against systemic pilocarpine.

2. Results

2.1. Fabrication of Electrospun Nanofiber Mats

After optimization, it was found that using acetone as the solvent gave the most homogeneous and stable polymer solution/emulsion, compared to other organic solvents tested. At PLGA concentration of <30% (*w*/*v*), the fibers produced were intertwined with unwanted particles. Changes in the collection height and voltage did not significantly change this outcome, though increasing the PLGA concentration from 10% to 25% (*w*/*v*) did augment the ratio of fibers to particles. Only at 30% (*w*/*v*)

PLGA concentration were uniform nanofibers with no more particles consistently observed (Figure 1A), and this was accomplished with electrospinning operating parameters of 0.3 mL/h flow rate, 11.0 kV voltage, and 10 cm height of collection. Our finding was consistent with the literature in that, in general, a lower polymer concentration favors the formation of particles while a higher polymer concentration favors fiber fabrication [23].

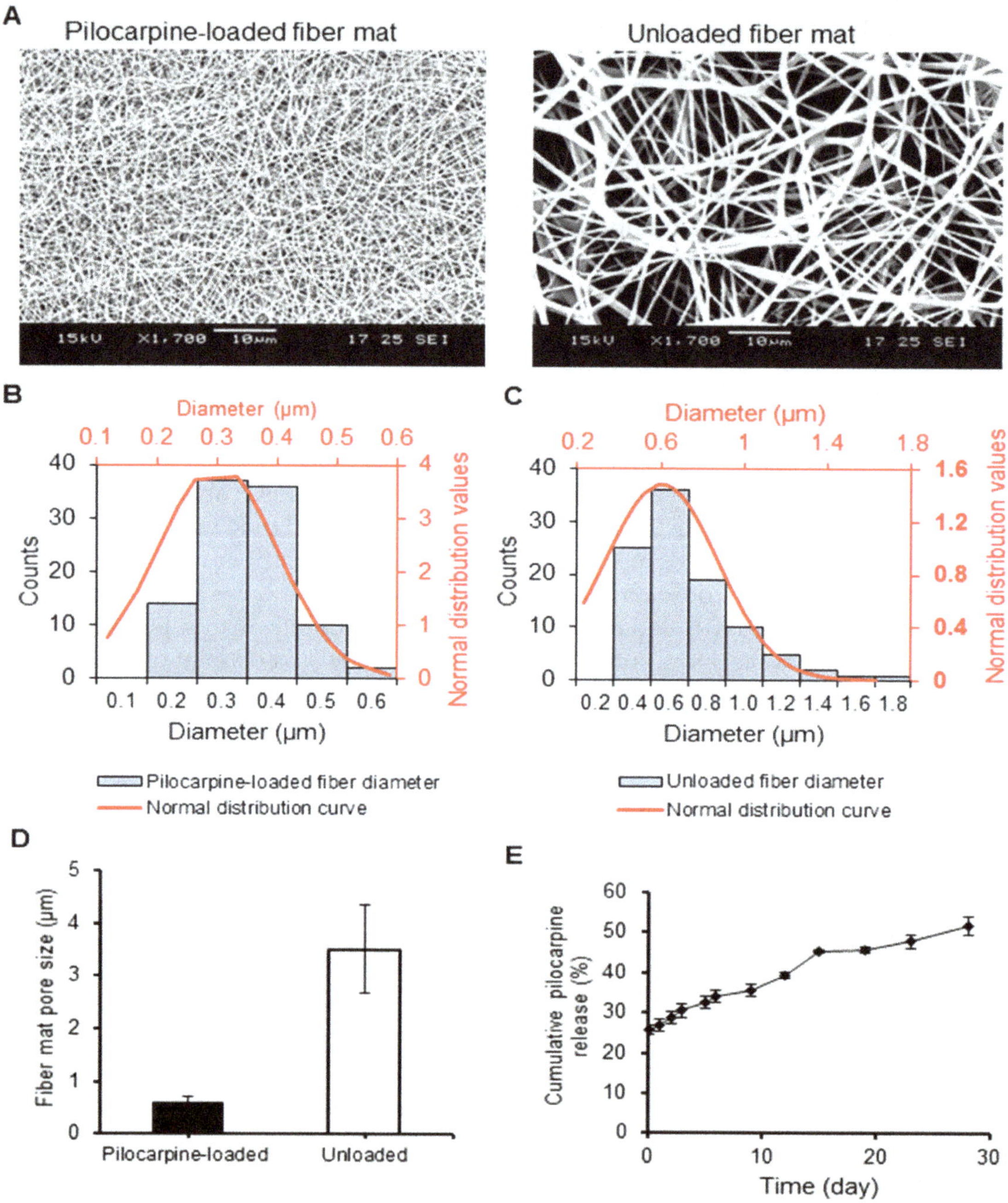

Figure 1. Structural and morphological comparison of pilocarpine-loaded and unloaded PLGA nanofiber mats, and in vitro pilocarpine release profile from pilocarpine-loaded mats. (**A**) Scanning electron microscopy (SEM) images at 1700× magnification. (**B–C**) Diameter distribution of the loaded (left) and unloaded PLGA fiber mats (right). (**D**) Mean porosity distribution of PLGA fiber mats. Error bars represent SD from $n = 10$. (**E**) Cumulative pilocarpine drug release from loaded PLGA nanofibers in the short and long term supported a steady pilocarpine release in vitro. The observed drug release profile was about 26% in the first 4.5 h, and increased steadily to 36% after 9 d, to 45% after 15 d, and to 52% after 28 d. This supports a steady pilocarpine release in vitro. Error bars represent SD from $n = 3$.

2.2. *Physical and Chemical Characterization of Nanofibers*

2.2.1. Scanning Electron Microscopy (SEM)

SEM images of the fabricated PLGA fiber mats (pilocarpine-loaded and unloaded) can be observed in Figure 1A. The average diameter and porosity of the fibers were determined for the loaded and unloaded formulations (Figure 1B,C, respectively). Well-distributed nano-scale fibers were observed for the pilocarpine-loaded fiber mat (diameter 384 ± 124 nm), and submicron fibers for the unloaded fiber formulation (diameter 936 ± 258 nm). The average porosity (pore size) of the pilocarpine-loaded fiber mat was significantly smaller as compared to the unloaded (611 ± 107 nm versus 3510 ± 838 nm) (Figure 1D). The porosity and diameter of the loaded nano-scale fiber mat was uniform as per its limited standard deviation.

2.2.2. Drug Loading Capacity, Encapsulation Efficiency, and Degradation

Next, the drug loading capacity of the loaded PLGA nanofiber mats as well as the encapsulation efficiency was calculated based on spectrophotometry results and standard theoretical formulas mentioned above. The drug loading capacity of the nanofibers was determined to be 0.84 ± 0.09% and the encapsulation efficiency was 81.1 ± 8.4%. For degradation studies of pilocarpine solution in different diluents (MilliQ water and 1× PBS), the optical densities of pilocarpine across a period from 4.5 h to 2 d did not change and were comparable for both diluents (results not shown), which indicates that no drug degradation occurred.

2.3. *Short- and Long-Term In Vitro Pilocarpine Release*

To determine the pilocarpine release from the PLGA nanofiber mats through time, we measured the pilocarpine released into a shaking PBS buffer from 4.5 h up to 28 d. In Figure 1E, the release curve showed an initial burst release of one-fourth of the encapsulated pilocarpine (25.7%) after 4.5 h, followed by a rather gradual and steady release of pilocarpine over time. After 15 d, almost 50% of encapsulated pilocarpine was released. Then, a slight plateau was noted from day 15 to day 19. After day 19, there was only a 6% increase up to day 28.

2.4. *Ex Vivo Studies in Hypofunctional Salivary Glands*

2.4.1. Cytotoxicity and ATP Activity of Pilocarpine

In order to test the cytotoxicity of pilocarpine in the SG organ, we cultured salivary glands ex vivo with media supplemented with this drug (Figure 2A) at a range of clinically relevant therapeutic concentrations, according to previous reports [24,25]. All pilocarpine concentrations, ranging from 0.1 to 20 μg/mL, supported the glandular growth through 48 h (Figure 2B and Figure S1), as well as the cellular metabolism as per stable ATP activity (Figure 2C). This indicated that no major organ cytotoxicity is induced by the pilocarpine solution within this clinical range. Therefore, the loaded nanofibers were fabricated to maximize the amount of pilocarpine up to 20 μg/mL.

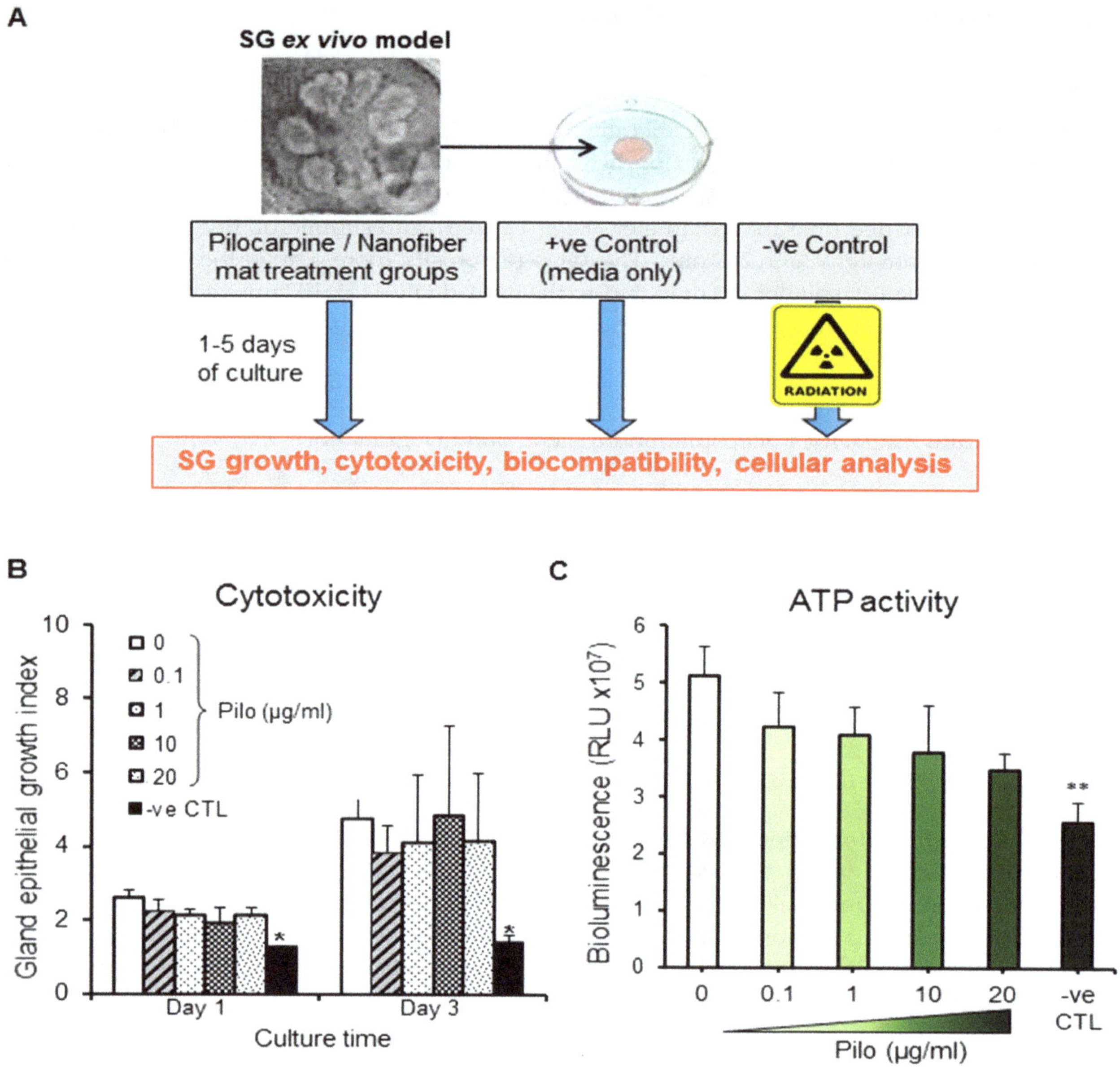

Figure 2. Biological effects in an ex vivo SG model. (**A**) Ex vivo SG model experimental set up used for testing the cytotoxicity of pilocarpine and biocompatibility of different nanofiber mats. (**B**) Glands were treated with therapeutic concentrations of pilocarpine (Pilo) ranging from 0.1 to 20 μg/mL. All gland growth index values at day 1 and 3 were normalized to time 0 (baseline). (**C**) ATP activity (a readout for gland viability) three days after glands were treated with therapeutic concentrations of pilocarpine (0.1–20 μg/mL). Error bars represent SD from $n = 4$. * $p < 0.05$ and ** $p < 0.01$ when compared to positive control without pilocarpine (0 μg/mL). Negative control (-ve CTL) represent glands damaged by gamma radiation.

2.4.2. Biocompatibility of Nanofiber Mats (Loaded and Unloaded)

To test the biocompatibility of the nanofibers, three different nanofiber discs were produced with different diameters and with a maximized concentration of pilocarpine (20 μg/mL), as shown in Figure S1. Then, ex vivo SG were cultured with media supplemented with pilocarpine-loaded and unloaded discs, and gland viability (a readout of epithelial growth) was quantified in the short and long term (Figure 3A,B). There was a steady increase in SG viability and growth in all treatment groups throughout the 5 d of culture. However, the 2 mm pilocarpine-loaded nanofiber mats produced a statistically significant lower gland viability across all culture days as compared to the gland with only media and no treatment provided (+ve CTL).

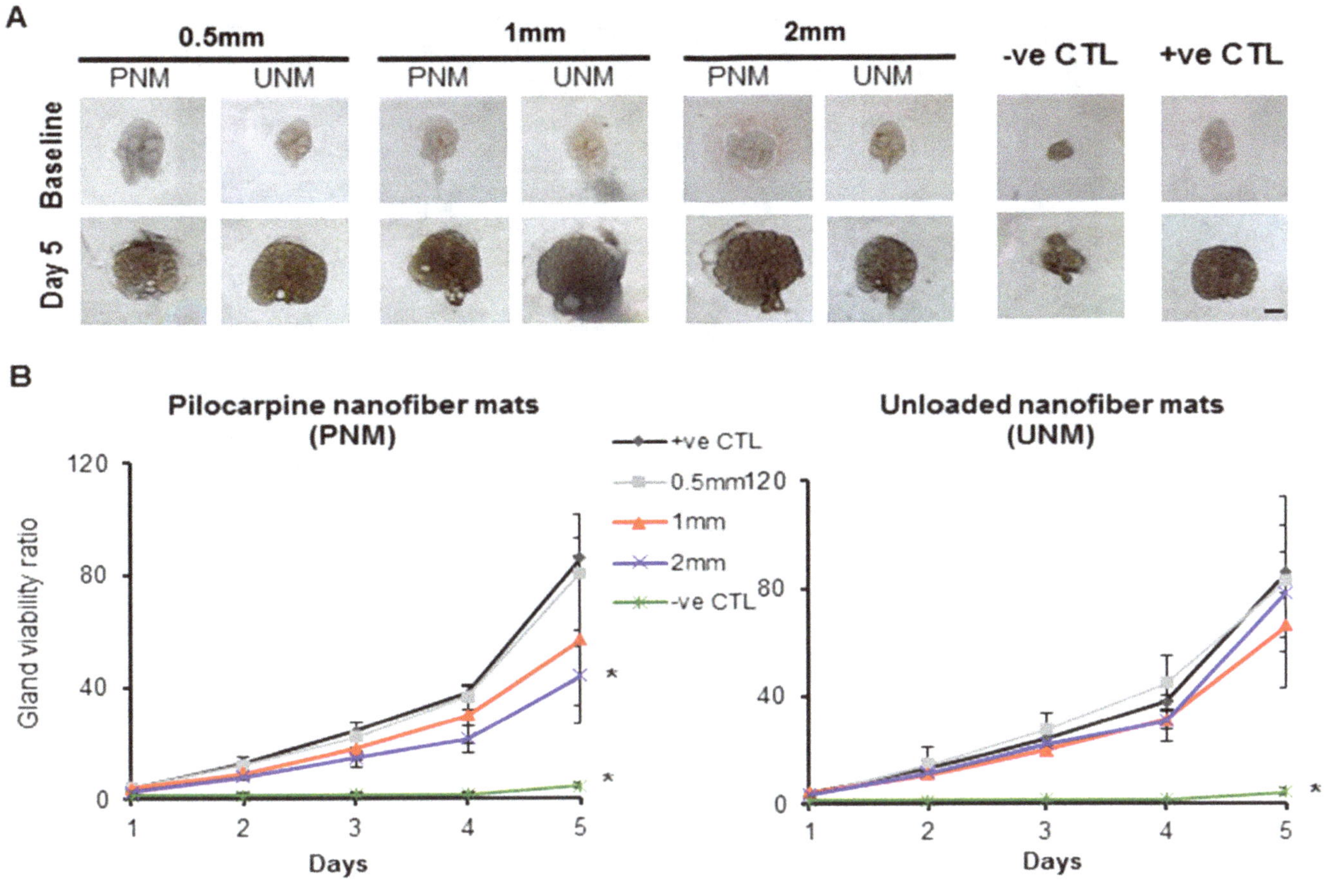

Figure 3. Biocompatibility of pilocarpine-loaded and unloaded nanofiber mats (PNM and UNM, respectively) in the ex vivo SG culture model. (**A**) Bright field images of the growing SG glands at 3.2× magnification. Scale bar: 400 µm. (**B**) SG epithelial viability (readout for organ biocompatibility) was supported by unloaded nanofibers and by 0.5 mm and 1 mm loaded nanofibers. Y axis is a ratio of epithelial bud number at a specific culture time relative to baseline. Error bars represent SD from $n = 4$–12. * $p < 0.05$, when compared to positive control without pilocarpine (+ve CTL) at every culture day; ns: not significant when compared to "+ve CTL". Negative control (-ve CTL) represent glands damaged by gamma radiation. PNM: Pilocarpine nanofiber mats. UNM: unloaded nanofiber mats.

2.4.3. Biological Effects of Pilocarpine-Loaded Nanofiber Mats in SG Cellular Compartments

Next, ex vivo salivary glands treated with pilocarpine-loaded nanofiber mats for 5 d were analyzed for the expression of cellular proliferation/pro-mitotic (Ki67) and pro-apoptotic (cleaved Caspase 3) markers, as seen in Figures 4 and 5, respectively. The Ki67 expression confirmed that the epithelial proliferation significantly decreased, in both the acinar branches and ductal networks, with 2 mm loaded discs (Figures 4 and 5). These cellular-based findings confirmed the outcomes from the previous organ toxicity experiments. As for cleaved Caspase 3, the expression of this pro-apoptotic marker was low (≤0.01%), and no statistical differences were observed between the loaded discs. This suggests that salivary gland pro-apoptosis is grossly absent in the presence of the pilocarpine-loaded mats ranging from 0.5 mm to 2 mm, regardless of the pilocarpine amount in such mats.

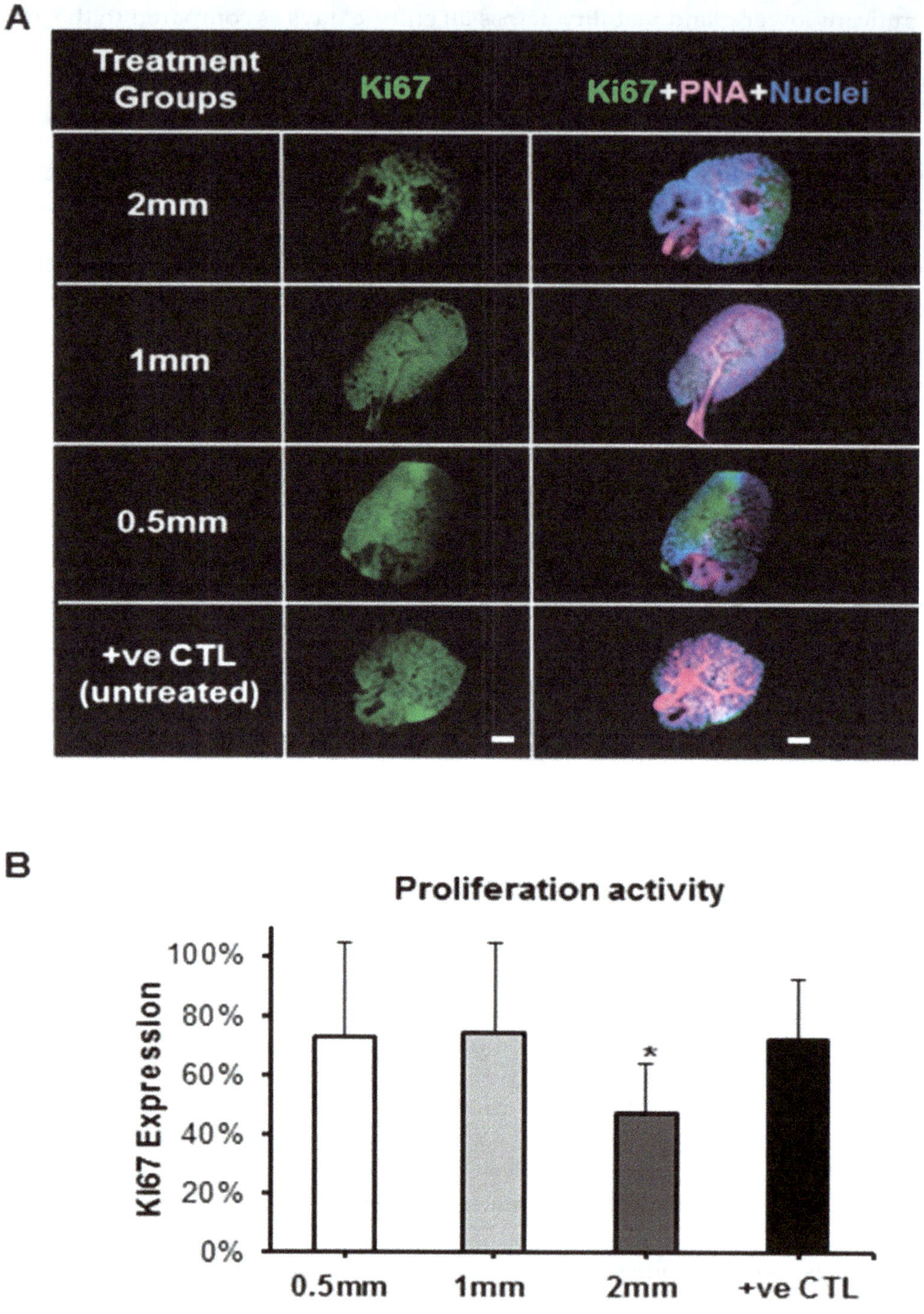

Figure 4. Expression of proliferation protein marker (Ki67) in SG after treatment with pilocarpine nanofiber mats after five culture days in the ex vivo SG model. (**A**) Fluorescence imaging after whole gland immunofluorescence staining showing expression of Ki67 in green (pro-mitotic marker), PNA in pink (peanut agglutinin staining the gland epithelial acini and ductal branched network) and nuclei in blue. (**B**) Expression of proliferation/pro-mitotic activity by quantification of Ki67 fluorescence after normalizing with nuclear counts. Error bars represent SD from $n = 4$. * $p < 0.05$ when compared to positive control. Positive control (+ve CTL) was not treated with nanofiber mats.

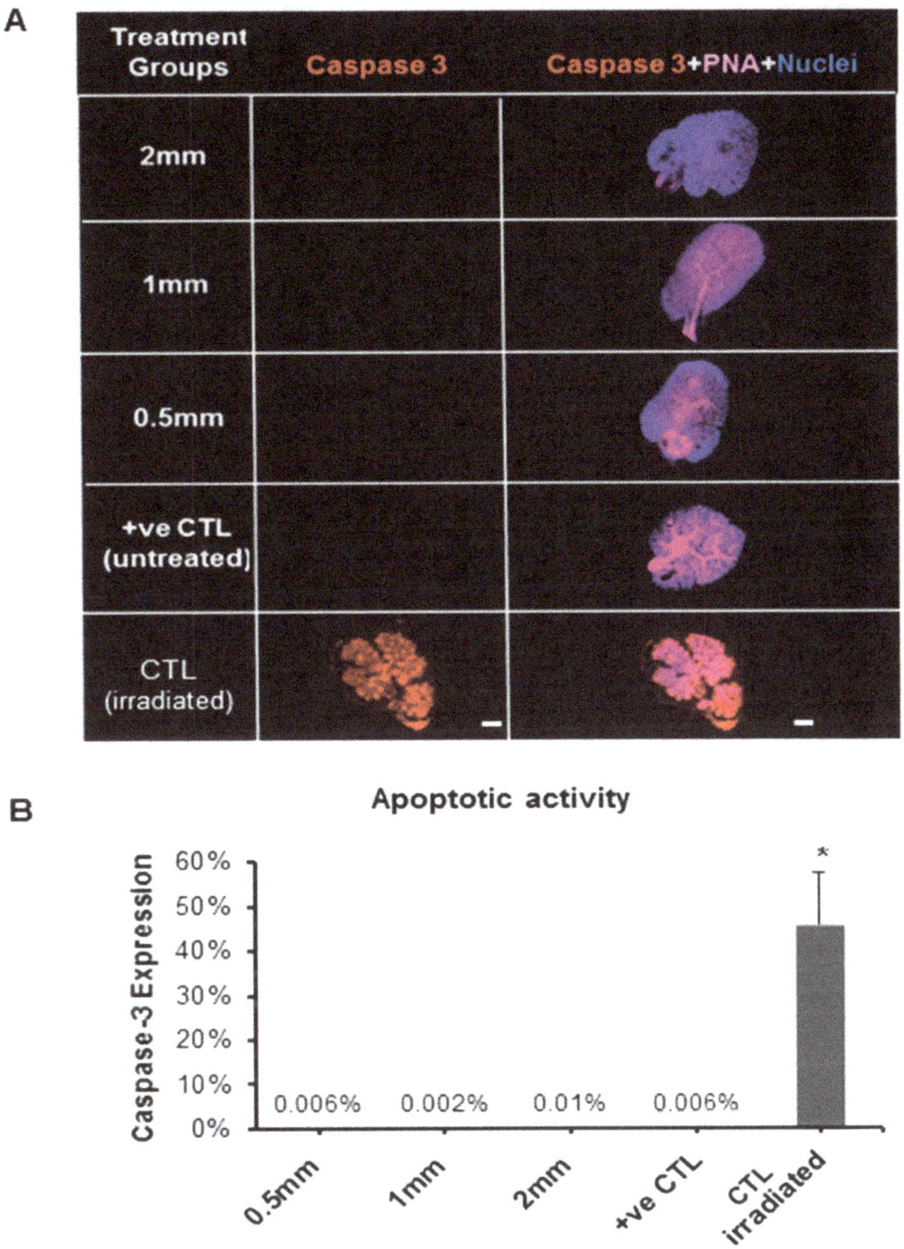

Figure 5. Expression of apoptotic protein marker (Caspase-3) in SG after treatment with pilocarpine nanofiber mats after five culture days in the ex vivo SG model. (**A**) Fluorescence imaging after whole gland immunofluorescence staining showing expression of Caspase-3 in red (apoptotic marker), PNA in pink (staining the gland epithelial acini and ductal branched network) and nuclei in blue. (**B**) Apoptotic activity by quantification of Caspase-3 fluorescence after normalizing with nuclear counts. Error bars represent SD from $n = 4$. * $p < 0.05$ when compared to positive control. Positive control (+ve CTL) was not treated with nanofiber mat and only had growth media. CTL (irradiated): gamma radiation treatment was used as a control for Caspase-3 staining since it induces apoptotic damage to the gland.

2.5. In Vivo Saliva Secretion after Intradermal Treatment with Pilocarpine-Loaded Nanofiber Mats versus Systemic Pilocarpine

Lastly, in vivo hypofunctional SG in an acute model (Figure 6A) were treated with intradermal applications of pilocarpine-loaded nanofiber mats (0.5 mm-diameter mats were selected based on high biocompatibility rates ex vivo) and compared with systemic pilocarpine (oral pilocarpine formulation could be used as per IACUC and mouse model limitations), and the salivary flow rate was determined to test our novel intradermal application formulation on a daily basis for 24 h (Figure 6B). After

4.5 h, SG with intradermal pilocarpine-loaded mats significantly increased the saliva secretion when compared to the systemic pilocarpine (Figure 6B). After 24 h, no difference was noticed between these two treatment formulations (Figure 6B). Furthermore, the whole gland weight was comparable between the two formulations indicating no gross changes in SG composition and cellular content (Figure 6C). Also, no histological differences were found between treatment groups.

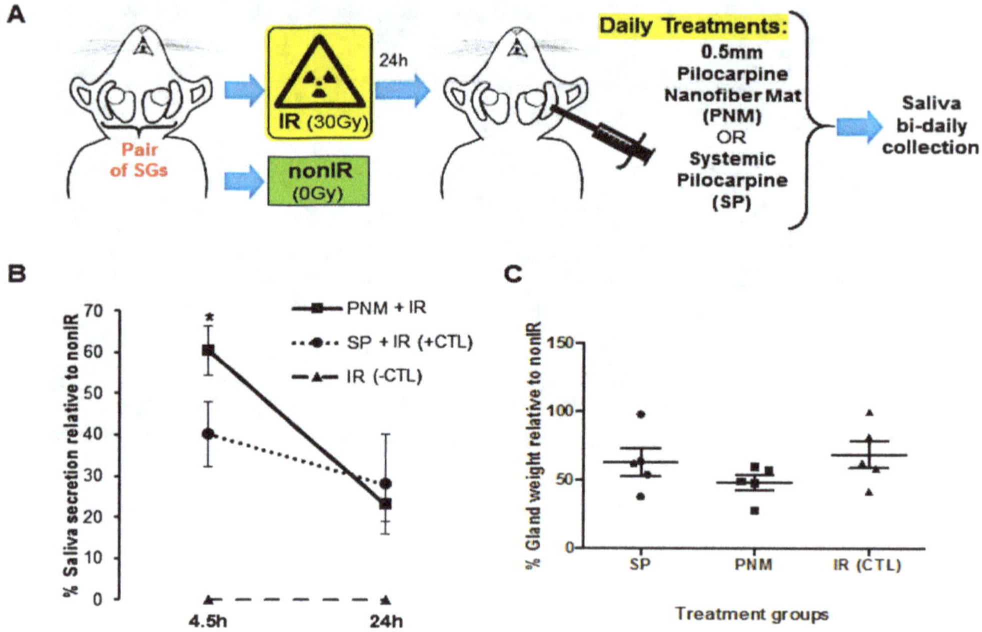

Figure 6. Treatment outcomes during daily intradermal applications of 0.5 mm pilocarpine nanofiber mats versus systemic pilocarpine in an acute in vivo SG model of SG hypofunction. (**A**) Schematic drawing of the in vivo SG hypofunction model to induce acute dry mouth for the daily proposed intradermal treatment with pilocarpine nanofiber mat and conventional systemic administration. (**B**) Saliva secretion rate during the first 24 h after daily intradermal application of 0.5 mm-diameter pilocarpine nanofiber mats (PNM) when compared to systemic pilocarpine (SP). (**C**) Salivary gland weight remained unchanged after intradermal application of 0.5 mm pilocarpine nanofiber mats. Error bars represent SEM from n = 4–5. * $p < 0.05$ when compared to irradiated group with systemic pilocarpine only (SP, which represents the positive CTL). IR: irradiated (negative CTL). nonIR: non-irradiated control group. SGs: salivary glands.

3. Discussion

This study developed a novel localized pilocarpine intradermal drug delivery system supporting the treatment of xerostomia at a greater extent than systemic pilocarpine. Our electrohydrodynamic atomization technique supported the production of a homogenous porous mats with a well-distributed network of electrospun PLGA/PEG nanofibers. Previous ophthalmic pilocarpine formulations used similar ingredients but a double emulsion fabrication method [24]. This latter method facilitated the fabrication of loaded nanoparticles, which possessed a pilocarpine encapsulation efficiency of only 57% as compared to 81.1% with our nanofibers. For double emulsion fabrication method, the chaotic liquid flow in the stirring region often results in spatially non-uniform stress and poor monodispersity, which is known to lead to low encapsulation efficiency [26]. In contrast, such stirring is not required in EHDA, and the fabrication is a one-step process as opposed to two-stage, hence minimizing the loss of drugs. This is also one key feature of the EHDA technique. Unfortunately, the oral/ophthalmic pilocarpine formulations could not be used in our mouse SG hypofunctional model as per local IACUC policies and unpredictable survival outcomes.

The nanofiber mats fabricated herein had a homogenous morphology, consistent diameter and porosity, alike other reports using electrospun fibers (Figure 1A–D) [27–29]. Other methodologies like the dropping method in a study by Kao and colleagues [25] revealed the difficulties in controlling the size of pilocarpine-loaded nanoparticles composed of chitosan and carbopol. In contrast, the nano-scale diameter of our fabricated pilocarpine-loaded mats was achievable with lesser difficulties probably due to salts present in the pilocarpine hydrochloride solution used. These salts might have enhanced the overall solution conductivity leading to nano-scale fiber formation when subjected to high voltage, as compared to the sub-micron scale of unloaded fiber mats [30].

As for the drug release profile (Figure 1E), a biphasic pilocarpine release in our nanofiber mats delivery system could be observed. The first phase consisted of an initial burst release of more than 25% within 4.5 h. This initial burst could be associated with the significant amount of drug just covering the outer surface of the nanofiber mats but not thoroughly encapsulated within, which can be easily solubilized in a favorable hydrophilic media like PBS. This initial burst may facilitate short-term localized and targeted formulations such as transdermal or topical (intra-oral as oral rinses). After 4.5 h, there was a slow and controlled drug release phase for up to 28 d of about 52% of pilocarpine. This secondary release phase may favor pilocarpine applications requiring a longer time in the mouth such as gel formulations to incorporate over stents or dentures.

Outcomes from the ex vivo study (Figures 3–5) revealed that when exposed to fiber mats, the gland cellular compartments were all found at a proliferative/pro-mitotic state with negligible pro-apoptotic activity, indicating that the toxicity of our fiber mats is low and that there is no impairment to the biocompatibility of the SG organ and its cellular compartment. Hence, this had a positive biological impact on the epithelial growth of our SG ex vivo model. These low cytotoxicity findings are also corroborated by other reports using similar materials [25,31].

Current pilocarpine systemic formulations require multiple intakes per day (three times at least) leading to poor patient adherence to this drug formulation [6,8,12]. On the other hand, our localized pilocarpine-loaded nanofiber mats could potentially be used as a single-dose daily formulation containing the therapeutic amount of pilocarpine to enhance saliva secretion when administered locally via an intradermal, as well as through subcutaneous, transdermal or topical applications (e.g., oral rinses or gels for dentures). Our in vivo study is the first comparing localized and systemic pilocarpine formulations for xerostomia (Figure 6). Applying these pilocarpine-loaded nanofiber mats locally via an intradermal route over the in vivo gland could greatly increase the saliva flow rate earlier on (4.5 h) when compared to systemic pilocarpine only (Figure 6B). Furthermore, both in vivo and ex vivo studies confirmed the biocompatibility of the nanofiber mats and supported the gland homeostasis and secretion. These outcomes make this pilocarpine-loaded nanofiber mats promising for clinical use once a day since they can readily increase saliva flow well before 24 h (4.5 h collection time). The long-term effects of these pilocarpine mats are to be explored in different in vivo SG hypofunction models using a clinically relevant radiotherapy fractionated dose regimen. Despite this, acute single-dose radiotherapy SG models, like the one used herein, can better induce epithelial damage promptly within 48 h [32], and are pertinent to study localized short-term effects for our proposed once daily pilocarpine intradermal mat administration. Pre-clinical trials determining the pilocarpine release pharmacokinetics are the next step if intradermal applications are to be tested. If transdermal applications are to be investigated, then further studies are necessary with skin adhesive patches to assess pilocarpine penetration, partitioning, diffusion and permeation properties [14].

4. Materials and Methods

4.1. Fabrication of Electrospun Nanofiber Mats

PLGA (50:50) (Lactel absorbable polymers, Birmingham, MI, USA) with an inherent viscosity of 0.26–0.54 dL/g was dissolved in acetone (VWR Chemicals, Fontenay-sous-Bois cedex, France) at 30% (*w*/*v*) overnight. A pilocarpine 2% solution (Alcon, Vilvoorde, Belgium) and polyethylene glycol-400 (PEG-400, Sigma-Aldrich, St. Louis, MO, USA) were added to the PLGA solution at PLGA: pilocarpine: PEG-400 volume ratio of 1: 0.1: 0.002 and the mixture was then sonicated at 30% amplitude (Vibra-cell

VCX 130, Sonics & Materials, Inc., Newtown, CT, USA) for a minute. For blank (unloaded) formulation, pilocarpine solution was replaced with distilled water. (Note: this final formulation was chosen after numerous rounds of optimization, using different solvents (dichloromethane (DCM), acetone, and ethanol) and mixing ratios/concentrations of each ingredients, to determine the most homogeneous and stable final polymeric solution/emulsion that does not phase separate. PEG known as a good surfactant was added to the solution to help increase the homogeneity and stability of emulsion.

After homogenization, solutions were loaded into a 5-mL syringe and the syringe was connected to the EHDA electrospinning setup to fabricate the fibers. The apparatus setup consisted of a stainless-steel needle/nozzle of inner diameter 0.72 mm (Popper and Sons, Lake Success, NY, USA), a syringe pump (KD Scientific, Holliston, MA, USA) to deliver polymer solution to the nozzle, a high voltage generator (Glassman High Voltage Inc., High Bridge, NJ, USA) to supply voltage to the nozzle via a crocodile clip, and a collecting stage at ground voltage. Upon steady state condition (i.e., the formation of Taylor cone at the tip of the nozzle), fiber sheets were collected in a glass Petri dish that was placed on the collecting stage. The dishes were subsequently wrapped with aluminum foil (since the drug is light-sensitive) and dried overnight in a vacuum oven to remove the residual solvent in the fibers. Next day, single-layer fiber sheets or mats were removed from the dishes and stored at 4 °C until use. Single-layer fiber mats were produced with different diameters (0.5, 1 and 2 mm) using a calibrated cylindrical puncher (Integra Miltex, Dutchess, NY, USA) as displayed in Table S1. This puncher allowed us to uniformly cut the mats to test the ex vivo biological effects with the different amounts/concentrations of biomaterials/pilocarpine, without changing their physical structure, fiber diameter, porosity and thickness.

4.2. Physical and Chemical Characterization of Nanofiber Mats

4.2.1. Scanning Electron Microscopy (SEM)

For SEM imaging, SEM metal stubs were placed directly under the Taylor-cone jet during electrospinning to collect representative fiber mat samples. The metal stubs were then sputter coated with Platinum (JFC-1300, JEOL, Tokyo, Japan) in vacuum at current intensity of 40 mA for 40 s. The coated samples were then viewed under the SEM (JEOL JSM 5600LV, Tokyo, Japan) to visualize the fibers morphology, distribution and pore size. To determine the diameter and porosity of the fibers, Image J software (NIH, Bethesda, MD, USA) was used.

4.2.2. Drug Loading Capacity and Encapsulation Efficiency

For this purpose, 10 mg of both unloaded and drug-loaded fiber mats were separately dissolved with 200 µL of DCM. Fibers were then vortexed for 30 s until full dissolution. Next, 5 mL of distilled water was added to the dissolved fibers, vortexed for 30 s, and centrifuged at 10,000 rpm for 10 min. Afterwards, the fibers were left for 1.5 h to allow for the separation of the organic and aqueous phases. Then, 3 mL of samples were collected from the aqueous phase. The samples were then analyzed for pilocarpine concentration by UV-Vis spectrophotometry (UV 1800, Shimadzu, Japan) at 215 nm (greatest sensitivity and maximum absorbance values; results not shown), with a standard curve having a good linear fitting (R^2 = 0.9965) within the pilocarpine concentration range of 5–40 µg/mL [33]. Unloaded fibers were used as the blank/reference in this analysis. These experiments were conducted in triplicate. Drug loading capacity was calculated using the following formula: (drug weight/(drug weight + PLGA weight + PEG-400 weight)) × 100%. The encapsulation efficiency (*EE*) was quantified using the following formula as per previous report (Kao, Lin et al. 2006): *EE* = [(Total pilocarpine-Free pilocarpine amount)/Total pilocarpine amount)] × 100%.

4.2.3. Degradation Studies for the Pilocarpine Solution

The pilocarpine solution was tested for degradation in diluents such as 1× phosphate buffered saline (PBS) and ultra-pure water (MilliQ water, Sigma-Aldrich, Saint Louis, MO, USA) as this is essential to validate the drug release experiments in vitro [33,34]. For this purpose, pilocarpine solution was dissolved in 5 mL MilliQ water and 1x PBS to have a final concentration of 40 µg/mL. Solutions were vortexed for 30 s and placed in the rotary incubator at 37 °C, 100 rpm. At pre-determined time intervals (4.5 h, 1 d, 2 d), 3 mL of the drug solutions (in the different diluents) were drawn and analyzed within a wavelength ranging from 200 nm to 300 nm in the UV-Vis spectrophotometer. Reference samples of pure MilliQ water and 1× PBS only were used to blank the pilocarpine containing solutions.

4.3. Pilocarpine Drug Release Analysis from Loaded Nanofiber Mats

Fabricated nanofiber mats (pilocarpine-loaded and unloaded) weighing 20 mg each were used to analyze the drug release in vitro in the short and long term. Then, 20 mg fibers were placed in 4 mL of 1× PBS (pH 7.4) in 15-mL Falcon tubes. Tubes were vortexed for 30 s and placed in an orbital shaker bath (GFLVR 1092, Burgwedel, Germany) at 37 °C, 100 rpm. At pre-determined time intervals (4.5 h, and 1, 2, 3, 5, 6, 9, 12, 15, 19, 23, and 28 d), the tubes were subjected to centrifugation at 10,000 rpm for 10 min. After centrifugation, the supernatant (3.3 mL) was carefully collected from each tube into a new tube and stored at −20 °C for further pilocarpine quantification. Fresh 1× PBS (3.3 mL) was then added to the original sample tubes, vortexed for 30 s and placed back in the incubator. This procedure was repeated for all collection time points. Three biological replicates were run for both unloaded and loaded nanofibers for each time point. The pilocarpine concentration in the collected samples was again measured by UV-Vis spectrophotometer as described above. For each collection time point, the average absorbance readings of the unloaded nanofiber were subtracted from each of the loaded nanofibers, and then these were added up to calculate the cumulative drug release since the first collection time at 4.5 h.

4.4. Ex Vivo SG Organ Culture Studies

4.4.1. SG Organ Culture Model

Pregnant ICR mice were used as per the approved National University of Singapore IACUC protocol no. 2014-00306. Mice at embryonic day 15, after epithelial differentiation occurs to become an adult organ, were selected. Major salivary glands including submandibular and sublingual glands were isolated from ICR mouse embryos using a microdissection technique under a stereozoom microscope (M80, Leica, Wetzlar, Germany) as per previous reports [35,36]. The glands were then placed onto polycarbonate filter papers (Whatman™ Nuclepore™ Track-Etched Polycarbonate Membrane Filter, Sigma-Aldrich, Saint Louis, MO, USA). A growth medium was added (200 µL per culture plate), which was composed of DMEM/F12 media, penicillin-streptomycin (1% *v*/*v*), vitamin C (0.2% *v*/*v*), and transferrin (0.02% *v*/*v*) (Thermo Fisher Scientific, Waltham, MA, USA). Four whole salivary glands were cultured per treatment group and incubated at 37 °C with 5% CO_2.

4.4.2. Cytotoxicity of Pilocarpine

The gland growth media of the ex vivo organ culture was supplemented with clinically relevant concentrations of pilocarpine ranging from 0.1 to 25 µg/mL. The cultures were then incubated as previously. Epithelial cellular growth was analyzed at baseline (t_0), day 1 and day 3 by taking bright field microscopy images at 3.2× magnification with the above stereozoom microscope set up. The total number of epithelial buds per gland was quantified from those images using Image J (NIH). The growth index for each gland was determined by normalizing the number of epithelial buds at day 1 and day 3 to the ones at baseline [36]. The growth index was used as a readout for organ cytoxicity. The positive control glands were those grown with the growth media only (without pilocarpine supplementation). The negative control glands were glands subjected to cytotoxic damage by gamma rays (7 Gy dosage) at baseline.

4.4.3. Biocompatibility of Nanofiber Mats

Punched nanofiber mats measuring 0.5, 1, and 2 mm were sterilize d under UV light for at least 6 h before utilization. To test the biocompatibility, mats were added to the growth media in the ex vivo SG organ cultures. These cultures were incubated for 5 d, and at each day, the viability index that measures epithelial cellular growth was determined for each gland as described above. Same positive and negative controls glands were used as before. Unloaded discs were used to make sure the unloaded nanofibers by itself are not causing any organ cytotoxicity. Three independent biological experiments were performed and four whole glands were used for each experiment.

4.4.4. Salivary Gland Cellular Analysis for Proliferation and Apoptotic Activity

Whole-mount immunofluorescence staining was used to evaluate and quantify the proliferative and apoptotic cell subpopulations in the ex vivo SG organ culture according to previous protocols [25,26]. Briefly, whole SG treated for 5 d with loaded nanofibers discs (0.5, 1, 2 mm in diameter) from the previous experiments were fixed in 4% paraformaldehyde followed by 1× PBS washing steps. Then, fixed glands were permeabilized, and blocked using 10% donkey serum and 5% bovine serum albumin for 2 h. This was followed by overnight incubation at 4 °C with primary antibodies anti-Ki67 (1:200 dilution, Cat no. 556003, BD Pharmingen, San Jose, CA, USA) and anti-cleaved Caspase 3 (1:200 dilution, Cat no. 9664S, Cell Signalling, Danvers, MA, USA). After washing, incubation with respective secondary antibodies followed (1:200 dilution, Alexa Fluor 488 and Alexa Fluor 635, Thermo Fisher Scientific). Rhodamine-labelled peanut agglutinin (1:200 dilution, Vector Lab, Burlingame, CA, USA) was used to stain the acinar and ductal branched epithelial structures of each gland. A nuclear fluorescent dye (Hoechst 33342, Invitrogen, Carlsbad, CA, USA) was used to counterstain the nuclei. Whole glands were then mounted on glass slides in resin mounting media using spacers to avoid gland crushing by glass slide. Slides were visualized, scanned and analyzed with Leica DMI-8 fluorescence microscope with a z-motorized axis and Leica LAS-X software (Leica Microsystems, Wetzlar, Germany) to obtain a z-stack of images for each gland with 20 μm z-steps. Maximum intensity projections were further produced at 10× and 20× magnifications. Automated cell counts for each gland z-stack were done using Image J (NIH, USA) for immuno-fluorescently labeled Ki-67+ and Caspase 3+ cells, and for all cells stained with the nuclear dye. Ki-67+ and Caspase 3+ cell counts for each gland were normalized to the total number of cells (stained with the nuclear dye).

4.5. In Vivo SG Hypofunctional Model

To generate hypofunctional SG with xerostomia measurable signs, a single acute dose of gamma radiation (30 Gy) was given to eight-week-old C57BL/6 mice as per a published protocol [37]. This protocol was approved by the National University of Singapore IACUC application no. 2014-00306. All in vivo experiments complied with the ARRIVE guidelines and were carried out in accordance with the National Institutes of Health guide for the care and use of laboratory animals (NIH Publications No. 8023, revised 1978). Animals were housed in a climate- and light-controlled environment and allowed free access to food and water at the bottom of the cage. One day after radiation was delivered, our localized pilocarpine nanofiber formulation was administered over the submandibular glands (via an intradermal route) and compared with systemic pilocarpine (via an intraperitoneal route, Sigma). The oral pilocarpine clinical formulation (available in the market) could not be given according to the IACUC committee, due to the unpredictability and life-threatening adverse side effects in rodents. The following experimental mouse groups were tested on a daily basis as per the acute SG dry mouth model: (A) Non-irradiated control (nonIR, n = 3); (B) Irradiated control (IR, n = 5); (C) Irradiated and treated daily with 0.5 mm diameter pilocarpine-loaded nanofibers (PNM, n = 5), the ones that performed effectively in the ex vivo biocompatibility tests; (D) Irradiated and treated daily with systemic pilocarpine as a positive/conventional control treatment (SP, n = 5). Intraperitoneal ketamine (10 mg/mL) and xylazine (1 mg/mL) were administered before the treatment was delivered to minimize animal discomfort. As for the nanofiber composition and formulation, the sterilized ones used in the abovementioned ex vivo studies were administered here: first these were placed in a syringe vessel with a 21G needle, and a sterile PBS 1× solution was added as a vehicle.

Whole stimulated saliva was collected at 4.5 h and 24 h after nanofiber administration. Saliva was extracted by capillarity every 3 min for 15 min using a 75-mm hematocrit tube (Drummond, Scientific Company, Broomall, PA, USA) [38]. These tubes were then placed in 1.5-mL pre-weight Eppendorf tubes, which were then weighed to determine the saliva secretion rate. To determine the percentage of secreted saliva relative to the control (NonIR), the saliva secretion rate was normalized to the average of saliva secreted by the NonIR group. Submandibular glands were surgically removed and freshly dissected in a stereozoom microscope and their weight was measured before fixation. Glands were then fixed with paraformaldehyde 4% overnight at 4 °C in a rotating shaker, followed by several washing steps with PBS and incubation with 30% cold sucrose (w/v) solution in 0.01 M PBS for 3–4 d. Then, after paraffin embedding, 4-μm gland sections were made and stained with hematoxylin and eosin and visualized with bright-field microscopy at 20–40× magnification.

4.6. Statistical Analysis

Data are presented as mean ± standard deviation (SD) from 3–12 independent samples, except for the in vivo experiments, where the standard error of the mean (SEM) was used. All statistical analyses were conducted using Prism version 6 (GraphPad Software, Inc., San Diego, CA, USA). All datasets were tested for normality. Student t-tests were performed for two-group comparison: unpaired with Welch correction for in vivo study outcomes, or paired for time-dependent experiments for drug release profile experiments. A one-way ANOVA with Dunnet post hoc tests for comparison of three or more experimental groups with a positive control for the case of ex vivo studies. The significance level for all experiments was set at $p < 0.05$.

5. Conclusions

In this study, the ultimate aim was to determine whether an intradermal pilocarpine-loaded PLGA/PEG nanofiber mat can be utilized to release pilocarpine while supporting the SG organ viability and stimulating saliva secretion.

The intradermal pilocarpine-loaded nanofiber mats ranging from 0.5 to 1 mm diameter induced the highest SG growth and cell proliferation with negligible cytotoxicity (apoptosis) in ex vivo SG models. In the acute dry mouth in vivo model, the daily intradermal application of 0.5 mm diameter pilocarpine-loaded nanofiber mats stimulated a higher saliva secretion before 24 h as compared to the conventional systemic pilocarpine. After 24 h, saliva secretion was comparable to systemic pilocarpine.

Thus, this pilocarpine delivery system is promising for potential clinical use as an intradermal formulation for the early and prompt treatment of xerostomia before and after 24 h of application. These formulations will be particularly useful in patients who have poor saliva secretion with conventional saliva stimulants.

Author Contributions: Conceptualization, P.D., C.-H.W. and J.N.F.; Methodology, W.C.N., P.D. and J.F; Validation, P.D., C.-H.W. and J.N.F.; Formal Analysis, S.M. and W.N.; Investigation, S.M., C.A., and K.K.N.; Resources, C.H.W. and J.N.F.; Data Curation, J.N.F.; Writing—Original Draft Preparation, S.M., W.C.N. and J.N.F.; Writing—Review & Editing, C.A., K.K.N., P.D., C.-H.W. and J.N.F.; Visualization, S.M., W.C.N., and J.N.F.; Supervision, C.A., K.K.N., P.D., and J.N.F.; Project Administration, J.N.F.; Funding Acquisition, C.-H.W. and J.N.F.

Acknowledgments: We thank Bruce Baum (National Institutes of Health) for his critical reading.

References

1. Barbe, A.G.; Bock, N.; Derman, S.H.; Felsch, M.; Timmermann, L.; Noack, M.J. Self-assessment of oral health, dental health care and oral health-related quality of life among Parkinson's disease patients. *Gerodontology* **2017**, *34*, 135–143. [CrossRef] [PubMed]
2. Gil-Montoya, J.A.; Barrios, R.; Sanchez-Lara, I.; Carnero-Pardo, C.; Fornieles-Rubio, F.; Montes, J.; Gonzalez-Moles, M.A.; Bravo, M. Prevalence of Drug-Induced Xerostomia in Older Adults with Cognitive Impairment or Dementia: An Observational Study. *Drugs Aging* **2016**, *33*, 611–618. [CrossRef] [PubMed]
3. Pajukoski, H.; Meurman, J.H.; Halonen, P.; Sulkava, R. Prevalence of subjective dry mouth and burning mouth in hospitalized elderly patients and outpatients in relation to saliva, medication, and systemic diseases. *Oral Surg. Oral Med. Oral Pathol. Oral Radiol. Endod.* **2001**, *92*, 641–649. [CrossRef] [PubMed]
4. Gil-Montoya, J.A.; Silvestre, F.J.; Barrios, R.; Silvestre-Rangil, J. Treatment of xerostomia and hyposalivation in the elderly: A systematic review. *Med. Oral Patol. Oral Cir. Bucal* **2016**, *21*, e355–e366. [CrossRef] [PubMed]
5. Napenas, J.J.; Brennan, M.T.; Fox, P.C. Diagnosis and treatment of xerostomia (dry mouth). *Odontology* **2009**, *97*, 76–83. [CrossRef] [PubMed]
6. Noaiseh, G.; Baker, J.F.; Vivino, F.B. Comparison of the discontinuation rates and side-effect profiles of pilocarpine and cevimeline for xerostomia in primary Sjogren's syndrome. *Clin. Exp. Rheumatol.* **2014**, *32*, 575–577. [PubMed]
7. Hendrickson, R.G.; Morocco, A.P.; Greenberg, M.I. Pilocarpine toxicity and the treatment of xerostomia. *J. Emerg. Med.* **2004**, *26*, 429–432. [CrossRef]
8. Davies, A.N.; Thompson, J. Parasympathomimetic drugs for the treatment of salivary gland dysfunction due to radiotherapy. *Cochrane Database Syst. Rev.* **2015**, *10*, CD003782. [CrossRef]
9. Kim, J.H.; Ahn, H.J.; Choi, J.H.; Jung, D.W.; Kwon, J.S. Effect of 0.1% pilocarpine mouthwash on xerostomia: Double-blind, randomised controlled trial. *J. Oral Rehabil.* **2014**, *41*, 226–235. [CrossRef]
10. Bernardi, R.; Perin, C.; Becker, F.L.; Ramos, G.Z.; Gheno, G.Z.; Lopes, L.R.; Pires, M.; Barros, H.M. Effect of pilocarpine mouthwash on salivary flow. *Braz. J. Med. Biol. Res.* **2002**, *35*, 105–110. [CrossRef]
11. Tanigawa, T.; Yamashita, J.; Sato, T.; Shinohara, A.; Shibata, R.; Ueda, H.; Sasaki, H. Efficacy and safety of pilocarpine mouthwash in elderly patients with xerostomia. *Spec. Care Dentist.* **2015**, *35*, 164–169. [CrossRef] [PubMed]
12. Spivakovsky, S.; Spivakovsky, Y. Parasympathomimetic drugs for dry mouth due to radiotherapy. *Evid. Based Dent.* **2016**, *17*, 79. [CrossRef] [PubMed]
13. Atkinson, J.C.; Baum, B.J. Salivary enhancement: Current status and future therapies. *J. Dent. Educ.* **2001**, *65*, 1096–1101.
14. Alkilani, A.Z.; McCrudden, M.T.; Donnelly, R.F. Transdermal Drug Delivery: Innovative Pharmaceutical Developments Based on Disruption of the Barrier Properties of the stratum corneum. *Pharmaceutics* **2015**, *7*, 438–470. [CrossRef] [PubMed]
15. Dhar, S.; Gu, F.X.; Langer, R.; Farokhzad, O.C.; Lippard, S.J. Targeted delivery of cisplatin to prostate cancer cells by aptamer functionalized Pt(IV) prodrug-PLGA-PEG nanoparticles. *Proc. Natl. Acad. Sci. USA* **2008**, *105*, 17356–17361. [CrossRef] [PubMed]
16. Bi, Y.; Liu, L.; Lu, Y.; Sun, T.; Shen, C.; Chen, X.; Chen, Q.; An, S.; He, X.; Ruan, C.; et al. T7 Peptide-Functionalized PEG-PLGA Micelles Loaded with Carmustine for Targeting Therapy of Glioma. *ACS Appl. Mater. Interfaces* **2016**, *8*, 27465–27473. [CrossRef]
17. Ranganath, S.H.; Fu, Y.; Arifin, D.Y.; Kee, I.; Zheng, L.; Lee, H.S.; Chow, P.K.; Wang, C.H. The use of submicron/nanoscale PLGA implants to deliver paclitaxel with enhanced pharmacokinetics and therapeutic efficacy in intracranial glioblastoma in mice. *Biomaterials* **2010**, *31*, 5199–5207. [CrossRef]
18. Davoodi, P.; Ng, W.C.; Yan, W.C.; Srinivasan, M.P.; Wang, C.H. Double-Walled Microparticles-Embedded Self-Cross-Linked, Injectable, and Antibacterial Hydrogel for Controlled and Sustained Release of Chemotherapeutic Agents. *ACS Appl. Mater. Interfaces* **2016**, *8*, 22785–22800. [CrossRef]
19. Feng, F.; Neoh, K.Y.; Davoodi, P.; Wang, C.H. Coaxial double-walled microspheres for combined release of cytochrome c and doxorubicin. *J. Control Release* **2017**, *259*, e30–e31. [CrossRef]
20. Davoodi, P.; Srinivasan, M.P.; Wang, C.H. Effective Co-delivery of Nutlin-3a and p53 genes via Core-shell Microparticles for Disruption of MDM2-p53 Interaction and Reactivation of p53 in Hepatocellular Carcinoma. *J. Mater. Chem. B* **2017**, *5*, 5816–5834. [CrossRef]

21. Xie, J.; Jiang, J.; Davoodi, P.; Srinivasan, M.P.; Wang, C.H. Electrohydrodynamic atomization: A two-decade effort to produce and process micro-/nanoparticulate materials. *Chem. Eng. Sci.* **2015**, *125*, 32–57. [CrossRef] [PubMed]
22. Davoodi, P.; Feng, F.; Xu, Q.; Yan, W.C.; Tong, Y.W.; Srinivasan, M.P.; Sharma, V.K.; Wang, C.H. Coaxial electrohydrodynamic atomization: Microparticles for drug delivery applications. *J. Control. Release* **2015**, *205*, 70–82. [CrossRef] [PubMed]
23. Xie, J.; Tan, R.S.; Wang, C.H. Biodegradable microparticles and fiber fabrics for sustained delivery of cisplatin to treat C6 glioma in vitro. *J. Biomed. Mater. Res. A* **2008**, *85*, 897–908. [CrossRef] [PubMed]
24. Nair, K.L.; Vidyanand, S.; James, J.; Kumar, G.S.V. Pilocarpine-loaded poly (DL-lactic-co-glycolic acid) nanoparticles as potential candidates for controlled drug delivery with enhanced ocular pharmacological response. *J. Appl. Polym. Sci.* **2012**, *124*, 2030–2036. [CrossRef]
25. Kao, H.J.; Lin, H.R.; Lo, Y.L.; Yu, S.P. Characterization of pilocarpine-loaded chitosan/Carbopol nanoparticles. *J. Pharm. Pharmacol.* **2006**, *58*, 179–186. [CrossRef] [PubMed]
26. Yuan, Q.C.; Williams, R.A. Precision emulsification for droplet and capsule production. *Adv. Powder Technol.* **2014**, *25*, 122–135. [CrossRef]
27. Chua, K.N.; Chai, C.; Lee, P.C.; Tang, Y.N.; Ramakrishna, S.; Leong, K.W.; Mao, H.Q. Surface-aminated electrospun nanofibers enhance adhesion and expansion of human umbilical cord blood hematopoietic stem/progenitor cells. *Biomaterials* **2006**, *27*, 6043–6051. [CrossRef]
28. Blakney, A.K.; Little, A.B.; Jiang, Y.; Woodrow, K.A. In vitro-ex vivo correlations between a cell-laden hydrogel and mucosal tissue for screening composite delivery systems. *Drug. Deliv.* **2016**, *24*, 582–590. [CrossRef] [PubMed]
29. Zeng, J.; Xu, X.; Chen, X.; Liang, Q.; Bian, X.; Yang, L.; Jing, X. Biodegradable electrospun fibers for drug delivery. *J. Control Release* **2003**, *92*, 227–231. [CrossRef]
30. Choi, J.S.; Lee, S.W.; Jeong, L.; Bae, S.H.; Min, B.C.; Youk, J.H.; Park, W.H. Effect of organosoluble salts on the nanofibrous structure of electrospun poly (3-hydroxybutyrate-co-3-hydroxyvalerate). *Int. J. Biol. Macromol.* **2004**, *34*, 249–256. [CrossRef]
31. Han, F.; Zhang, H.; Zhao, J.; Zhao, Y.; Yuan, X. Diverse release behaviors of water-soluble bioactive substances from fibrous membranes prepared by emulsion and suspension electrospinning. *J. Biomater. Sci. Polym. Ed.* **2013**, *24*, 1244–1259. [CrossRef] [PubMed]
32. Varghese, J.J.; Schmale, I.L.; Mickelsen, D.; Hansen, M.E.; Newlands, S.D.; Benoit, D.S.W.; Korshuno, V.A.; Ovitt, C.E. Localized Delivery of Amifostine Enhances Salivary Gland Radioprotection. *J. Dent. Res.* **2018**, *97*, 1252–1259. [CrossRef] [PubMed]
33. Agban, Y.; Lian, J.; Prabakar, S.; Seyfoddin, A.; Rupenthal, I.D. Nanoparticle cross-linked collagen shields for sustained delivery of pilocarpine hydrochloride. *Int. J. Pharm.* **2016**, *501*, 96–101. [CrossRef] [PubMed]
34. Saleh, N.; Al-Handawi, M.B.; Al-Kaabi, L.; Ali, L.; Salman Ashraf, S.; Thiemann, T.; Al-Hindawi, B.; Meetani, M. Intermolecular interactions between cucurbit [7]uril and pilocarpine. *Int. J. Pharm.* **2014**, *460*, 53–62. [CrossRef] [PubMed]
35. Adine, C.; Ng, K.K.; Rungarunlert, S.; Souza, G.R.; Ferreira, J.N. Engineering innervated secretory epithelial organoids by magnetic three-dimensional bioprinting for stimulating epithelial growth in salivary glands. *Biomaterials* **2018**, *180*, 52–66. [CrossRef] [PubMed]
36. Ferreira, J.N.; Zheng, C.; Lombaert, I.M.A.; Goldsmith, C.M.; Cotrim, A.P.; Symonds, J.M.; Patel, V.N.; Hoffman, M.P. Neurturin Gene Therapy Protects Parasympathetic Function to Prevent Irradiation-Induced Murine Salivary Gland Hypofunction. *Mol. Ther. Methods Clin. Dev.* **2018**, *23*, 172–180. [CrossRef]
37. Lin, A.L.; Johnson, D.A.; Wu, Y.; Wong, G.; Ebersole, J.L.; Yeh, C.K. Measuring short-term gamma-irradiation effects on mouse salivary gland function using a new saliva collection device. *Arch. Oral Biol.* **2001**, *46*, 1085–1089. [CrossRef]
38. Baum, B.J.; Afione, S.; Chiorini, J.A.; Cotrim, A.P.; Goldsmith, C.M.; Zheng, C. Gene Therapy of Salivary Diseases. *Methods Mol. Biol.* **2017**, *1537*, 107–123. [PubMed]

Permissions

All chapters in this book were first published by MDPI; hereby published with permission under the Creative Commons Attribution License or equivalent. Every chapter published in this book has been scrutinized by our experts. Their significance has been extensively debated. The topics covered herein carry significant findings which will fuel the growth of the discipline. They may even be implemented as practical applications or may be referred to as a beginning point for another development.

The contributors of this book come from diverse backgrounds, making this book a truly international effort. This book will bring forth new frontiers with its revolutionizing research information and detailed analysis of the nascent developments around the world.

We would like to thank all the contributing authors for lending their expertise to make the book truly unique. They have played a crucial role in the development of this book. Without their invaluable contributions this book wouldn't have been possible. They have made vital efforts to compile up to date information on the varied aspects of this subject to make this book a valuable addition to the collection of many professionals and students.

This book was conceptualized with the vision of imparting up-to-date information and advanced data in this field. To ensure the same, a matchless editorial board was set up. Every individual on the board went through rigorous rounds of assessment to prove their worth. After which they invested a large part of their time researching and compiling the most relevant data for our readers.

The editorial board has been involved in producing this book since its inception. They have spent rigorous hours researching and exploring the diverse topics which have resulted in the successful publishing of this book. They have passed on their knowledge of decades through this book. To expedite this challenging task, the publisher supported the team at every step. A small team of assistant editors was also appointed to further simplify the editing procedure and attain best results for the readers.

Apart from the editorial board, the designing team has also invested a significant amount of their time in understanding the subject and creating the most relevant covers. They scrutinized every image to scout for the most suitable representation of the subject and create an appropriate cover for the book.

The publishing team has been an ardent support to the editorial, designing and production team. Their endless efforts to recruit the best for this project, has resulted in the accomplishment of this book. They are a veteran in the field of academics and their pool of knowledge is as vast as their experience in printing. Their expertise and guidance has proved useful at every step. Their uncompromising quality standards have made this book an exceptional effort. Their encouragement from time to time has been an inspiration for everyone.

The publisher and the editorial board hope that this book will prove to be a valuable piece of knowledge for researchers, students, practitioners and scholars across the globe.

List of Contributors

Angelika Rauch, Sebastian Hahnel, Elena Günther, Wolfgang Bidmon and Oliver Schierz
Department of Prosthodontics and Materials Science, University of Leipzig, Liebigstr. 10, Haus 1, 04103 Leipzig, Germany

André Edelmann, Lisa Riedel and Ralf Hellmann
Applied Laser and Photonics Group, University of Applied Sciences Aschaffenburg, 63743 Aschaffenburg, Germany

Salvatore Sauro
Applied Laser and Photonics Group, University of Applied Sciences Aschaffenburg, 63743 Aschaffenburg, Germany
Department of Therapeutic Dentistry, Sechenov University Russia, 119435 Moscow, Russia
Departamento de Odontología, Facultad de Ciencias de la Salud, Universidad CEU-Cardenal Herrera, C/Del Pozos/n, Alfara del Patriarca, 46115 Valencia, Spain
Tissue Engineering and Biophotonics Research Division King's College London Dental Institute (KCLDI), London SE1 9RT, UK
Institute of Dentistry, I. M. Sechenov First Moscow State Medical University, 119146 Moscow, Russia

Vicente Faus-Matoses and Vicente Faus-Llácer
Departamento de Estomatología, Facultad de Medicina y Odontología, Universitat de Valencia, 46010 Valencia, Spain

Irina Makeeva
Department of Therapeutic Dentistry, Sechenov University Russia, 119435 Moscow, Russia
Institute of Dentistry, I. M. Sechenov First Moscow State Medical University, 119146 Moscow, Russia

Juan Manuel Nuñez Martí, Raquel Gonzalez Martínez and José Antonio García Bautista
Applied Laser and Photonics Group, University of Applied Sciences Aschaffenburg, 63743 Aschaffenburg, Germany

Izabela Barszczewska-Rybarek
Department of Physical Chemistry and Technology of Polymers, Silesian University of Technology, 44-100 Gliwice, Poland

Grzegorz Chladek
Institute of Engineering Materials and Biomaterials, Silesian University of Technology, 44-100 Gliwice, Poland

Han Xie and Tong Cao
Faculty of Dentistry, National University of Singapore, 9 Lower Kent Ridge Road, Singapore 119085, Singapore

Alfredo Franco-Obregón
Department of Surgery, Yong Loo Lin School of Medicine, National University of Singapore, NUHS Tower Block, Level 8, IE Kent Ridge Road, Singapore 119228, Singapore
BioIonic Currents Electromagnetic Pulsing Systems Laboratory, BICEPS, National University of Singapore, MD6, 14 medical Drive, #14-01, Singapore 117599, Singapore

Vinicius Rosa
Faculty of Dentistry, National University of Singapore, 9 Lower Kent Ridge Road, Singapore 119085, Singapore
Department of Materials Science and Engineering, National University of Singapore, Blk EA, #03-09 9 Engineering Drive 1, Singapore 117575, Singapore
Centre for Advanced 2D Materials and Graphene Research Centre, National University of Singapore, 6 Science Drive 2, Singapore 117546, Singapore

Susanne Jung, Lauren Bohner, Marcel Hanisch, Johannes Kleinheinz and Sonja Sielker
Department of Cranio-Maxillofacial Surgery, Research Unit Vascular Biology of Oral Structures (VABOS), University Hospital Muenster, 48149 Muenster, Germany

Diana A. Cunha, Nara S. Rodrigues and Lidiane C. Souza
Post-Graduate Programme in Dentistry, Federal University of Ceará, Rua Monsenhor Furtado S/N, Rodolfo Teófilo, Fortaleza 60430-355, Ceará, Brazil

Diego Lomonaco
Post-Graduate Programme in Dentistry, Federal University of Ceará, Rua Monsenhor Furtado S/N, Rodolfo Teófilo, Fortaleza 60430-355, Ceará, Brazil
Department of Organic and Inorganic Chemistry, Federal University of Ceará, Fortaleza 60440-900, Ceará, Brazil

Flávia P. Rodrigues
Post-Graduate Programme in Dentistry, Federal University of Ceará, Rua Monsenhor Furtado S/N, Rodolfo Teófilo, Fortaleza 60430-355, Ceará, Brazil
School of Dentistry, Paulista University – UNIP, R. Dr. Bacelar 1212, Vila Clementino, São Paulo 04026-002, SP, Brazil

Felipe W. Degrazia and Fabrício M. Collares
Laboratório de Materiais Dentários, Faculdade de Odontologia, Universidade Federal do Rio Grande do Sul, Rua Ramiro Barcelos, 2492, Rio Branco, Porto Alegre 90035-003, Rio Grande do Sul, Brazil

Vicente P. A. Saboia
Post-Graduate Programme in Dentistry, Federal University of Ceará, Rua Monsenhor Furtado S/N, Rodolfo Teófilo, Fortaleza 60430-355, Ceará, Brazil

Prakan Thanasrisuebwong
Department of Oral and Maxillofacial Surgery, Faculty of Dentistry, Mahidol University, Bangkok 10400, Thailand
Ph.D. program in Oral Biology, Faculty of Dentistry, Mahidol University, Bangkok 10400, Thailand

Rudee Surarit
Department of Oral Biology, Faculty of Dentistry, Mahidol University, Bangkok 10400, Thailand

Sompop Bencharit
Department of General Dentistry, School of Dentistry, Virginia Commonwealth University, Richmond, VA 23298, USA
Department of Biomedical Engineering, College of Engineering, Virginia Commonwealth University, Richmond, VA 23298, USA

Nisarat Ruangsawasdi
Department of Pharmacology, Faculty of Dentistry, Mahidol University, Bangkok 10400, Thailand

Luiz Filipe Barbosa-Martins and Jossaria Pereira de Sousa
Department of Pediatric Dentistry, Piracicaba Dental School, State University of Campinas, Piracicaba 13414-903, Brazil

Lívia Araújo Alves
Department of Oral Diagnosis, Piracicaba Dental School, State University of Campinas, Piracicaba 13414-903, Brazil

Robert Philip Wynn Davies
Division of Oral Biology, School of Dentistry, Faculty of Medicine & Health, University of Leeds, Leeds LS9 7TF, UK

Regina Maria Puppin-Rontanti
Departments of Pediatric Dentistry and Restorative Dentistry, Piracicaba Dental School, University of Campinas, Piracicaba 13414-903, Brazil

Takeo Karakida, Mari M. Saito, Risako Chiba, Ryuji Yamamoto and Yasuo Yamakoshi
Department of Biochemistry and Molecular Biology, School of Dental Medicine, Tsurumi University, 2-1-3 Tsurumi, Tsurumi-ku, Yokohama 230-8501, Japan

Kazuo Onuma
Department of Biochemistry and Molecular Biology, School of Dental Medicine, Tsurumi University, 2-1-3 Tsurumi, Tsurumi-ku, Yokohama 230-8501, Japan

Toshie Chiba
Research Center of Electron Microscopy, School of Dental Medicine, Tsurumi University, 2-1-3 Tsurumi, Tsurumi-ku, Yokohama 230-8501, Japan

Yukihiko Hidaka, Keiko Fujii-Abe and Hiroshi Kawahara
Department of Dental Anesthesiology, School of Dental Medicine, Tsurumi University, 2-1-3 Tsurumi, Tsurumi-ku, Yokohama 230-8501, Japan

Faisal D. AlQarni and Yousif A. Al-Dulaijan
Department of Substitutive Dental Sciences, College of Dentistry, Imam Abdulrahman bin Faisal University, Dammam 34212, Saudi Arabia

Thomas W. Oates and Mary Anne S. Melo
Department of Advanced Oral Sciences and Therapeutics, University of Maryland School of Dentistry, Baltimore, MD 21201, USA

Hockin H. K. Xu
Center for Stem Cell Biology & Regenerative Medicine, University of Maryland School of Medicine, Baltimore, MD 21201, USA
Ph.D Program in Dental Biomedical Sciences, University of Maryland School of Dentistry, Baltimore, MD 21201, USA
Department of Advanced Oral Sciences and Therapeutics, Division of Biomaterials and Tissue Engineering, University of Maryland School of Dentistry, Baltimore, MD 21201, USA
University of Maryland Marlene and Stewart Greenebaum Cancer Center, University of Maryland School of Medicine, Baltimore, MD 21201, USA

Raphael Pilo, Sharon Agar-Zoizner, Shaul Gelbard and Shifra Levartovsky
Department of Oral Rehabilitation, The Maurice and Gabriela Goldschleger School of Dental Medicine, Tel-Aviv University, Tel -Aviv 6997801, Israel

Mar Gonzálvez-García
Cell Therapy Unit, IMIB-University Hospital Virgen de la Arrixaca, Faculty of Medicin, University of Murcia, 30120 Murcia, Spain
Service of Oral and Maxillofacial Surgery, Clinical University Hospital Virgen de la Arrixaca, 30120 Murcia, Spain

Carlos M. Martinez
Inflammation and Experimental Surgery Unit, CIBERehd, Institute for Bio-Health Research of Murcia, Clinical University Hospital Virgen de la Arrixaca, 30120 Murcia, Spain

Victor Villanueva
Service of Oral and Maxillofacial Surgery, Clinical University Hospital Virgen de la Arrixaca, 30120 Murcia, Spain

Ana García-Hernández, Miguel Blanquer, José M. Moraleda and Luis Meseguer-Olmo
Cell Therapy Unit, IMIB-University Hospital Virgen de la Arrixaca, Faculty of Medicin, University of Murcia, 30120 Murcia, Spain

Ricardo E. Oñate Sánchez
School of Dentistry, University of Murcia, 30003 Murcia, Spain

Francisco Javier Rodríguez-Lozano
Cell Therapy Unit, IMIB-University Hospital Virgen de la Arrixaca, Faculty of Medicin, University of Murcia, 30120 Murcia, Spain
Unidad de Pacientes Especiales y Gerodontología, Universidad de Murcia, IMIB-Arrixaca, Hospital Morales Meseguer, 30008 Murcia, Spain
School of Dentistry/Cellular Therapy and Hematopoietic Transplant Unit, Hematology Department, Virgen de la Arrixaca Clinical University Hospital, IMIB-Arrixaca, University of Murcia, 30120 Murcia, Spain
School of Dentistry, Hospital Morales Meseguer 2pl. Av. Marqués de los Vélez s/n, University of Murcia, 30008 Murcia, Spain

Enrico Conserva, Pierantonio Bellini and Ugo Consolo
Department of Surgery, Medicine, Dentistry and Morphological Sciences with interest in Transplant, Oncology and Regenerative Medicine, University of Modena and Reggio Emilia, 41125 Modena, Italy
Operative Unit of Dentistry and Maxillofacial Surgery, Department Integrated Activity-Specialist Surgeries, University-Hospital of Modena, 41125 Modena, Italy

Alessandra Pisciotta, Laura Bertoni, Giulia Bertani, Aida Meto, Bruna Colombari, Elisabetta Blasi, Anto de Pol and Gianluca Carnevale
Department of Surgery, Medicine, Dentistry and Morphological Sciences with interest in Transplant, Oncology and Regenerative Medicine, University of Modena and Reggio Emilia, 41125 Modena, Italy

Carmen Llena and Leopoldo Forner
Department of Stomatology, University de Valencia, 46010 Valencia, Spain

Mar Collado-González, Christopher Joseph Tomás-Catalá, David García-Bernal and Ricardo Elías Oñate-Sánchez
School of Dentistry/Cellular Therapy and Hematopoietic Transplant Unit, Hematology Department, Virgen de la Arrixaca Clinical University Hospital, IMIB-Arrixaca, University of Murcia, 30120 Murcia, Spain

Federico Foschi and Massimo Giovarruscio
Institute of Dentistry, I. M. Sechenov First Moscow State Medical University, 119146 Moscow, Russia
Departamento de Estomatología, Facultad de Medicina y Odontología, Universitat de Valencia, 46010 Valencia, SPAIN

Paula Maciel Pires
Departamento de Odontologia, Facultad de Ciencias de la Salud, Universidad CEU Cardenal Herrera, 46115 Valencia, SPAIN
Department of Pediatric Dentistry, Federal University of Rio de Janeiro, 21941-617 Rio de Janeiro, Brazil

Maria Elisa Martins Moura
Departamento de Odontologia, Facultad de Ciencias de la Salud, Universidad CEU Cardenal Herrera, 46115 Valencia, SPAIN
Materiais Dentários, Universidade Federal do Ceará, Fortaleza, 60430-355 Ceará, Brazil

Aline Almeida Neves
Department of Pediatric Dentistry, Federal University of Rio de Janeiro, 21941-617 Rio de Janeiro, Brazil

Maria Salem Ibrahim
Ph.D Program in Dental Biomedical Sciences, University of Maryland School of Dentistry, Baltimore, MD 21201, USA
Department of Preventive Dental Sciences, College of Dentistry, Imam Abdulrahman Bin Faisal University, Dammam 34212, Saudi Arabia

Ahmed S. Ibrahim
Medical Microbiology Department, Health Monitoring Centers, Ministry of Health, Jeddah 21176, Saudi Arabia

Abdulrahman A. Balhaddad
Ph.D Program in Dental Biomedical Sciences, University of Maryland School of Dentistry, Baltimore, MD 21201, USA
Department of Restorative Dental Sciences, College of Dentistry, Imam Abdulrahman Bin Faisal University, Dammam 34212, Saudi Arabia

Michael D. Weir
Ph.D Program in Dental Biomedical Sciences, University of Maryland School of Dentistry, Baltimore, MD 21201, USA
Department of Advanced Oral Sciences and Therapeutics, Division of Biomaterials and Tissue Engineering, University of Maryland School of Dentistry, Baltimore, MD 21201, USA

Nancy J. Lin
Biosystems and Biomaterials Division, National Institute of Standards and Technology, Gaithersburg, MD 20899, USA

Thomas W. Oates
Department of Advanced Oral Sciences and Therapeutics, Division of Biomaterials and Tissue Engineering, University of Maryland School of Dentistry, Baltimore, MD 21201, USA

Franklin R. Tay
Department of Endodontics, The Dental College of Georgia, Augusta University, Augusta, GA 30912, USA

Mary Anne S. Melo
Ph.D Program in Dental Biomedical Sciences, University of Maryland School of Dentistry, Baltimore, MD 21201, USA
Division of Operative Dentistry, Department of General Dentistry, University of Maryland School of Dentistry, Baltimore, MD 21201, USA

Sujatha Muthumariappan, Christabella Adine and Kiaw Kiaw Ng
Department of Oral and Maxillofacial Surgery, Faculty of Dentistry, National University of Singapore, Singapore 119085, Singapore

Wei Cheng Ng, Pooya Davoodi and Chi-Hwa Wang
Department of Chemical and Biomolecular Engineering, National University of Singapore, Singapore 117585, Singapore

Joao N. Ferreira
Department of Oral and Maxillofacial Surgery, Faculty of Dentistry, National University of Singapore, Singapore 119085, Singapore
Faculty of Dentistry, Chulalongkorn University, Bangkok 10330, Thailand
National Institute of Dental and Craniofacial Research, National Institutes of Health, Bethesda, MD 20892-4370, USA

Index

www.ingramcontent.com/pod-product-compliance
Lightning Source LLC
LaVergne TN
LVHW060528210926
848485LV00005B/1169